Praise for Never Fear Cancer Again

"Raymond Francis lifts the veil no ⋯ ⋯s cancer treatments but on the mystery of ⋯ f cancer and, most importantly, arms the re ⋯ prevent and reverse this scourge."

⋯hneider

⋯⋯, Comedian, Screenwriter, and Director

"*Never Fear Cancer Again* can only be described as a masterpiece. This book explains the cancer process, the various causes, and, most importantly, the best weapons for not only prevention and early cancer treatment but for treatment of advanced cancers as well. This is a very important book that should be read by everyone."

—Russell L. Blaylock, M.D., CCN
Neurosurgeon (Ret)
Visiting Professor Biology Belhaven University
Author, *Natural Strategies for Cancer Patients*

"Raymond Francis gave me a new lease on life. I am a medical doctor with an almost four-year history of stage IV metastatic kidney cancer who had exhausted the standard treatment protocols for treating my cancer. After a PET scan revealed progression of my cancer, my oncologist suggested I contact hospice. By chance, I met Raymond Francis who listened to my story, shared with me his theory of disease, and encouraged me to start an alternative course to treat and reverse my cancer. I read Raymond's book *Never Be Sick Again* and started on the path to regaining my health. Seven months later, my last scan showed dramatic reductions in the size of my tumors. They have almost completely disappeared, my health has returned, and I am back to work. Reading *Never Fear Cancer Again* could save your life!"

—Ronald L. Greene, M.D.

"Because of his twenty-five plus years of experience healing people of all kinds of chronic degenerative conditions, I was delighted when Raymond told me he was writing a book on cancer healing. This man is better qualified than anyone I know to write such a book. If you want to understand this epidemic condition that is spreading like wildfire throughout the civilized world—why it happens, how to avoid it, and how to heal it—you need to read this book. Don't procrastinate. Purge your fear of the word *cancer* by reading Raymond's clear, concise information on it. Get this information to your loved ones. We all need it."

—Bill Henderson
Author, *Cure Your Cancer* and *Cancer-Free*

"Raymond Francis explains the causes of cancer with clarity and compassion. Science has confirmed that healthy people make and elimnate cancer cells every day. Only when intrinsic anti-cancer mechanisms are disabled can cancer grow. Raymond offers insights into keeping inner anti-cancer mechanisms strong. He also offers guidance on how to restore or strengthen them if they are weak. *Never Fear Cancer Again* is for everyone who seeks a cancer-free life."

—Russell Jaffe, M.D., Ph.D.
Fellow, Health Studies Collegium

"As Raymond Francis so clearly states, 'You don't have to be a helpless victim. *If you can turn cancer on, you can turn cancer off.*' In a sea of misinformation and self-serving interests, this book is a lifeline to help you understand and overcome barriers to cancer prevention and healing."

—Hyla Cass, M.D.
Author, *8 Weeks to Vibrant Health*

"*Never Fear Cancer Again* is the light of hope for people with cancer. This book will transform your thinking on cancer, change your views on health and wellness, and unlock your inner potential to get well and triumph over this deadly disease. Raymond Francis, in his simple style, gives you a holistic roadmap to health. This book is filled with priceless, cutting-edge information that could save your life."

—Suprabha Jain, M.D.
Medical Director, Mt. Diablo Wellness Center
www.mdiwellness.com

"Wise and provocative words from a learned and gifted expert on health and well-being."

—Edgar Mitchell, Ph.D., Sc.D.
Apollo 14 Astronaut, founder Institute of Noetic Sciences

"Raymond Francis is a visionary who sends a simple message that all can understand—you can do more for yourself than any doctor. A very important work."

—Frank D. Wiewel
Former Chairman, Pharmacological and Biological Treatments Committee,
National Institutes of Health (NIH), Founder, People Against Cancer

"Raymond Francis's bold explanation for the reasons why we get cancer and how we can eliminate it awakens even the most skeptical thinker. In *Never Fear Cancer Again*, Francis's clear and easy to understand style challenges us with shocking data from mainstream-medical research. This landmark book is a must read for every medical doctor and every person who has or knows someone who has cancer. This is an outstanding contribution!"

—Len Saputo, M.D.
Author of *A Return to Healing*
www.doctorsaputo.com

"Raymond Francis is a brilliant and advanced thinker and practitioner in the health field. Personally, as a practitioner of Integrative and Preventive Medicine for forty years, I can appreciate when complicated issues are made simple. Raymond Francis does that in his new book. *Never Fear Cancer Again* provides the concepts and solutions to keep this life-threatening disease away. Staying healthy is our best defense."

—Elson M. Haas, M.D. (www.elsonhaas.com)
Integrated Medicine Physician, Preventive Medical Center of Marin
Author of many books, including *Staying Healthy with Nutrition*

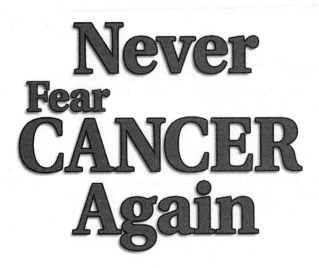

Never Fear CANCER Again

How to Prevent and Reverse Cancer

Raymond Francis, M.Sc.
Author of the Bestseller *Never Be Sick Again*

Foreword by Harvey Diamond
Coauthor of the #1 *New York Times Bestseller Fit for Life*

Health Communications, Inc.
Deerfield Beach, Florida

www.hcibooks.com

Never Fear Cancer Again and the information contained in this book are not intended as a substitute for the advice and/or medical care of the reader's physician, nor are they intended to discourage or dissuade the reader from the advice of his or her physician. The reader should regularly consult with a physician in matters relating to his or her health, especially with regard to symptoms that may require diagnosis. Any eating, exercise, or lifestyle regimen should not be undertaken without first consulting the reader's physician.

Library of Congress Cataloging-in-Publication Data

Francis, Raymond, 1937-
    Never fear cancer again : how to prevent and reverse cancer / Raymond Francis;
[foreword by] Harvey Diamond.
        p. cm.
    Includes bibliographical references and index.
    ISBN-13: 978-0-7573-1550-3 (pbk.)
    ISBN-10: 0-7573-1550-X (trade paper)
    ISBN-13: 978-0-7573-9190-3 (e-book)
        1. Cancer—Prevention—Popular works.   I. Title.
    RC268.F73 2011
    616.99'405—dc23

                                                                2011021214

©2011 Raymond Francis

Publisher: Health Communications, Inc.
            3201 S.W. 15th Street
            Deerfield Beach, FL 33442–8190

R-10-11

Cover design by Larissa Hise Henoch
Interior design by Lawna Patterson Oldfield
Interior formatting by Dawn Von Strolley Grove

I dedicate this book to the loving memory of my brother Bernard. An inspiration to anyone suffering with cancer, in 1991 Bernie was diagnosed with inoperable prostate cancer that had metastasized to his lymphatic system. Conventional medicine had little to offer, and his projected life expectancy ranged from six months to an optimistic three years. Not liking those numbers, Bernie had the wisdom and courage to seek out alternative treatments. He radically changed his diet, reduced his toxic exposures, and took the nutritional supplements that I recommended. He succeeded in putting his cancer into remission. His perplexed physicians called him "the miracle patient." Bernie lived an additional two decades of very high quality life. He died on April 9, 2011, at the age of eighty, having outlived the average American male by five years.

Contents

Acknowledgments

My abundant gratitude goes to all those dedicated scientists who came before me to help us understand the biological process we call cancer. I thank my publisher, Health Communications, Inc., for making this book possible and to its entire staff, who contributed to its success. Special thanks go to my editor Allison Janse, who has been a friend, a guide, and an inspiration, and has had the grace and the patience to suffer through three of my books.

Many thanks also to the friends who have spent many hours of their time reading and critiquing to help make the book more readable and meaningful to the average reader. Of special note is my friend Norman Hawker, who went way beyond the call of friendship and spent countless hours patiently editing, researching, and offering suggestions for improvement. Thanks, Norman! Thanks also to Dr. Linda Howard for making all those cuts that were painful at the time, but made for a better, higher quality manuscript. Thanks also to Dr. David Rovno, Joan Carole, Pamela Strong, Stacy Jett, and Austin Jett. Your contributions have been meaningful, and they are appreciated. Most importantly, the reader has a more useful product because of your thoughtful attention and comments.

Foreword

The words, "You have cancer" can be devastating and land with a thud in your heart, producing shock and terror. This deadly disease appears to be something over which we have very little control. It seems to strike innocent victims for no apparent reason, like a cruel game of chance with the highest of stakes. Contributing to the anxiety and distress associated with a diagnosis of cancer are particularly aggressive treatments that are themselves quite frightening while yielding extremely meager results.

But it doesn't have to be this way.

Raymond Francis breaks the mold while intelligently and convincingly setting the record straight on the true reasons why cancer shows up in some people and not in others. *Never Fear Cancer Again* explains that cancer is not something to be poisoned, burned, or cut out of the body, but rather a process that needs to be recognized and shut down. The cancer process requires a certain environment in the body to sustain itself. The surest and safest way to prevent or evict cancer from the body is to stop creating the conditions that allow it to thrive.

Never Fear Cancer Again takes the mystery and fear out of cancer by shining the light of knowledge on it, revealing how cancer is caused, and how to implement its reversal and prevention. Raymond Francis takes the best that science has to offer and reduces it to simple language, providing readers with what they need to know to become well, stay well, and remain cancer free. Using his simple, yet profound concept that there's really only one disease and two causes of disease, Francis redefines health and disease, opening the door and leading the way to an entirely new and effective way of practicing medicine. He explains complex science in easy-to-understand language, empowering readers to help themselves. This revolutionary book is decades ahead of the approach of most doctors, and may very well rank among the most significant and practical books ever written on the subject of cancer. Given conventional medicine's abysmal success rate with cancer, this book is not only a timely contribution but also heralds in new and real hope for those either in the grip of cancer or those desiring to optimize their chances of its prevention.

The reason people fear cancer so is because conventional cancer treatments are both brutalizing and ineffective. Conventional treatments are harmful, damaging the body's natural ability to fight cancer while actually producing more cancer in the process. The failure of the standard approach to cancer can be directly traced to the unfortunate and ineffectual tradition of treating only the symptoms while ignoring the causes, allowing the cancer process to continue unchecked. Most people think of cancer as a mysterious monster over which they have little or no control. Not so! The knowledge that already exists is sufficient to end this epidemic. In fact, a growing body of scientific evidence clearly shows that the vast majority of cancers can be prevented with changes in diet and lifestyle. All that is needed is to put the knowledge we already have to good use, which is exactly what this groundbreaking book succeeds in doing.

Cancer can be prevented, and it can be reversed.

Raymond Francis, a graduate of the Massachusetts Institute of Technology (M.I.T.), has been cited as "one of the few scientists to achieve a breakthrough understanding of health and disease." With backgrounds in both science and engineering, he employs that rare combination of scientific rigor and the practicality of an engineer. In *Never Fear Cancer Again,* Francis lives up to his well-earned reputation for insightful, breakthrough thinking. He is a master at taking complex science, understanding its implications, and then reducing it to practical concepts that almost anyone can use to acquire and maintain health and well-being. After decades of extensive research and observation, Francis presents us with the tools we need to end this out-of-control scourge.

While the knowledge to end this epidemic already exists, the problem is that it is not being assembled and packaged into something we can use. In this eye-opening book, that's what Francis so eloquently succeeds in doing, and that's why it is a must-read for anyone seeking to prevent or reverse cancer. It is well researched, with an extensive bibliography, and is easy to understand. Francis exposes how cancer survival statistics have been manipulated to the point of being meaningless, with the real cancer survival rates being no better than they were in the 1950s. He explains why conventional cancer treatments fail, pointing out how they actually contribute to the cancer process, often killing the patient faster than if they had no treatment at all!

The real power of *Never Fear Cancer Again* is that it presents a simple, yet comprehensive and holistic program for preventing and reversing cancer. Francis's Beyond Health Model of One Disease, Two Causes, and Six Pathways to health or disease provides a roadmap for creating health and shutting down the cancer process. Francis uses the analogy of switching on and driving a cancer to switching on and driving a car. Just as you can learn to control your car, you can learn to control cancer. He even shows you how to keep cancer locked in the garage so it can't go anywhere and do harm. Francis demonstrates why the Standard American Diet is actually a cancer-causing diet. He outlines the critical role of environmental toxins. With his holistic approach, he shows how your thoughts and emotions, lack of sleep, not enough exercise or sunlight, malfunctioning genes and even common medical treatments can cause cancer.

Armed with the knowledge contained in this book, you can take control of your life by supporting your body's natural ability to prevent and reverse cancer. Instead of being at the mercy of an uncontrollable threat, you can move forward confidently knowing that you are doing everything possible to make your body a place where cancer cannot take hold.

Never Fear Cancer Again is science based, decades ahead of conventional medicine, well written, and easy to understand. Best of all—it works! We should all be thankful there are dedicated individuals such as Raymond Francis out there, committed to revealing much needed health truths to a deserving populace.

Harvey Diamond
#1 *New York Times* Bestselling Author
Fit for Life: A New Beginning

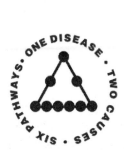

Introduction

Each patient carries his own doctor inside him. We are at our best when we give the doctor who resides within a chance to go to work.

—Albert Schweitzer, M.D., Nobel Laureate and medical missionary

As Albert Schweitzer advises above, give the doctor within a chance to go to work. The purpose of this book is to help you do that. We already know how to prevent and reverse cancer. This knowledge exists—all you have to do is learn it and apply it. The problem is that today we are so inundated in information, much of it conflicting and false, that even the well-educated are not sure what to think, believe, or do. People are lost, confused, and frustrated. My goal is to cut through the confusion, and turn that information into practical knowledge that you can use to take control of your health, just as I did for myself.

In 1985, I almost died. I started out complaining of fatigue and allergies, and after a series of catastrophic misdiagnoses and mistakes by my physicians, I came close to death from liver failure caused by taking an antibiotic drug that was known to be toxic to the liver. My condition deteriorated to a point where I was reduced to a human skeleton and the doctors said nothing further could be done for me. Facing imminent death, I was forced to use my knowledge of biochemistry to save my life. What seemed like a nightmare at the time turned out to be one of the best things that ever happened to me, because it began an odyssey of learning about health and teaching it to others that continues to this day.

At the age of forty-eight, it took two years of study and hard work to bring myself from the brink of death and restore normal function. During that time, I made some amazing discoveries about how to get well and stay well that took me from death's door to living in extraordinary health. Today, at age seventy-four, I have boundless energy, a sharp mind, and I never get sick (I have had only one cold in the last twenty-four years). I have brought the biological age of my arteries down to that of someone in his mid-twenties, and my goal is to have the arteries of a teenager by the time I'm eighty. It has been a truly joyful experience helping people all over the world to learn how to get well and stay well, and now I want to share this knowledge with you—particularly about the disease we fear the most: cancer.

As a chemist by training and a graduate of the Massachusetts Institute of Technology (M.I.T.), I accessed cutting-edge science to unravel the mystery of my illness. By understanding my problems on a cellular level, I learned how I, like most people, had unwittingly created my health problems through decades of poor choices. My symptoms included chronic fatigue, extreme chemical sensitivities, allergic reactions to almost everything, lupus, Hashimoto's thyroiditis, Sjogren's syndrome, fibromyalgia, vision problems, digestive problems, skin rashes, headaches, brain fog, dizziness, and grand mal seizures. Fortunately, I found that by changing my daily choices regarding diet and lifestyle, I could reverse the disease process and achieve optimal health.

The body wants to be well, it knows how to be well, and it will be well if only we give it a chance. To give it a chance, our job is to give the body what it needs and then not interfere with its work. Unfortunately, few people—including doctors—know how to do this. When I was sick, the physicians I hoped would heal me almost killed me instead. They didn't know any better! These well-meaning, highly educated professionals had been taught a hopelessly outdated, unscientific system of medicine. Our physicians learn that drugs and surgery are the answers to disease. They are taught a "disease-care" model of health that is incapable of either preventing or curing disease, when the real answer is giving body cells what they need to do their jobs and reducing their toxic burdens.

Conventional medicine doesn't attempt to prevent disease; it only springs to action after signs of disease have appeared. Then instead of curing disease, it addresses only the symptoms and not the causes. This approach keeps people sick, and comes at enormous personal and economic cost. In fact, we don't have a healthcare industry, we have a "disease industry" that is totally dependent on millions of people getting sick and staying that way. Unfortunately, this ineffective, expensive, and dangerous approach to health care is the norm in our society. Even worse than keeping people sick, it does so much damage that medical intervention has become a leading cause of disease and the single largest cause of death in America.

Word of my recovery got around among the support groups I had belonged to, and people began to seek me out for advice. With my new science-based understanding of health and disease, I helped people with all kinds of problems to reverse their diseases and restore their health. What I came to realize is that it doesn't matter what your health problem is, you really have only one choice—get well! The way to get well is to give the doctor within a chance to go to work.

As I witnessed how many seriously ill people I helped to get well, I became determined to use the remainder of my life to share my new knowledge with others. I wrote two books, *Never Be Sick Again* and *Never Be Fat Again*, and I give workshops and seminars all over the world, helping people everywhere to get and stay well. I am also the founder of The Project to End Disease (TPED), whose mission is to end the epidemic of chronic disease by teaching people around the world how to get well and stay well. My approach has succeeded in reversing cancer in hundreds of "incurable" cases in varying stages. Consider LeRoy as an example.

In 2005, LeRoy was diagnosed with non-Hodgkin's lymphoma and went through eight months of chemotherapy. His cancer went into remission. Unfortunately, as usual with chemotherapy, the cancer came back. In December of 2009, he was sent to the Mayo Clinic where they did twelve biopsies and three PET (positron emission tomography) scans. The doctors confirmed that the lymphoma had returned with lesions in his neck and chest, and a large one in his abdomen. More chemotherapy was recommended.

LeRoy knew that his situation with multiple metastases was grave, and by this time he had learned that, given his situation, conventional medicine could not save him. He started searching for alternatives. In January of 2010, LeRoy purchased a copy of *Never Be Sick Again*. He radically changed his diet and went on a supplement program. He called me for guidance and started taking about forty different supplements per day. By March, LeRoy felt better and knew that something good was happening in his body. In July, he had more PET scans and his doctor could not believe the results:

- The lesion in his neck was significantly smaller.
- The lesion in his chest had disappeared.
- The large lesion in his abdomen had disappeared.

As of this writing, LeRoy is continuing to rebuild his health. He used to run marathons, and he is back to running and lifting weights, and doing things he had been unable to do since his original cancer treatment in 2005. In LeRoy's words:

I was very skeptical when I started supplements, but I did not want to go through chemo again. When I had chemo the first time, my doctor told me that he did not think I would make it. But here I am. I guess Mr. Francis is right, that cancer is reversible. I am living proof.

Cancer is America's most expensive disease, and it will soon become our leading cause of death. The death toll is rising; cancer is striking its victims at an alarming rate, and the treatments are worse than the disease. Close to half of all Americans will develop diagnosable cancer in their lifetime, and conventional medicine has been unable to stem this epidemic.

Here is the good news: *You don't have to be a victim!*

Despite official pronouncements to the contrary, we already have sufficient knowledge to prevent and reverse cancer; all we have to do is put it to use. This revolutionary book will teach you what you need to know to get your health back. You will learn a new way of thinking that will fundamentally change your understanding of health and disease. If you embrace this information and realize how extraordinary it is to have bodies that are designed to keep us well, you will be able to reverse and prevent cancer.

Because cancer is a process and not a thing, attempting to surgically remove it, poison it with chemotherapy, or burn it with radiation doesn't work. The cancer will likely come back because the process of producing cancer is still operating. To win, you have to switch the process off. This is why, for those three-out-of-four cancer patients whose cancer has already metastasized by the time they are diagnosed, standard cancer therapy has a success rate of less than 1 percent—a fact the cancer industry would rather you didn't know and is successful in obscuring.

Never Fear Cancer Again teaches you how to turn cancer off for good by addressing the causes at the cellular level. By addressing what has gone wrong and learning how to restore the normal biological balance in your cells, you can make cancer disappear.

If every cell in your body is functioning normally, you can't be sick. There are only two reasons why cells malfunction: *deficiency* and *toxicity*. When cells don't get what they need to function properly or when they get too much of something that interferes with their operations, they'll malfunction.

When cells malfunction, thousands of symptoms can be produced. Which symptoms depend on your particular combination of deficiencies and toxicities and your unique genetic makeup. Physicians misinterpret these as thousands of different diseases. In truth, they are merely different symptoms produced by cells that are malfunctioning due to deficiency and toxicity. What we call cancer is merely a certain class of these symptoms—cells in different parts of the body, such as the breast, lung, or liver, keep growing and don't stop. To get well and stay well, it is necessary to remove the deficiencies and toxicities and restore cells to normal function. Whenever you do this, no disease can persist—not even cancer.

Most people think of cancer as a mysterious, all-powerful disease that is associated with extraordinary suffering, pain, and death.

Even occasional reading of newspapers and magazines will give the impression that *everything* causes cancer and that nothing cures it. You get the feeling that you have no control, and you just give up control to your doctor. Yet there is a reason why cancer is the diagnosis people fear the most: conventional cancer treatments don't work.

Health is *your* responsibility, and you have more control over your health than you can imagine. The doctor within is very powerful! Because health occurs naturally and responds to the laws of nature, all we have to do is obey nature's laws. Obeying those laws and keeping ourselves in good health is a duty—a personal responsibility. For those willing to accept responsibility for their health, miracles happen. I invite you to participate in this process of relearning what health is and thinking about disease in a different way. Cancer can be prevented and reversed! I will show you how.

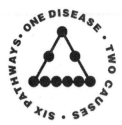

1

AN OVERVIEW
OF CANCER

Cancer is potentially the most preventable and
most curable of the major life-threatening diseases facing humankind.

—Dr. John R. Seffrin, CEO American Cancer Society

Most cancer patients in this country die of chemotherapy. . . .
Chemotherapy does not eliminate breast, colon, or lung cancers. . . .
Yet doctors still use chemotherapy for these tumors. . . .
Women with breast cancer are likely to die faster with chemo than without it.

—Alan Levin, M.D., Clinical Ecologist, San Francisco

"You have cancer." These are some of the most terrifying words
you will ever hear. They will change your life in an instant, turning your world upside down. Cancer is officially the second leading

cause of death in the United States, and is on its way to becoming the leading cause of death—but you don't have to live in fear. Most cancer occurs needlessly, and can be turned off like a light switch.

People fear cancer for the same reason children fear the dark. It is not the darkness itself that is feared, but the uncertainty of not knowing what is there, and imagining what might be there. Cancer is scary, especially when hearing the diagnosis for the first time. It causes large uncertainties: how long will you live, how will it affect your family, your job, and so forth? This book shines light into that darkness with knowledge that reveals what cancer is, how it is caused, and how to reverse it. Eliminate the darkness of ignorance and you will never have to fear cancer again.

Preventing and Reversing Cancer

The truth is cancer cells are always being produced in the body. It is an ongoing process; some researchers estimate that we all produce from several hundred to several thousand cancer cells per day. Historically, this hasn't been a problem because our immune systems were designed to seek these cells out and destroy them. However, beginning in the mid-twentieth century we started to dramatically increase the number of cancer cells we are producing. What is driving this explosion? Our junk-food diets, living in a sea of manmade toxins and electromagnetic fields, high-stress lifestyles, lack of exercise, exposure to artificial light, and health-damaging medical treatments.

All the above have impaired our immune systems, and we are now creating more cancer cells than our overworked and depleted immune systems can destroy. These same factors also shift the body's internal environment to one that promotes the growth of cancer. This is why almost all of us, especially those over age fifty, now have small clusters of cancer cells throughout our bodies. The chances are, if you are over age fifty, you already have cancer! Fortunately, these cancer cells won't bother you—unless you switch them on and drive them to grow and metastasize—and you have control over whether this happens. You don't have to be a helpless victim. *If you can turn cancer on, you can turn cancer off.*

We have to remind ourselves that historically cancer was a rare disease. It is only since the early part of the twentieth century, and especially over the last half century in the industrialized nations, that cancer has increased dramatically. Why is this happening? What have we changed?

We have changed what we eat and how we live. What we call "modern civilization" has fundamentally changed our *diet*, our *environment*, and our *lifestyle*. These changes have reduced the amount of essential nutrients available to our cells, filled our bodies with toxins, exposed us to radiation, caused massive disruption to our normal biorhythms, and impaired our bodies' internal communication, self-regulation, and self-repair—that's a lot of change.

Changes in farming, food distribution, food processing, and animal management have reduced the nutritional content of our food, altered the ratios of critical nutrients, changed the chemistry of the fats and oils in our diet, and added thousands of unnatural, man-made chemicals. Large quantities of refined sugar and refined oils have been added to our diet. In fact, more than half our calories now come from foods that didn't even exist when our genes were developing. These are: refined sugar, bleached flour, and processed oils. We are now consuming a diet filled with low quality food that is woefully deficient in life-supporting nutrients while being loaded with toxins.

We live in an invisible sea of toxic chemicals, most of which didn't exist prior to World War II, and our bodies are absorbing these chemicals like sponges. Hundreds of them are bioaccumulating in our cells and tissues, building up to levels that cause serious malfunction, weakening our immune systems, and making us sick. Once sick, we are treated with drugs made of toxic synthetic chemicals, which make our bodies even more toxic and therefore sicker.

Our lifestyles expose us to unprecedented amounts of radiation; we live sedentary lives, have disrupted our sleep patterns, don't get enough sunlight, and are chronically stressed. When you think about it, it's amazing we are functioning as well as we are, but then more than three out of four of all Americans suffer from at least one diagnosable chronic disease.

To make sense of our unprecedented epidemic of chronic and degenerative disease, you have to understand that, in a relatively short period of time, we have fundamentally changed the parameters of human existence—our diet, environment, and lifestyle. These changes are having a catastrophic impact on our ability to maintain health. The reality is this: *We are now eating a diet, functioning in an environment, and living a lifestyle that promotes cancer.* Cancer has become normal given the way we live! Fortunately, all we need to do is remove the conditions that allow it to develop in the first place.

Problems get solved when you address the cause. If you want to end cancer, at least in your own body, you have to reverse the conditions that allowed your cancer to develop by making different choices. You must change your internal environment into one that supports health rather than one that promotes cancer. You must learn how to give your cells the nutrients they need, how to reduce your toxic load, and how to live a lifestyle that supports health rather than disease.

Nobody knows everything there is to know about cancer, and

most likely, a lot of what we think we know is wrong. However, we don't need to know everything to prevent cancer or make it go away. What we already know is sufficient. Science has already provided a good understanding of what makes cancer grow and metastasize, so you can learn how to make choices in your daily living that prevent cancer from growing and metastasizing. We really don't need to spend billions more trying to find a cure for cancer.

To help you make the right choices, I have created a simple model of health, which I call the Beyond Health Model, based on the concept of *One Disease, Two Causes*, and *Six Pathways*. I also use a simple analogy between driving your car and driving cancer. Take your foot off the accelerator, apply the brake, turn the ignition switch off, and your car stops. In much the same way, you can stop cancer.

Martha's Experience

In 2006, Martha was diagnosed with a malignant lump growing in her neck that was affecting her facial nerves. Doctors surgically removed the lump and deemed the operation a success but, as usual with conventional treatment, the patient wasn't cured. A little more than a year later, Martha was diagnosed with five lesions in her lungs and a lesion on one arm. Her cancer had metastasized. She knew how much trouble she was in. Martha had already learned enough on her own to know that she would not survive if she continued to pursue conventional treatments with her metastasized cancer. She decided to help herself by choosing to get well. She took personal responsibility for her health, and learned how to turn her cancer switches off and to stop driving her cancer.

After reading *Never Be Sick Again,* Martha contacted me for help to get on the best diet and supplement program. She eliminated sugars, grains, processed oils, dairy, and animal protein. She added fresh organic fruits as well as large quantities of vegetables in the form of juices. She also started on a program of high-quality, anti-cancer supplements. After only a few weeks, Martha went for her scheduled surgery to have her lung removed, but after repeated scans on her lungs, the doctors couldn't find any lesions. They thought there was something wrong with the machine. In disbelief, they sent her home. The doctor who was supposed to remove the cancer on her arm kept calling, wanting to schedule surgery to remove the lesion that was no longer there, even though he had been told it was gone.

Martha is far from alone with such an experience. Her cure was not miraculous, nor was it an isolated, random incident without a cause. Martha's experience has been shared by countless other individuals who have had more faith in the body's ability to heal itself than in conventional medicine's toxic treatments. Cancer can be prevented and reversed by addressing the underlying causes. Martha now understands that the changes she made to reverse her cancer were the very same ones that could have prevented it in the first place. She has now permanently changed her diet and lifestyle to make sure the cancer never returns—she is choosing health instead of disease.

Even better than reversing cancer is preventing it. Prevention is the ultimate answer to cancer. It is far easier to prevent cancer than to fix it after it happens. Dr. Samuel Broder, former director of the National Cancer Institute, once said, "Each time a patient comes in and needs cancer therapy, you could say it was a failure of prevention." The most promising approach to controlling our cancer epidemic is a commitment to prevention—anyone can make this commitment.

Cancer is easier to prevent than to reverse. Isolated cancer cells are easy to keep under control, but once they start growing, they create their own support system with their own blood supply that provides tremendous amounts of sustenance to the growing tumor. An effective prevention program would virtually eliminate cancer. There are simple choices anyone can make to dramatically reduce their risk of developing cancer—these same simple choices can also reverse cancer. You can learn how to keep yourself cancer free. You can switch cancer on or you can switch it off. The choice is yours.

Medicine's Misunderstanding of Cancer

Conventional medicine fails to appreciate that cancer is not a thing. Cancer is a process. When you have cancer, the problem is not confined to one area of the body: it is everywhere. It's a systemic disease—a whole body problem. Abnormal metabolism sets the stage for cancer throughout the body. Doctors give different names and classifications to cancer. They try to remove or kill the cancer in your breast, prostate, or lung, but it's like treating only muscle aches when somebody has the flu. The flu affects everything in your body, not just the muscles. Focusing on where the tumor is makes no sense, and it has proven to be a losing strategy. *Cancer is not a thing you can cut, poison, or burn—it is a biological process affecting the entire body.*

To make cancer happen, you have to turn on a number of biological switches, and then you have to drive the process forward. Where the cancer shows up doesn't matter. Cancer is cancer no matter what body part is involved. There is only one cancer—in fact, there is only one disease: malfunctioning cells. Removing body parts with surgery, poisoning your body with toxic chemicals, or destroying tissue with cancer-causing radiation will not solve your problem—the cancer will come back because the process is still operating. If you want to get rid of cancer, *you have to turn the process off.*

A Brief History of Cancer

Many people think the amount of cancer we are experiencing is normal. It is not normal. Although cancer has been around as long as we have, it was once a rare disease. Today it is an epidemic. In the nineteenth century, cancer affected only one out of a thousand people. By the early 1900s, it affected thirty out of a thousand. Right now, increasing at an alarming rate, close to 500 Americans out of a thousand will be diagnosed with cancer in their lifetime. Since 1940, cancer has increased rapidly in all the industrialized nations, and the trend has accelerated even more since 1975. From 1950 to 2001, national cancer statistics show that the incidence for all types of cancer increased by 85 percent in the United States. Cancer has been rising so dramatically that right now more Americans die of cancer *each year* than all the servicemen and women who lost their lives in World War II, Korea, and Vietnam put together.

We have been conditioned to believe the myth that cancer is a disease of aging. It is not. Old people don't have cancer because they are old. Cancer was unknown in traditional societies, such as the Hunza, where just 100 years ago the average age at death was about 120 versus our 78. The Hunza lived far longer than we do, and they didn't have any cancer. If cancer is a disease of aging, how do we explain the absence of cancer among these old people, and how do we explain the fact that cancer is increasingly affecting our young people? In fact, the *fastest growing incidence* of cancer for any age group is among children. After accidents, cancer is the leading cause of death for children and those in their twenties and thirties. Nearly half of all deaths from eight categories of cancer, including bone, cervix, and thyroid, occur in those under thirty-four years of age. Clearly, cancer is not a disease of aging.

Many think that cancer is caused by inherited genes. It is not. Sometimes we see cancer appear to run in families, but we fail to appreciate that diet and lifestyle also run in families. Inherited genes can't explain the explosion of cancer we have experienced over the last half century. Our genes have changed little for thousands of years. Think about it: Asians have lower cancer rates than Americans, but when Asians move to the U.S. and adopt our diet and lifestyle, their cancer rates soon become the same as ours. If you want to get cancer, move to America!

Since 1971, when President Nixon declared "war" on cancer by signing the National Cancer Act, the United States has spent hundreds of billions of dollars on cancer research and trillions on cancer treatment. In 1971, it was proclaimed that we could have a cure within five years—in time for our 1976 Bicentennial. Needless to say, despite all the research, conventional medicine hasn't found a cure for cancer. More than one person every 30 seconds is being diagnosed with cancer—and more than one person dies every minute. Meanwhile, the cancer industry continually issues claims that we are winning the war on cancer. After all those years and dollars spent, the evidence is overwhelming that the cancer death rate is continually climbing despite propaganda to the contrary.

Most cancer research dollars have been wasted. They have been spent trying to find new moneymaking treatments for cancer rather than finding its causes and discovering natural cures. Only 3 percent of the money allocated to cancer research has been spent to discover what causes cancer. Yet 97 percent is spent on developing new ways to diagnose cancer, after it already exists, and to treat it in ways that don't cure it. To justify all this wasted money, new cancer treatments are constantly being developed, highly publicized, and tested—but none of them work. This has been going on for decades. We keep throwing good money after bad, hoping that the "big breakthrough" is just around the corner. Cancer researchers are asking the wrong questions, looking in all the wrong places, and recycling the same failed approaches while expecting different results. As Albert Einstein is thought to have said, "The definition of insanity is doing the same thing over and over again and expecting different results." When people die from their cancer, 90 percent of the time what kills them is metastasis—aggressive cells spreading to other areas of the body. Yet, according to an editorial in a 2010 *European Journal of Cancer Research,* only about five percent of total cancer research funding is spent on investigating metastases in Europe, and in the U.S., it's even worse with only one half of 1 percent spent to research metastasis.

Cancer research has become a massive, self-perpetuating, moneymaking industry. Little progress is made because research and publishing has become an end in itself. Every study ends with the conclusion that "further study and more research are required." It is like a government jobs program. Research laboratories are kept going year after year, focusing on studies that are highly unlikely to make any significant progress in finding a cure for cancer. Meanwhile, the people who allocate the funds continue to approve the same failed approaches, rehashing the work of others. This is unproductive and a waste of money. The researchers make money and the institutions they represent make money, but *you* end up with little to show for it.

In truth, what we already know is sufficient to end the cancer epidemic—no further research is required!

So many billions are spent and there's so little to show for it. There is a reason for this. There is little money to be made in preventing or curing cancer. The money is in diagnosing and treating cancer. That's where all the research dollars go. Robert Ryan, author of *Cancer Research—A Super Fraud?*, quoted chemist and Nobel Laureate Linus Pauling as saying:

Everyone should know that most cancer research is largely a fraud and that the major cancer research organizations are derelict in their duties to those that support them.

Conventional Treatments Fail

Conventional cancer treatments damage your health, cause new cancers, lower your quality of life, and decrease your chances of survival. They are both ineffective and dangerous. Today, most people who die from cancer are not dying from cancer. *Most cancer patients die from their treatments.*

Most oncologists know from the statistics that their treatments don't work. In the next century, medical historians will look back at these inhumane and barbaric slash, burn, and poison treatments and wonder if we were all crazy. Published research has shown that a substantial number of oncologists would not use chemotherapy on themselves or their loved ones because they consider it to be ineffective and dangerous. Perhaps it is not a coincidence that more than half of all oncologists say they are emotionally exhausted, expressing feelings of low personal accomplishment. How can you feel accomplishment when the body of knowledge you learned in school is wrong, the tools you were taught to use don't work, you are killing your patients with deadly treatments, and you are not allowed to find better solutions?

If conventional treatments are useless and dangerous, and scientific research supports a less invasive and more effective approach, why not put that knowledge to use? There are many factors inhibiting changes in the way we treat cancer. One is that the cancer industry attacks and vigorously suppresses every effective solution. Cancer patients themselves contribute to this problem. They think that if there were a way to cure cancer, their doctor would know about it, so they assume a cure doesn't exist. Both cancer patients and their physicians are ignorant of what can be done to restore good health and fearful of trying something new.

On April 9, 2011, my brother Bernie died at the age of eighty. He outlived the average American male by five years. What is more significant about his death is that two decades prior Bernie was diagnosed with "inoperable," advanced prostate cancer. Bernie was informed that his cancer had metastasized throughout his body, and that there was little that could be done for him—a death sentence. His life expectancy was estimated to be anywhere from six months to an optimistic three years. With little to lose he decided to seek my guidance in trying alternative treatments, which included daily meditation, a complete change in diet, and taking dozens of dietary supplements. Bernie succeeded in putting his cancer into remission. To the amazement of his physicians—they called him their miracle patient—he lived a very high-quality life for two decades after his diagnosis. He traveled all over the world, learned to fly, got a pilot's license, and continued to do engineering consulting work.

In the years after his diagnosis, Bernie lost five friends to prostate cancer, including his best friend, Dan. Bernie, an advertisement for alternative approaches to cancer, tried to convince each of his friends to do as he had done. Their doctors actively discouraged them from trying anything unconventional. Out of fear and ignorance, both doctors and patients went the way of traditional treatments. Bernie visited Dan one day in the hospital. Dan took Bernie by the hand, looked him in the eye and said, "Well, your way worked and mine didn't." Dan died a few days later. All five friends pursued conventional treatments. All five said they trusted their doctor's advice, and all five died within three years of their diagnosis.

Having lost his friends, Bernie learned of a neighbor who was diagnosed with prostate cancer. He did the neighborly thing and walked down the street and knocked on the door. He spent two hours with this man, telling him of his experiences and offering to help him explore the option of alternative solutions to his problem. The man expressed interest and asked for more information. Bernie left saying he would put a package of information together.

The next morning the phone rang. It was the neighbor's wife. She thanked Bernie for his offer to help and then informed him that they trusted their doctor and had no interest in pursuing alternative approaches. She asked that he please never again speak to her husband about such matters. Obviously, the woman thought she was protecting her husband from some kind of quackery, but in reality, she closed the door on what could have healed him.

Beyond fear and ignorance, there are *legal factors* inhibiting cancer patients from getting well. Even though they are dangerous and mostly ineffective, the conventional cancer treatments—surgery, chemotherapy, and radiation have been *written into the law* in about half the states. For example, in California it is a felony for a physician to use any other treatment for cancer. That's a powerful disincentive for doctors who want to use a treatment that is safer and more effective! They could lose their license or go to jail if they do. Then there are insurance regulations that prohibit an oncologist from suggesting alternative cancer treatments to their patients. These legal strongholds make progress in cancer treatment not only difficult but next to impossible.

In addition, there is an economic impediment to progress in how we treat cancer. With about half of all Americans expected to get cancer in their lifetime, the cancer industry is huge and growing, amounting to hundreds of billions of dollars per year. Too many people depend on this industry for their living. *Preventing cancer and adopting a simple, inexpensive cure would be devastating to the cancer industry.* Even the American Cancer Society is at best indifferent, and at worst hostile, to cancer prevention. Their focus is on the cancer-industry standard of diagnosing and treating cancer, not on preventing and reversing it. If cancer were eliminated, a lot of people would lose their jobs. There would be no need for the American Cancer Society, the National Cancer Institute, or any other such organization. As journalist Upton Sinclair once observed, "It's difficult to get a man to understand something when his salary depends upon his not understanding it."

It is painfully ironic that the very professionals who are supposed to help you have their hands tied behind their backs. But *your* hands are not tied. You can take action now by following the principles in this book to support your body's natural defenses against all types of cancer. Nothing you would choose to do is dangerous or illegal, nor does anything recommended in this book undermine any conventional treatment you might choose to undergo.

Why Conventional Treatments Don't Work

Conventional cancer treatments have failed us. A study in a 2000 issue of the *Journal of the American Medical Association* concluded that the five-year survival rate for most forms of cancer was the same in 1995 as they were in 1950. Another example of this failure was highlighted in a 2002 *New England Journal of Medicine* study, where it was determined that twenty years of clinical trials using chemotherapy on advanced lung cancer have yielded survival improvement of only two months. Why? *Cancer is a biological process.* What we call cancer, usually a tumor, is merely a symptom—a product of that process. Yet *all* the attention goes to the symptom. *You can cut, poison, and burn the symptom all you want, but unless you turn the cancer process off—you still have cancer and it will come back.* The return of cancer is usually what happens with conventional treatments.

Conventional cancer treatments can actually make matters worse. In the majority of cases, cancer has already metastasized prior to diagnosis. Once this happens, conventional treatments have a success rate of less than 1 percent, and some researchers believe the true success rate to be zero. This makes conventional treatments useless, but even worse, they can hasten death. At least three major scientific studies, including a 1991 analysis in the *Lancet* by Dr. Ulrich Abel, have concluded that a patient who does nothing will have a better combination of longer life and higher quality of life than those who choose conventional treatment. *You can actually live longer and better if you do nothing* because "doing nothing" does no further damage to your already sick cells.

Conventional cancer treatments can remove or reduce the size of a tumor, but here is the problem—they do nothing to address the cause. Worse, they can make cancer spread, creating entirely new tumors. There are times when surgery may be necessary: for example, a large tumor impinging on another organ and threatening near-term death. If such is not the case, think twice about your options. Surgery is known to promote the spread of active cancer cells throughout the body by a process called *tumor spillage*. Even a diagnostic needle biopsy can spill cancer cells into the bloodstream or lymphatic system and spread active cancer cells throughout the body. Surgery also creates another problem. Removing a primary tumor reduces the body's natural production of cancer-fighting substances. The tumor stimulates the production of antitumor chemicals; removing the tumor stops their production. This can have an unfortunate side effect. The growth of distant clusters of inactive cancer cells is no longer inhibited, allowing whole new cancers to grow.

Chemotherapy and radiation are especially dangerous because they damage healthy cells, unnecessarily causing harm to critical tissues and doing long-term damage to the liver, kidneys, heart, nerves, and immune system. In addition, *chemotherapy drugs and radiation are themselves carcinogenic, causing entirely new cancers a few years later*. Chemotherapy drugs are some of the most powerful carcinogens known, and according to Dr. Samuel Epstein, as recorded in the *Congressional Record* of September 9, 1997, chemotherapy and radiation can increase the risk of developing a second cancer by up to 100 times. Surgery, chemotherapy, and radiation all suppress the immune system, and cancer grows and metastasizes when the body's natural immune defenses are depressed. Immune suppression alone is a powerful argument for not using these dangerous and ineffective treatments. It is well known that cancer survival is directly dependent on the strength of your immune defenses. A fully functional immune system is critical to preventing and reversing cancer.

The human body was designed to cure itself when left to its own natural devices. By depressing your immune system, chemotherapy virtually eliminates the possibility of using it to overcome your cancer; that's why chemotherapy increases your risk of dying from cancer as well as from infection. In addition, chemotherapy does something else that you should know about. It kills only the cancer cells that are the most susceptible to the drug. The tumor shrinks, and your doctors declare success. However, the cancer cells that are more drug resistant don't die. They continue to multiply and the cancer comes roaring back. This makes shrinking the tumor a second or third time much more difficult, and even impossible, because the tumor is now made of drug-resistant cancer cells. In almost all cases, conventional treatments actually make matters worse and work against your long-term recovery. *Conventional medicine has little to offer the cancer patient except high costs, pain, and perhaps a few additional weeks of miserable, low-quality life*—yet doctors are telling us it is effective.

What do they mean by effective? The U.S. Food and Drug Administration (FDA), which approves all new chemotherapy drugs, defines "effective" as achieving a 50 percent or more reduction in tumor size for twenty-eight days. Does that sound effective to you? According to a December 2004 study in the journal *Clinical Oncology*, chemotherapy has an average five-year survival success rate of about *2 percent* for all cancers. However, even in those very few cases where chemotherapy appears to work, alternative treatments would have worked even better. Yet this tiny success rate continues to fuel the use of chemotherapy. Chemotherapy is routinely prescribed for advanced lung cancer where the success rate is *less than 1 percent*.

One is reminded of bloodletting, a standard medical practice for more than 2,000 years despite the fact it was useless and dangerous. Over the centuries many people, including George Washington, were bled to death by their physicians. Bloodletting was used because physicians did not understand the causes of disease. I believe today's conventional cancer treatments will someday appear just as illogical as bloodletting.

Writing in the medical journal *Lancet* in 1991, Albert Braverman, M.D., professor of oncology at the State University of New York, said:

> *Many medical oncologists recommend chemotherapy for virtually any tumor, with a hopefulness undiscouraged by almost invariable failure. Most cancer patients in this country die of chemotherapy. Chemotherapy does not eliminate breast, colon, or lung cancers. This fact has been documented for over a decade, yet doctors still use chemotherapy for these tumors.*

That was written in 1991—yet they are still doing it! Despite the fact it has been known for decades that chemotherapy doesn't work, neither doctors nor patients seem prepared to give it up.

Cancer Statistics Are Misleading

A few years ago headlines screamed, "U.S. Cancer Deaths Decline for First Time Since 1930." The decline, by the way, amounted to just 369 fewer deaths in 2003 than in 2002, out of more than a half million deaths. The American Cancer Society issued statements saying that they expected the trend to continue. Projections were made for 2006 saying that while the actual number of new cancer cases was expected to increase, the death rate was expected to continue its decline due to earlier detection and better treatments. The sad truth is cancer deaths have not declined.

Conventional cancer treatments have been a colossal failure, and more people are dying from cancer and its treatments than ever before. This is why the cancer industry has resorted to outright fabrications to make you believe otherwise and to justify the hundreds of billions they have wasted on cancer research. The cancer industry will tell you that more people are surviving longer than ever before. But, on average, they are surviving only a few months longer, and as you will see, even those few months are fictitious. Long-term survival rates for advanced cancers have barely budged, and in fact, survival rates are worse than ever because so many people are dying from their treatments, and these deaths do not get recorded as cancer deaths. Because the truth is so outrageous, cancer survival statistics have been manipulated to the point of being meaningless. If people knew the truth, few would use conventional treatments. *If your cancer has metastasized, and most have by the time they are diagnosed, you need to know that conventional treatments will not help you.*

If we look at the real statistics instead of the propaganda, it is easy to understand why the advertised cancer survival rates are misleading. Consider this: You often hear or read that cancer can be cured if caught early. Cure rates of 40 to 50 percent are often quoted. Is this true? Look around you and judge for yourself. Is 40 to 50 percent of cancer being cured? When you see how many people are dying, does it look that way? It isn't happening! The following are a few examples of how the statistics are being falsely manipulated:

Lung cancer is the top cause of cancer death in the United States. In fact, lung cancer kills more people than colorectal, breast, and prostate cancers combined. So you would expect lung cancer to be part of the survival statistics, right? Think again. Deaths from lung cancer are not included in the statistics. When you exclude the leading cause of cancer death, the survival rates are going to look a lot better. Non-white Americans have lower cancer-survival rates than white Americans. So guess what? Non-whites are not included in the statistics—survival rates are looking even better. Simple skin cancers are *not* life threatening, but they *are* included in the survival statistics—looking better still. Other non-life-threatening, precancerous conditions, such as ductal carcinoma-in-situ, are also included in the survival statistics. No wonder they can claim cancer deaths are declining and 40 to 50 percent of cancers are being cured!

Then there is the problem of what is "survival." To hide medicine's colossal failure to deal with cancer, the American Cancer Society, the FDA, the National Cancer Institute, and other mainstream organizations involved with recording or publishing cancer statistics have invented an entirely new definition for the word "cure." For cancer patients, "cure" is arbitrarily defined as being alive *five years after diagnosis*. This means that if you die five years and one day after diagnosis, you have been cured. Surviving five years is hardly a cure, and almost all of the people who have been cured eventually die of their cancer. This phony definition is deliberately deceptive. It makes the survival statistics look better, and fools a lot of people into thinking that conventional cancer treatments can help them. What it really represents is the admission that they don't know how to cure cancer.

Early diagnosis contributes to these misleading survival statistics. Due to recent advances in diagnostic technology, cancer is being diagnosed an average of about six months earlier. Since cure is defined as survival for five years after diagnosis, diagnosing cancer six months earlier puts more people in the category of living longer than five years after diagnosis. This makes it appear as though people are surviving longer, but they aren't. The true death rate has not improved at all. A 2000 study in the *Journal of the American Medical Association* concluded that *the only reason cancer patients appear to be living longer is because of earlier diagnosis.* According to this study, the five-year survival rates for most forms of cancer were the same in 1995 as they were in 1950. The increased survival rates touted by the cancer industry have nothing to do with advances in medicine. Cancer patients are no better off today than they were in 1950! In fact, they are worse off because, as mentioned before, so many people are now dying from their treatments, which are *not recorded as cancer deaths.*

The fact that most cancer patients die from their medical treatments ironically improves the survival statistics. Conventional cancer treatments, especially radiation and chemotherapy, depress immunity. Knowing this, you have to ask: Why would any rational person want to wipe out the very system that the body uses to prevent and eliminate cancer? As a result of collapsed immune systems, cancer patients develop infections, such as pneumonia, and many die from these infections. The death is then recorded as being from pneumonia or some other infection, and not from the cancer or the toxic chemotherapy drug that actually killed them by depressing their immunity. By recording that people have died from infections instead of cancer, it helps the cancer survival rates look better—a lot better.

There has been a very real reduction in breast-cancer mortality, and the cancer industry is taking credit for it. But—is this a triumph of modern medicine? Here is the truth: According to a 2006 study reported in *Science Daily,* this decline is the direct result of a reduction in the number of physicians prescribing *hormone replacement therapy.* This common menopause therapy, routinely prescribed for millions of women, was found to be causing Alzheimer's, strokes, heart attacks, lung cancer, and *breast cancer*. The reduction in breast cancer mortality is happening because fewer doctors are *giving* their patients breast cancer!

To hide its failure, the extent of the deception in the cancer industry is so colossal that even clinical-trial studies on cancer are rigged to give misleading results. For example, say there is a ninety-day trial of a new chemotherapy drug. People in the chemotherapy group who die before the end of the ninety-day period are dropped from the study and their deaths are not recorded. Such people could be dying from the chemotherapy drug or from the cancer itself. Meanwhile, anyone in the control group who dies within the ninety-day period is listed as a cancer death. This deceptive practice helps to get dangerous cancer drugs approved.

You get the picture. Published cancer statistics are fictitious, and the cancer death rate is not going down. If you have cancer that has metastasized, conventional medicine is not going to save you—you need to take control of your own recovery.

Introducing a Bright New Chapter in the History of Cancer

If your cancer has metastasized, there are much safer alternatives to chemotherapy, radiation, and surgery that are not debilitating. They are far more effective because they address *causes*.

When cancer goes away without medical treatment, such cures are called "spontaneous remission." This is medical terminology for the unexplained and sudden disappearance of all signs and symptoms of cancer. Many cases of spontaneous remission have been recorded in conventional medical literature, but almost all of them go unrecorded. Rarely is any attempt made to identify and document the possible reasons for the remission. Physicians are mystified by these cures. But are they really mysterious?

Consider the 1988 study in the *International Journal of Biosocial Research* by Dr. Harold Foster. Foster studied 200 cases of spontaneous remission. What he found was that every one of these "mysterious" remissions had a good explanation. Almost 90 percent of these people had made major changes to their diet. The remainder had undergone detoxification programs or went on supplement programs. The fact is all 200 had done something substantial to alter their cell chemistry, turning off the switches and shutting down the drivers that were promoting their cancer—not so mysterious after all. By reactivating genes through good nutrition and detoxification, these people were able to restore apoptosis (natural cell death) in their cancer cells, causing the cells to die and their cancer to disappear. These patients did what their doctors could not do—cure their cancer. You can do the same. In fact, given that most people have cancer cells in their body, yet not everyone gets cancer, spontaneous remission may be the norm with millions of people having experienced it without ever knowing it.

Meanwhile, in the face of these sudden unexplained cures, most physicians remain bewildered. They often try to explain them by saying the patients were misdiagnosed and didn't have cancer after all or by saying that previous conventional treatments had finally kicked in and worked. But in truth, the mechanisms of spontaneous remissions are well enough understood that we can put them to work for the good of all.

The body wants to be well, it knows how to be well, and it will be well if you give it the physical and mental support it needs. *The key to eliminating cancer, or any other disease, is to create health by giving your body what it needs to function normally and to protect it from anything that interferes with the body's natural control mechanisms.* It's that simple.

Paul's Experience

Paul was athletic and a successful corporate CEO in his mid-forties. He consumed an average American diet and thought of himself as healthy. Then one day he got the shock of his life.

Paul had started to feel ill. He went to his doctor, and after extensive testing, he was diagnosed with kidney cancer. One kidney was surgically removed and Paul received chemotherapy. His body was devastated by these treatments, which didn't work. Then he got the really bad news—Paul's cancer had spread throughout his body. Paul was released from the hospital and was told that there was nothing medical science could do for him. He was sent home to die.

Fortunately, Paul was a dynamic, take-charge personality who wasn't going to go without a fight. Instead of accepting his death sentence, he sought out alternative health information and purchased a copy of *Never Be Sick Again*. He completely overhauled his diet and lifestyle. These changes shut the cancer process down, and a few months later he was cancer free.

Paul has now been cancer free and in vigorous health for eight years. Not bad for someone with terminal cancer who was supposed to be dead within months. Instead of trying to kill the cancer, he chose to turn his cancer off by addressing its causes, giving his body what it needed to get well. By turning cancer's switches and drivers off, Paul chose an approach to his problem that was safer, less expensive, not debilitating, and, most importantly, more effective. He saved himself from medically certain death. Anybody *can* do this. The body knows how to heal itself, and it will. All you have to do is support rather than hinder the healing process. The human body is a miraculous thing, if we give the healer within a chance to do its work.

Once you understand that cancer is not a thing to be killed with poison or surgically removed, but a process that can be switched on or off like a lamp in your living room, a new world of possibilities opens. What we already know about this process is sufficient to intervene effectively to prevent and reverse almost all cancer. Once you learn about cancer's switches and drivers, you can stop driving your cancer and switch it off. You are in charge.

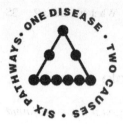

ONE DISEASE · TWO CAUSES · SIX PATHWAYS

2

WHAT IS DISEASE?

Simplicity is the ultimate sophistication.

—*Leonardo da Vinci*

The specific disease doctrine is the grand refuge of weak,
uncultured, unstable minds . . . There are no specific diseases.

—*Florence Nightingale*

H ere is what you need to know about disease: The science
is there and the facts are indisputable. When correctly
understood at the cellular and molecular level, virtually
all disease can be prevented and reversed. The purpose of this chapter is to use the available science to give you a basic understanding
of how to prevent and reverse disease—an understanding your physician most likely doesn't have.

Making Disease Simple

This chapter presents you with a truly revolutionary and profound new understanding of health. You already have the power to create health in your life, thereby eliminating disease, including cancer. You don't have to be good at science, nor do you have to know all there is to know, so long as what you know is sufficient to keep you in good health.

Knowledge is power, and if you can understand what causes disease, you have the power to end it. To the average person, sickness is something mysterious and often frightening. We don't know why it happens. Why do you have a cold? Why do you have cancer? Why did my husband have a heart attack? Why does Mother have Alzheimer's? Even our physicians don't understand what causes disease at the cellular level or how to reverse it, so they resort to toxic drugs and invasive surgery, not to cure disease, but merely to suppress its symptoms. In truth, no one fully understands disease because human biology is almost infinitely complex. Yet nothing happens without a reason, and even our incomplete understanding of disease is sufficient to put an end to our epidemic of chronic disease and cancer—if only we apply what we already know.

The enormous amount of disease in America today is truly astonishing. Compared to other industrialized countries, we rank near the bottom in overall health and longevity. Despite the fact that we spend more than twice as much as any other country, the World Health Organization (WHO) ranks the U.S. as only thirty-seventh in terms of overall health. More than three out of four Americans have a diagnosable chronic disease; more than half of our children will experience a chronic disease; more than two out of three are overweight; less than 1 percent of the population can be considered healthy, and it is getting worse every year. Our young people are in such poor health that medical journals are projecting life expectancy in America to trend downward after two centuries of increases. Given the money we spend on health care, we have the worst performing health care system in the world. Since the health-care system isn't delivering, we need to provide our own health care. *This is why we need to simplify.*

The One Disease

How is this for simplicity? *There is only one disease.* Yet practitioners of conventional medicine continue to believe there are thousands of diseases, and they keep inventing new ones. No one can cope with thousands of diseases, so we abdicate our responsibility for our own health and put our faith in the experts to save us. But even the experts can't cope with thousands of diseases, so they keep breaking medicine up into more and more medical specialties. However, once you understand there is only one disease, this takes the complexity out of disease—it makes most specialists obsolete. This simple concept of one disease puts the power over disease into *your* hands.

What is this one disease? *Malfunctioning cells!* Each of us starts life as a single cell in our mother. That one cell grows into a community of tens of trillions of cells communicating and cooperating with each other. All tissues and organs are made of cells; all bodily functions are carried out by cells, and these cells are specialized depending on which function they perform.

Diseases originate inside of cells. If each of your individual cells is functioning normally, all of your cells will be communicating with each other and your body will be self-regulating, self-repairing, and balanced.

When your body is in balance, you are healthy and *you cannot be sick*. This balanced state is called "homeostasis." When you are in homeostasis, your body will regulate its internal conditions, regardless of outside conditions. A simple example of homeostasis is the body's ability to maintain its internal temperature within a narrow range, despite large variations in the outside temperature. When your body is in balance, you are healthy. When cells malfunction and the body's ability to communicate, self-regulate, and self-repair is impaired—you are sick. We put a lot of wear and tear on the body every day, and if your body is not fully self-repairing daily, you will develop repair deficits. Your body will soon let you know. Any illness is a sign that you need repairs that your body isn't making. Repair deficits in your car make it age, break down, and end up in a junkyard. Your body is no different. Repair deficits manifest as aging, disease, and disability—people end up sick, frail, and in nursing homes, unable to care for themselves. They are falling apart from lack of repair. In fact, all chronic disease involves repair deficits, and this is why they are degenerative. Whichever disease label your physician has slapped on you, whether it's allergies, arthritis, diabetes, cancer, Alzheimer's, or osteoporosis, all are due to cellular malfunction that results in repair deficits.

Getting well involves shifting the body back into the normal repair mode. To do this, you have to eat a good diet and take high-quality supplements so you can give your cells all the repair materials they need to do their job, *and* you must keep your cells free of toxins that can interfere with their communications or shut down your repair machinery. When you give the doctor within the chance to go to work, and your body is once again communicating, self-regulating, and self-repairing, you will become biologically younger, happier, mentally sharper, stronger, healthier, and disease free.

Once you understand the concept of malfunctioning cells and only one disease, you'll see that all the thousands of other so-called "diseases," including cancer, do not exist. So if they don't exist, why does diabetes look different from Alzheimer's and heart disease look different from cancer? It's because these so-called diseases are merely different symptoms produced by cells in different tissues that are malfunctioning for different reasons in different ways—*but it is all cellular malfunction.*

Disease cannot happen unless cells malfunction. Alzheimer's disease is cells that are malfunctioning in the memory part of the brain. Parkinson's disease is cells malfunctioning in the motor part of the brain. Macular degeneration is cells malfunctioning in the eye. Breast cancer is cells that are malfunctioning in the breast. In each case, we have cells malfunctioning in a different part of the body, but to think of them as different diseases is self-defeating and indicates a lack of understanding of the true causes of disease. To empower ourselves to prevent and reverse all disease, we need to focus on what is common to each disease, not on what is different.

Cellular malfunction is the essence of every so-called disease. Unless cells malfunction, there can be no disease—*disease is cellular malfunction.* Either your cells are functioning as they should, or they are not. It's that simple. If they are not functioning as they should, you can exhibit thousands of symptoms. Our physicians call them thousands of diseases, but if cells were not malfunctioning, there would be no symptoms. *No matter what the symptoms, if you restore cells to normal function, the symptoms go away.*

What we call "cancer" is cells that are malfunctioning in a way that interferes with their normal communication and growth-control mechanisms, so the cells grow uncontrollably. Cancer, like any disease, is cellular malfunction. When cells malfunction, different symptoms are produced depending on a number of factors, including your unique genetic makeup. To give different names to different symptoms may be useful for discussion purposes, but it is counterproductive for treatment purposes. The name of your disease doesn't matter because there is only one disease and only one treatment.

Cellular malfunction is the one disease, which causes all symptoms. The one treatment is restoring cells to normal function, which eliminates all symptoms.

You can call certain symptoms cancer if you like, but how does that help you? Does it tell you how you got the cancer? Does it tell you how to prevent cancer or how to reverse cancer? Don't be confused by the name. Once you know that cancer is caused by cellular malfunction it is simple to treat.

To reverse cancer, all you have to do is change from the conditions that favor the cancer process to those that favor health. Make your cells healthy and the cancer goes away. We already know how to do this—so much for cancer being a mysterious, life-threatening monster.

To reverse disease, you have to restore malfunctioning cells to normal. You prevent disease by preventing cellular malfunction. This is the same no matter what your disease is called.

The Two Causes of Disease

As we have just seen, there is only one disease: cellular malfunction. *There are only two causes of cellular malfunction: deficiency and toxicity. Therefore, there are only two causes of disease.* Either cells are getting *too little* of what they need or *too much* of something they don't need. The common denominators of all cellular malfunctions are deficiency and toxicity. Cancer does not cause people to become sick. Deficiency and toxicity cause people to become sick. What we call cancer is just one set of symptoms that can be produced by cellular deficiency and toxicity. *To shut down the cancer process, cancer treatment must focus on removing these two causes of cellular malfunction.*

Are you having a problem embracing this simplicity? Are you asking, "Doesn't stress cause disease?" It sure does, but through the same two causes—deficiency and toxicity. Manufacturing stress chemicals depletes the body of critical nutrients, causing deficiency. Chronic stress causes a buildup of stress chemicals in the body, and the excess of stress chemicals has a toxic effect on the body. Even infectious and genetic diseases manifest because of deficiency and toxicity. When genes malfunction, they are not producing what they should be producing or are producing too much of something they should not be producing—deficiency and toxicity. In every case you might think of, it always comes back to deficiency and toxicity—the two causes that are common to all disease.

Want to talk about miracles? Think of each single cell in your body as a vast industrial park containing thousands of factories, producing tens of thousands of life-sustaining chemicals every day. Some of these chemicals are hormones to help regulate your body, neurotransmitters to enable you to learn, think, and remember, and antibodies to keep you free of infection. Each cell contains hundreds of powerhouses, called mitochondria, to produce the "energy of life." There are also warehouses, a central computer, traffic directors, communications systems, raw material delivery systems, waste disposal systems, security systems and much more. All of this metabolic machinery knows how to function perfectly when the right raw materials are available and toxic substances are not interfering with normal operations.

If even one raw material (nutrient) is chronically lacking, your body will not be able to make enough of the right chemicals. Without all the essential nutrients and all the metabolic machinery working smoothly and being given the correct operating instructions, your body will be unable to keep you in good repair or to build those hormones that are so necessary to keep the body balanced, the neurotransmitters so critical to your brain function, or those antibodies to keep your immune system strong. In each cell, every second, there are about 100,000 chemical reactions taking place with literally trillions of individual activities occurring. Our job is to support all this. When we don't, we get sick.

A chronic deficiency of even one nutrient will make us sick. The average American is chronically deficient in at least several essential nutrients. We know that *even one toxin can disable critical metabolic machinery or give incorrect instructions to the machinery, creating chaos in the cells and the body.* The average American is in toxic overload with hundreds of toxins accumulating in their tissues. Studies show that combinations of toxins acting together can be thousands of times more damaging than any one of them acting alone—sometimes unbelievably more damaging. Given our state of deficiency and toxicity, it is no wonder cancer is an out-of-control epidemic.

Suppose you go to your doctor with the following three complaints: asthma, arthritis, and depression. Suppose the doctor examines you and determines that you also have high blood pressure and osteoporosis. According to conventional medicine's view of disease, you now have five diagnosable diseases. You may be referred to different specialists. Perhaps you will see a pulmonary specialist for your asthma, a psychiatrist for your depression, and a bone specialist for your osteoporosis. You will almost certainly end up on a number of drugs: perhaps a bronchodilator and a corticosteroid for your asthma, acetaminophen for your arthritis, several drugs for your hypertension, Fosamax for your osteoporosis, and Zoloft for your depression. *None of these drugs will cure you!* On the contrary, the combination of them will be so toxic that you are virtually guaranteed to develop entirely new diseases. So as not to alarm you that you are now much sicker than when you started, physicians don't call these new problems "diseases." They obscure this reality by calling them "side effects." Additional drugs may be prescribed to suppress the symptoms of these newly created problems, but since drugs are toxins, and toxins cause disease, the more drugs you take the sicker you will get.

There is only one disease, but a conventionally trained physician will think you have five diseases, so it is virtually certain you will be treated incorrectly, creating even more disease. In reality, you have only one disease. What you have is a large number of malfunctioning cells, causing a lot of different symptoms. In the case above, the cells are malfunctioning because they are toxic with too much mercury. Mercury is a toxic heavy metal that, even at extremely low doses, can cause *all* of the above so-called diseases, at the same time, in the same person. In addition, mercury's toxicity causes many deficiencies. Once again, it always comes back to deficiency and toxicity and only one disease, not five. All five will disappear when you address the true cause—excess mercury. Sources of mercury include dental amalgam fillings, vaccinations, and seafood.

You might be wondering, *how does mercury toxicity cause deficiencies?* Here is how. Enzymes are special protein molecules that facilitate the building of essential molecules that your body needs such as hormones and neurotransmitters. They also act to break down molecules, for example, in the digestive process. There are many enzymes in the body; each is designed to do a specific task, and each is an essential part of your body's metabolic machinery. Mercury reacts with enzymes and disables them, blocking their function. This happens even at extremely low concentrations. Since most people have a deficiency of essential minerals in their diet, the toxic effects of mercury will be even greater because of these deficiencies. Disabled enzymes can no longer facilitate the building of hormones, neurotransmitters, and other essential molecules, nor can they break down molecules in the digestive process. This disruption causes a deficiency of critical body chemicals, seriously impairing the functional activity of critical organs and tissues. This can cause many different symptoms to appear, which conventional medicine then groups together into so-called "diseases."

Depending on which enzymes are being disabled, a deficiency of biologically active enzymes can cause any number of symptoms. When you disable enzymes that break down chemicals that raise blood pressure, blood pressure increases. Disabling enzymes in your brain reduces the supply of critical neurotransmitters (chemicals that transmit nerve impulses), causing depression, learning disabilities and other mental problems. Mercury can disable energy-producing enzymes in your mitochondria, causing fatigue. (Mitochondria are sometimes described as "cellular power plants" because their primary purpose is to manufacture adenosine triphosphate, or ATP, which is used as a source of energy.) Digestive enzymes can be disabled, causing poor digestion. Enzymes in your thyroid can be disabled, causing thyroid insufficiency and any number of thyroid-related problems. Mercury's combination of toxicity and induced deficiencies causes all of the above so-called diseases plus many more, including cancer.

To reverse the above "diseases," you have to first understand there is only one disease—malfunctioning cells. Next you have to address what is causing them to malfunction. In this case, identify the mercury toxicity and get rid of the mercury. Once you do this, all of the diseases will disappear—a far better option than taking toxic drugs to treat the symptoms, which will not only keep you sick, but make you even sicker.

We have just looked at a partial list of the number of so-called diseases that just one toxin can cause. A deficiency of even one nutrient can cause a similar list of diseases. Given that Americans are chronically deficient in at least several essential nutrients and they are accumulating hundreds of toxins resulting in thousands of "diseases" for which thousands of toxic drugs can be prescribed, the result is more toxicity and more disease. The prostate gland is a zinc-rich tissue; a zinc deficiency will cause prostate problems. The thyroid gland is an iodine-rich tissue; an iodine deficiency will cause thyroid problems. The cervix is a vitamin C- and folate-rich tissue; women with low vitamin C intake have a substantially higher cervical cancer risk. Thousands of so-called diseases can be produced by deficiencies, and you can be sure that conventional medicine will treat almost all of them incorrectly because our physicians have not been trained to understand this: *There is only one disease and only two causes of disease—deficiency and toxicity.*

The Promise of Health

It is possible to cure "incurable" diseases. It is possible to get well, stay well, and never be sick again. It is possible to reduce your biological age and become physically younger. All these things are possible because the human body is a truly magnificent self-regulating, self-repairing, and self-healing machine. We only have to help the doctor within, and let the body do what it already knows how to do.

We can do this by supplying cells with all the nutrients they need and keeping them free of toxins that can interfere with their proper functions.

The body makes about 10 million *new* cells every second and almost a trillion new cells every day. Most of the cells in your body are replaced in one year. Here are questions you need to ask yourself:

- Are the millions of cells I am now making better than the ones they are replacing?
- Am I supplying high quality building materials to make the new cells?
- Am I supplying these cells with the nutrients they need to operate normally?
- Am I keeping them free of toxins that will poison them?

When you replace old, sick cells with new healthy cells, you are shifting your body into repair mode. This creates health; you get well and become biologically younger. If every new cell is better than the one it's replacing, you are creating a new you—you are growing younger and healthier!

The problem for most of us is this: our new cells are no better than our old ones, and frequently are even worse. New cells can only be created with the building materials you are supplying through your diet. You cannot get well when you make your new cells out of the same nutritionally deficient, toxic junk foods that made you sick in the first place. This will create new cells that are lacking the critical nutrients required for healthy function and load them with toxins that interfere with their function. Your new cells will be created with improperly constructed cell membranes, damaged energy-producing systems, disabled metabolic machinery, and unrepaired

DNA damage. They cannot and will not function normally. Unless you consistently supply your body with high-quality nutrition—you will get sick, and you will stay sick.

You can get well, stay well, and even reverse the aging process by learning how to keep your body in good repair—by making sure that every new cell you create is better than the one it's replacing. If you are going to repair something, you have to fix what's broken. A deficiency of even one nutrient, a single toxin, chronic stress, negative thoughts, lack of exercise, lack of sunlight, genetic mutations, and exposure to electromagnetic radiation will all contribute to cellular malfunction and disease. Each of these factors will be operating in different ways, to a larger or lesser extent, in each individual. One person may need more nutrition, another more detoxification, and another more love in their life. Only by taking a comprehensive approach to illness can you make sure all of the potential causes are being addressed.

The Six Pathways to Health or Disease

There are six major pathways to health and disease by which we can either become deficient and toxic or avoid becoming deficient and toxic. Think of it this way: There are two major cities—Health and Disease. There are six major highways connecting these two cities. If you are traveling on all major highways toward Health, guess where you will end up? In Health. On the other hand, if you are traveling toward Disease on all the highways, you will end up in Disease. Most Americans are heading toward Disease because they don't know any better, but you don't have to be one of them. There are daily choices we all make that determine where we are on each pathway, in which direction we are heading, and how fast we are going. The choice between health and disease—between cancer and no cancer—is yours. Get yourself moving toward health on all Six Pathways and you will have a winning strategy—a strategy that addresses every aspect of your life that affects your health.

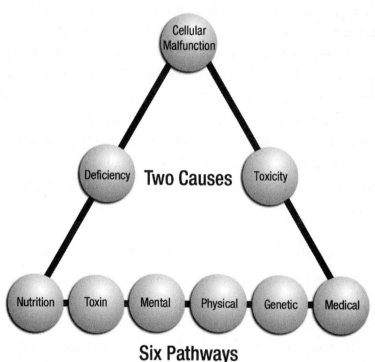

One Disease

Cellular Malfunction

Deficiency **Two Causes** Toxicity

Nutrition Toxin Mental Physical Genetic Medical

Six Pathways

The Nutrition Pathway

To be healthy, the exquisitely complex metabolic machinery in your cells must be provided with the nutrients they need to function properly. The Nutrition Pathway is about learning how to give your cells what they need on a daily basis. In most cases, this means changing what you eat. There is so much confusion regarding nutrition because most of the nutritional advice in the popular press is wrong. Here we will tell you how to select, prepare, and combine foods, what to order at restaurants, and which supplements you should take to enhance your health. In the Nutrition Pathway chapter (Chapter 4) you'll learn how to make nutritional choices that will support health and discourage disease—choices that will help to prevent and reverse cancer by shutting down the cancer process. If you eat junk, you will deliver junk to your cells and they will malfunction. If you eat healthy foods, tumors will shrivel up and die.

The Toxin Pathway

Toxicity is one of the two causes of all disease. To get well and stay well, you must minimize your toxic load by learning how to dramatically reduce your toxic exposures, how to support your body's detoxification system, and how to get rid of previously stored toxins. In the Toxin Pathway chapter (Chapter 5) you will learn how toxins both cause and drive the cancer process, and what you need to do to prevent and reverse that process.

The Mental Pathway

What you put into your mind every day is even more important than what you put into your body. Every thought has a biological consequence. *Putting thoughts into your mind every waking hour is one of the most important activities of your life.*

Thoughts can change your body chemistry, for better or for worse, in a matter of seconds. Each and every thought has a physical effect. In fact, it is not possible to have a thought without a physical effect. Thoughts affect our genes and our immune, hormone, digestive, and other body systems. You can think your way into cancer, and you can think your way out of it. Every thought is a cause, and if you want to change the effects, you have to change the causes—you have to change your thoughts. In the Mental Pathway chapter (Chapter 6), you will learn how to use this incredible power to prevent and reverse cancer.

The Physical Pathway

To be healthy, we must give our cells all the nutrients they need and keep them free of toxins that can harm them. To function optimally, they also need something else—to be moved and stretched. Movement helps deliver nutrients and remove toxic waste products from cells. Physical movement is a necessity for healthy life, and believe it or not, anyone can get the movement they need—almost effortlessly, if they're taught how.

Cells need to be protected from physical harm. This includes being protected from the cancer-causing harm of medical x-rays. The body also needs to be exposed to adequate amounts of sunlight in order to function properly. These and more, such as the effects of sleep and noise are covered in the Physical Pathway chapter (Chapter 7).

The Genetic Pathway

Most of us think that genes run our lives, and it's true. Genes do run our lives, but guess what? We run the genes! Cancer results from changes in how genes function, which alter the way cells behave. Genes don't cause cancer, but they play a vital role in the cancer process. Our job is to prevent damage to our genes, quickly repair any damage that occurs, and give our genes the proper instructions so they will work for our greatest good. (See Chapter 8.)

The Medical Pathway

If you have an acute medical emergency, such as a heart attack or a traumatic injury, conventional medicine will offer your best option for care. However, if you have a chronic illness, such as cancer, conventional medicine will be of little help, will probably make you sicker, and might even kill you. So-called "modern" medicine has failed to put into clinical practice the enormous advances in science over the last century. As a result, most conventional treatments are unscientific and hopelessly outmoded—the modern day equivalent of bloodletting. In the Medical Pathway chapter (Chapter 9), you will learn how to choose medicine's benefits and how to avoid its harm, especially regarding cancer.

Takeaway Tips

- Chronic disease is epidemic. People are getting sicker and the costs are escalating out of control. Given what we get for what we spend, we have one of the worst performing healthcare systems in the world. Conventional medicine has failed us.

- There is a need to simplify. By using cutting-edge science to understand what has to go wrong at the cellular level for disease to happen, we place ourselves in the position of being able to effectively intervene to prevent and reverse almost all disease.

- There is only One Disease, Two Causes of disease, and Six Pathways to health or disease, and you are in charge.

- While it appears that there are thousands of different diseases, these "diseases" are just symptoms of cellular malfunctions. It is your unique set of deficiencies and toxicities, all acting through a unique set of genes that produces the symptoms physicians call a disease.

- Disease can only be prevented and reversed by addressing the underlying causes. But there is no magic bullet. Each person is different. This is why you need to follow all Six Pathways to make sure all your issues are being addressed.

- The body has an almost endless capacity for healing. Give cells the nutrients they need, eliminate their toxic load, and they will function normally. Almost anyone can do this and enjoy disease-free living with boundless energy, without medical bills, and without drugs and surgery. Give the doctor within the chance to go to work.

Even if you have a history of eating the wrong foods and exposing yourself to toxins, you can reverse most of the damage. In the following chapters, you will discover how you can make this knowledge work for you, so you can prevent and reverse cancer.

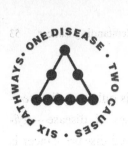

ONE DISEASE · TWO CAUSES · SIX PATHWAYS

3

UNDERSTANDING CANCER

It will not be long before the entire population will have to decide whether we will all die of cancer or whether we will have enough wisdom, courage, and will power to change fundamentally all our living and nutritional conditions.

—*Dr. Max Gerson, developer of the Gerson Cancer Therapy*

As a chemist trained to interpret data, it is incomprehensible to me that physicians can ignore the clear evidence that chemotherapy does much, much more harm than good.

—*Alan Nixon, Ph.D., past president, American Chemical Society*

I n the last chapter you learned that there is only one disease—*malfunctioning cells*—and only two causes of disease—*deficiency* and *toxicity*. Like any other so-called disease, cancer is nothing more than malfunctioning cells caused by deficiency and toxicity. To triumph over cancer, we need to understand which deficiencies and toxicities cause the malfunction we call cancer. There are literally thousands of ways in which cells can malfunction, producing thousands of symptoms. We need to know what is special or unique about cancer cells. What are the particular deficiencies, toxicities, and cellular malfunctions that are responsible for switching on and driving the cancer process? Once you know this, you will be able to prevent that process from turning on, and you will even be able to turn it off.

In this chapter, my objective is to identify the best science and translate that into simple actionable information, so that in most cases, you can keep yourself cancer free.

Cancer is the result of a staggering number of biological and genetic malfunctions with many contributing factors. This complexity has conventional medicine utterly baffled; it views cancer as a collection of more than one hundred separate and distinct diseases because it is always looking for what is different. This only adds to confusion. Since there is only one disease, how can there be over a hundred kinds of cancer? If we look at the whole picture, what we find is that all of these so-called different kinds of cancer share common biological malfunctions. It is these common abnormalities that create what we call cancer. It is not in what is different, but in what is common, that we will find the answer to cancer.

What Is Cancer?

Cancer begins as a single abnormal cell that begins to multiply out of control. To keep itself in good repair, the body produces more than 10 million new cells every second—almost a trillion new cells every day. New cells develop only from preexisting cells, as needed. Two new cells will be produced from one parent cell through a process of cell division called "mitosis." Cancer happens when mitosis goes out of control and cells experience abnormal, rapid growth. Cancer cells divide endlessly, forming tumors. Some of these cancer cells break away from the parent tumors and metastasize (spread) throughout the body, forming new tumors.

Healthy cells have mechanisms that control and regulate their growth. For example, when a cell divides more than it should, neighboring cells become aware of this and send messages to slow the growth. Good cellular communications are critical to keeping the body cancer free. For cancer to happen, communications must be disrupted. Another important control mechanism is *apoptosis* (often called "cell suicide"). Apoptosis is genetically programmed into every cell, killing off damaged cells and preventing uncontrolled growth that can lead to tumors. When this control mechanism breaks down, cells don't die when they are supposed to. Uncontrolled growth invades local organs and then distant organs through metastasis. Invasion of multiple organs impairs critical body functions; unable to carry on essential functions, we die.

In 1997, a report from Columbia University School of Public Health in New York stated that 95 percent of all cancer is caused by diet and environment. Cancer doesn't just happen! It doesn't fall out of the sky and hit you over the head. By learning how and why cancer develops, you can learn how to support your cells to prevent and reverse cancer. Even if cancer is highly advanced in your body, it is never too late to start the process of restoring health.

Indeed, there is only *one* solution to *any* health problem—*restore health*. To restore health, cells must be returned to normal function by addressing their deficiencies and toxicities. Drugs, radiation, and surgery are not the answer; they damage the body and make you less healthy. Today we live in a stressful world filled with cancer-causing toxins and radiation. These, combined with our poor diets and overworked and weakened immune systems, allow cancer to thrive in our bodies.

Given the reality that cancer is a complex disease with numerous factors playing a role, no one fully understands it all, but we don't have to. We just need to know what is sufficient to prevent and reverse the disease. If we can discover something common to every cancer cell, interfering with this common element would be a powerful tool to help us prevent and reverse the cellular malfunction we call cancer. Using the analogy of driving a car, there are a lot of ways in which you can interfere with driving a car. You can fail to turn the ignition on, fail to put the car in gear, fail to release the parking brake, or even fail to put fuel in the tank. Cancer is the same way; it's complex and there are a lot of ways to intentionally screw it up. You are about to learn how to do that. I recommend doing everything possible that interferes with the cancer process. Numerous factors can contribute to the deficiency and toxicity that cause disease. Every time you do even one thing that helps your body to function at a higher level, you are creating health and adding to your defenses against disease.

We must ask what turns cancer on and what fuels and drives cancer. By identifying and learning how to interfere with the known mechanisms upon which the cancer process depends, you will have specific directions to help you prevent and reverse cancer in yourself and in those you love and care about. This chapter covers the major switches and drivers that enable cancer, and outlines a comprehensive approach for controlling the cancer process. In truth, there are a number of safe, natural, and effective treatments for cancer, but only a few people are using them. Most people don't even know about them or are too frightened to try them for fear they might not work. Instead, they turn to conventional treatments that we know with certainty do not work.

Researchers tell us that cancer cells are produced in our bodies on a regular basis, yet only a tiny percentage of cells in every person turn cancerous. Normally, the body has the capacity to neutralize these cancer cells before they do harm. Too many of us are now exceeding our body's capacity to neutralize these cells. Living in our cancer-promoting society with poor diets, toxic overload, viruses, carcinogens, health-damaging medical treatments, and radiation, our immune systems have become significantly overworked and weakened. It's so bad that, after age fifty, 40 percent of American men have prostate cancer and 40 percent of women have breast cancer. In truth, almost every American over age fifty has microscopic clusters of cancer cells (microtumors) throughout their bodies just waiting for the opportunity to grow. Fortunately, the body has a number of ways for keeping these cells under control and inhibiting their growth. Even though most of us have cancer cells in our bodies, *if they don't grow, it's not a problem.*

One of the most important things we can do to prevent cancer from growing is to maintain a strong immune system. Unfortunately, today most of us have overworked and weakened immune systems. It is well known that survival rates among cancer patients are directly proportional to the strength of their immune systems.

According to George C. Pack, M.D., a cancer specialist at Cornell Medical School, "The only real defense against cancer is the immune system. Everyone produces cancer every day, but if the immune system is where it should be, those cancer cells are eliminated and we never know it."

Dr. Pack went on to say, "*Once a person has developed cancer, even though treatments get it into remission, it will recur again unless the body conditions that allowed it to develop in the first place are corrected.*" Remember cancer is not a thing. It is a biological process that requires certain conditions for the process to operate. Tumors are products of this process—they are a symptom. Cancer is not the tumor; cancer is the process that created the tumor. Consider that by the time a tumor is diagnosed, you have already had cancer for years or perhaps even decades. What is important is the process that is producing the tumor, not the tumor itself. This is why you can't win by removing or trying to kill the tumor. To win, you have to shut down the process. To do that, you have to change the conditions that allow it to happen, including strengthening the immune system. Conventional treatments only suppress the symptoms while weakening the immune system and contributing to the cancer process. The cancer comes back, usually worse than before.

A 2000 study in the *New England Journal of Medicine* helps us to understand how cancer evolves. The study concluded, "Cancer results from the accumulation of mutations in genes that regulate cellular proliferation." Many forms of cancer are thought to be the result of reactions between free radicals and DNA, resulting in mutations. Cells contain genes that can be switched on as required when a cell needs to divide. These genes turn on briefly to do their job and then turn off. Problems arise when the genes become damaged (mutated) or are given incorrect instructions. As the number of problem genes accumulates, the risk of cancer increases. When too many growth-control genes become damaged or otherwise reprogrammed, the resulting programming errors cause cells to lose control over their growth rate and they continue to divide, thereby forming tumors.

It is normal for some genes to be damaged by free radicals, which are produced through a number of normal body functions as well as when the body is subjected to infections or toxic environmental exposures. A free radical is an atom or group of atoms that has at least one unpaired electron, causing it to become highly chemically reactive. Electrons like to travel in pairs, so free radicals with unpaired electrons attack the nearest stable molecule, "stealing" its electron. When the "attacked" molecule loses its electron, it becomes fundamentally changed. It now becomes a free radical itself, beginning a chain reaction that can cascade, finally resulting in the disruption of a living cell. Critical molecules can be damaged, preventing them from doing their important jobs, like maintaining the integrity of a cell membrane. When free radicals react with DNA (a nucleic acid that contains the genetic instructions), this changes how the DNA functions, and the accumulation of damage over time ages us and causes disease, including cancer.

The body is designed to handle the free radicals produced by its normal metabolism, but if antioxidants are unavailable, or if the free-radical production becomes excessive, damage will occur. Of particular importance is that free radical damage accumulates with age.

Genes don't have to be damaged to malfunction; they can be reprogrammed by changes in cell chemistry and exposure to environmental toxins. For example, a single gene can be capable of producing thousands of different proteins. These proteins have many critical functions in maintaining and regulating the body. How does a cell know which one of the thousands to make and when to make it? The internal mental and physical environment you create for your genes provides the instructions and determines how they will express. Changes in cell chemistry due to deficiency and toxicity can give genes improper instructions. This can cause the cell-growth on/off switch to turn on, resulting in uncontrolled growth. Genes are obedient servants, and do what they are asked to do. This is why it is important to maintain a normal, healthy environment inside your cells so that your genes are provided with instructions that support health rather than disease. Such an environment cannot be maintained if you eat the nutrient-deficient Standard American Diet, keep increasing your toxic load, or continually hold negative thoughts.

Genes also control critical cell-to-cell communications that help to control growth, yet these critical communications are being increasingly compromised. A 1982 study in *Carcinogenesis* found that common environmental chemicals can cause cancer simply by interfering with cell-to-cell communications. Almost every American is in toxic overload, with hundreds of these toxic chemicals bio-accumulating in our cells and tissues. This is why we need to learn how to limit our toxic exposures and how to reduce the toxic burden we have already accumulated.

Genes are more likely to suffer damage if you eat a diet and live a lifestyle that encourages the production of free radicals. This same kind of diet is usually lacking in antioxidants that protect against free-radical damage. An antioxidant is a nutrient or chemical that reacts with and neutralizes free radicals, protecting you from their damage. The combination of excess free-radical production plus poor antioxidant defenses makes genes highly susceptible to free-radical damage and mutation. The American diet and lifestyle significantly promote free-radical production and create woeful deficiencies in antioxidants—a perfect combination for creating cancer. Further, more than two out of three Americans are overweight, and fat cells produce a constant flood of inflammatory chemicals that result in free-radical damage to genes. This is one reason why overweight people age faster, experience more disease, have more cancer, and die younger.

Clearly, every practical step should be taken to prevent gene mutations. It is not possible to prevent all gene mutations, and this is why we have DNA repair systems to repair the damage. However, there is a limit to the number of gene mutations that can be repaired. We can minimize DNA damage by avoiding those factors that create excess free-radical production, such as eating sugar or wheat, consuming the wrong oils, being overweight, or allowing excessive exposure to radiation and environmental toxins. Then we must nutritionally support our DNA repair systems with a good diet and nutrient supplementation. We must also increase the antioxidants in our diet to help neutralize free radicals by eating more fresh fruits and vegetables and taking high quality supplements. Supplementing with antioxidant vitamins and minerals, such as vitamins C and E, and carotenes and selenium, will help to prevent DNA damage. Once damage has occurred, vitamins B3, B6, B12, folate, zinc, and L-carnitine will support DNA repair. Repairing DNA damage before cells divide prevents the damage from becoming permanent.

The Prime Cause

Thousands of studies have indicated that cancer has endless causes, including damaged genes, carcinogenic chemicals, nutritional deficiencies, electromagnetic fields, radiation, stress, and viruses. However, none of these are the *prime cause* of cancer. A prime cause is something that must be *acting in every case*. For example, we know genes play an essential role in cancer, but the same genetic mutations are not found in every cancer cell. We know that toxins and nutritional deficiencies contribute to cancer, but the same combinations are not acting in every case. What then, if anything, can be found in every cancer cell? In searching for the prime cause, only one thing has been found that is common to all cancer cells: *a deficiency of oxygen metabolism in the cell*. Oxygen metabolism is the combining of oxygen with a fuel in a cell to create heat and energy.

Oxygen deficiency—insufficient oxygen metabolism in a cell—is the prime cause of cancer. Therefore, preventing and reversing cancer must be about preventing and reversing impaired oxygen metabolism. All disease is caused by deficiency and toxicity. Different combinations of deficiencies and toxicities create different symptoms. Our physicians give the symptoms different names. The symptoms they call cancer are the result of cellular malfunctions caused by oxygen deficiency in different areas of our bodies—*cancer is an oxygen deficiency disease.*

Healthy cells create energy through *oxygen respiration*. Oxygen respiration is a process where oxygen is brought into the cell and combined with a fuel (sugar or fat). Think of it as burning fuel to keep your body warm and supply you with energy, just as you burn gasoline in your car.

Oxygen respiration is dependent on bringing adequate oxygen into the lungs, transferring that oxygen from the lungs into the bloodstream, and combining it with hemoglobin in the blood cells. The red blood cells then transport the oxygen around the body to where it is needed. When arriving at cells that need oxygen, the oxygen must then detach from the hemoglobin, be transported across the cell membrane, and finally react with a fuel in the cell to produce heat and energy.

The process of taking oxygen from the air, attaching it to hemoglobin, transporting it to a cell, and metabolizing it inside the cell is very complex, requiring successful completion of numerous biological steps. Unless all these steps are successfully executed, oxygen metabolism inside the cell may not be sufficient to maintain healthy life. There are many ways in which we can interfere with these steps and give ourselves what we call cancer. We do this through poor nutritional choices, exposure to environmental toxins, and causing programming errors in genes that regulate respiration.

Respiration will be impaired when there is a lack of oxygen in the cell. However, even in the presence of sufficient oxygen, respiration will be impaired if the metabolic machinery to process the oxygen is compromised. When oxygen respiration is significantly impaired, cells are less able to generate the energy required to sustain life and they may die. Without sufficient oxygen or working machinery, in order to prevent the death of cells, some cells alter their genetic programming and revert to a different way of producing energy—*fermentation*, which allows the cell to continue living, but is ultimately destructive.

Sugar fermentation will produce energy in the absence of oxygen. This allows cells to create enough energy to survive, but this survival mechanism can cost you your life. As oxygen respiration in a cell decreases, the amount of fermentation increases to compensate for the loss of energy production from oxygen respiration. When the loss of energy from oxygen respiration reaches a critical point and fermentation takes over, fundamental changes take place in the way the cell operates.

Normal cells are highly differentiated, performing many specialized tasks the body needs to function as a whole. Think of brain cells, eye cells, different types of blood cells, skin cells, muscle cells, bone cells, liver cells, pancreatic cells, and so forth. Each type of cell does something special that other cells don't do. When cells get their energy through fermentation, there is no longer sufficient energy to perform the usual tasks, so genetic programming is changed and differentiation is lost. The cell is transformed into a more primitive form of life where it no longer performs specialized tasks and is no longer able to communicate effectively with other cells. Its only remaining function is to survive and grow—*this is cancer*!

The Cancer Process

This underlying common denominator of all cancer—insufficient oxygen metabolism—was discovered early in the twentieth century by German chemist Otto Warburg. Warburg first published on this subject in 1910, and he won his first Nobel Prize in Physiology/Medicine in 1931 for proving that oxygen deficiency will cause cancer.

We have known Warburg's critical, life-saving information for over 100 years. Warburg actually won *two* Nobel Prizes for his work proving that cancer is caused by a lack of oxygen respiration in cells and replacement by sugar fermentation. The fermentation process changes the chemical environment in cells. The changed environment alters instructions given to the genes, and cells lose control over their growth.

Warburg determined that cancer cells were fundamentally different from normal cells. Normal cells combine fuel with oxygen to produce energy. Cancer cells produce energy by fermenting sugar in the absence of oxygen, and a 35 percent reduction in cellular oxygen levels is sufficient to trigger the shift toward fermentation. The less oxygen we have, the more energy is produced by fermentation until the cell finally becomes a cancer cell. In a paper titled "The Prime Cause and Prevention of Cancer," which he presented in lecture at a meeting of Nobel Laureates on June 30, 1966, Warburg stated, "The cause of cancer is no longer a mystery; we know it occurs whenever any cell is denied 60% of its oxygen requirements." Warburg concluded that *the primary cause of cancer is oxygen deficiency and the replacement of oxygen respiration in normal cells with the fermentation of sugar to create energy.*

Despite his two Nobel Prizes for discovering the cause and treatment for cancer, the medical establishment dismissed Warburg's work as too simplistic. Nevertheless, Warburg's conclusions have never been proven wrong. To the contrary, recent research supports Warburg's discoveries. Experiments at the National Cancer Institute have found that cancers with the highest growth rates had the highest fermentation rates. In fact, since Warburg's discovery, the lack of oxygen respiration has remained the most fundamental difference consistently found between normal cells and cancer cells. In 2008, Boston College biology professor Thomas Seyfried and colleagues published new evidence in support of the century-old work of Warburg in the *Journal of Lipid Research*. These researchers concluded that now that we understand the sugar fermentation defects of cancer cells, this presents a weakness that we can use in our fight against cancer without harming normal body cells. Numerous other studies have also supported Warburg's findings that oxygen deficiency and fermentation of sugar are the hallmark of cancer cells. Despite the constant validation of Warburg's findings, they are still not being used in clinical practice. Because they are so simple, they could endanger the survival of the entire cancer industry.

Cancer cells need a low oxygen environment in order to survive; *increasing the amount of oxygen in a cancer cell will kill the cell.* Increasing the amount of oxygen in a cancer cell is inexpensive, safe, and effective. It addresses the prime cause of cancer rather than treating the symptoms. Once you understand this about cellular oxygen, it is easy to see why conventional cancer treatments fail. They not only fail to address the cause of cancer, they actually promote cancer.

Conventional cancer treatments promote the underlying cancer-causing conditions, making cancer more aggressive and more likely to metastasize. This explains why most people who choose conventional treatments die sooner than if they had done nothing. Chemotherapy and radiation drastically lower blood oxygen levels. Making matters even worse, these conventional treatments shut down the cellular machinery needed for oxygen respiration. Chemotherapy and radiation overload cells with toxins, which inactivates critical respiratory enzymes. When normal cells are damaged this way, they are more likely to develop into cancer cells. Thus chemotherapy and radiation increase the risk that new cancer will develop, and this is usually what happens—the cancer comes roaring back. To protect yourself, think twice about such dangerous and ineffective treatments, and instead change your internal environment to one in which cancer cannot thrive.

Switches and Drivers

Now that you know what causes cancer—insufficient oxygen metabolism in the cell—you can learn how to prevent and reverse it. As previously stated, almost all older Americans have small clusters of cancer cells throughout their bodies from consuming a cancer-promoting diet and living a cancer-promoting lifestyle. However, these cancer cells are *not* a threat to your life—*unless* they grow and travel to other parts of your body (metastasize).

To make cancer simple, refer again to the analogy between driving cancer and driving your car. Think of microtumors as cars in a garage. To make the cars go somewhere, you have to activate switches and then drive the car. Driving a car recklessly can kill you. Those microtumors are no different. You have to switch them on and drive them. If you drive them recklessly, you can end up dead. Once a tumor is out of the garage, it can grow slowly, rapidly, or even go back to the garage, depending on how you drive it. The point being, you are in control of cancer just as much as you are in control of your car.

Carrying the analogy further, before you can get in the car, you have to activate a switch that unlocks the door. Then you have to put the key in the ignition and switch the engine on. Even with the engine on, the car still isn't going anywhere until you switch the transmission out of park and into drive or reverse. Next, you have to drive the car by pressing on the accelerator, turning the steering wheel, and occasionally applying the brake. You can press lightly on the accelerator and drive slowly, or you can floor it and drive fast. You can drive responsibly, making correct turns and stops, or you can drive recklessly. All of the above are under your control. In order to make a car go somewhere, you have to activate a number of switches in the proper sequence, and you have to drive the car. To get cancer to grow and travel to other parts of the body, you have to activate biological switches and drive the cancer. We do this by living recklessly. Unfortunately, the diet we eat, the products we use, and our lifestyle are so normal to us that we don't think of them as reckless.

Everything happens for a reason; cancer is no different. Cancer is a complex disease and it is not easy to make it happen. The reason cancer was a rare disease historically is because it is so difficult to make it happen. You have to do a lot of things *just right* to get cancer. A series of biological switches have to be turned on in the correct sequence, and then you have to drive this complex process. The problem is that modern living has made it real easy to do everything just right. That's why cancer has gone from being a rare disease to being an epidemic, affecting almost half the American population. Fortunately, the need to do everything just right presents a marvelous opportunity for doing it wrong—*interfering with the cancer process gives you the power to prevent or reverse cancer.*

We all know if you took your car out of gear while driving it, turned the ignition off or ran out of fuel, no matter how fast you were going, the car would eventually stop. If you applied the brake, it would slow down. If you drove it very slowly, it wouldn't go anywhere fast. As you see, there are a number of actions you can take that will slow or stop your car—similarly, we know how to slow or stop cancer.

If you keep your car in the garage with the engine turned off, the brake on, the gear in park, the fuel tank empty, and the door locked, you can be sure your car isn't going anywhere. Similarly, if you help your body create conditions that do not feed cancer and that shut it down, you won't have to worry about cancer.

In order to control cancer's switches and drivers, you need to learn how cells become oxygen deficient. There are a number of reasons why cells can become poorly oxygenated. To take oxygen from the air, put it into the blood, and transport it to individual cells, and to have it be metabolized inside the cells is a biologically complex process. All these complex actions need to be done correctly, and you may be amazed to see what can go wrong and how all the pieces need to fit together.

Switching Cancer On or Off

Most of cancer's switches and drivers are controlled by what you eat. Yet most physicians tell cancer patients they can eat anything they want. As you will see, this advice is totally irresponsible and deadly wrong. The wrong foods will drive cancer so powerfully that nothing can stop it. Let's explore some of cancer's on switches and drivers, as well as how to turn them off or keep them off in the first place.

Processed Oils

Processed oils switch cancer on and drive it. In fact, *processed oils (virtually all the oils you buy in a supermarket) may be the single largest cause of cancer. If you have cancer, you need an oil change.*

Our cancer epidemic is being caused by the fundamental changes we have made in our diet over the last century. One of the biggest changes we have made is the kind of fats and oils we consume. This is critical because the cell membrane (the wall surrounding each cell) is constructed mostly of oils, but if the membrane is not constructed of the right oils, it will inhibit oxygen from getting into the cell and, as you'll recall, this will cause cancer. Through clever advertising and massive misinformation campaigns, Americans have been hoodwinked into consuming large quantities of all the wrong oils. This is causing an epidemic of chronic disease from diabetes to cancer. In fact, if you eat the Standard American Diet, it is impossible to get a sufficient quantity and balance of the correct oils. *More than 90 percent of all Americans are deficient in essential fatty acids (EFAs)—the results are catastrophic.* It is one reason we have so much obesity. EFA deficiency can cause constant hunger and carbohydrate cravings. This adds on pounds, and the resulting fat helps to cause and drive cancer. EFA deficiency is a major reason, if not the major reason, why we have so much cancer and why EFA supplementation is essential.

It is not a coincidence that for a half century, German chemist Johanna Budwig, author of *Flax Oil As a True Aid Against Arthritis, Heart Infarction, Cancer and Other Diseases,* successfully treated thousands of cancer patients with a diet rich in high doses of flaxseed oil. Budwig was considered one of the world's leading authorities on fats and oils. She clearly demonstrated the devastating effects of consuming commercially processed oils on the integrity of cell membranes, lowering the voltage of the cells and inhibiting the transport of oxygen into the cells. By changing their oils, cancer patients were able to restore cell membrane integrity, enhance oxygen respiration and cure their cancers.

The wrong oils help to switch the cancer process on, and the right oils help to prevent and reverse it. Even if you don't have cancer, if you have been eating processed oils you most likely need an oil change. In Chapter 4, the Nutrition Pathway, we will talk more about how to avoid the bad oils and how to put good ones into your diet so you can keep this cancer switch turned off.

Acidic pH

Do you know what your body pH is? The pH balance in the body is one of our most important biochemical balances, and altering your pH has profound biological effects. Even a small change in pH can have a large effect on the oxygen-carrying capacity of the blood and the transport of oxygen into the cells. pH also controls enzyme activity in the body. It activates and deactivates pH-dependent enzymes, controlling the production and speed of critical biochemical reactions. Plus, pH also plays a role in gene expression, with different pH levels giving different signals and instructions to the same genes. This is why every cancer patient, and for that matter every chronic disease patient, *must* pay attention to normalizing their pH levels. Your pH is measured on a scale from zero to 14. A pH of 7 is neutral, while numbers above 7 are alkaline and below 7 are acidic. Normal pH inside a cell is slightly alkaline at about 7.4. You can check your pH level using pH paper that you wet with first-morning urine and match the resulting color to the chart included with the paper to determine the corresponding pH.

Acidosis, making the body too acidic, is a huge contributor to our cancer epidemic. Cells and body fluids that are too acidic drive cancer. Excessive alkalinity can also support cancer, but most cancer patients are too acidic. To prevent and reverse cancer, you must normalize your cellular pH to slightly alkaline.

One of the fundamental changes we have made in our diet is to shift from a primarily alkalizing diet of fresh vegetables and fruits to an acidifying diet of sugar, grains, excessive animal protein, and sodas containing phosphoric acid. Making the body's cells too acidic increases the production of free radicals that damage DNA, cells, and tissues. *An acidic pH changes your internal environment to one that supports cancer.*

Dramatic things happen when you change the normal, slightly alkaline pH of the cell. An alkaline pH is important for oxygenation of body tissues because a slightly alkaline solution can absorb over 100 times as much oxygen as a slightly acidic solution; acidic body fluids will not support the oxygen-rich environment that the body needs for good health. When the fluid inside and outside the cells becomes too acidic, cell walls begin to lose their integrity. This not only damages the ability to transport oxygen into cells, it also allows carcinogenic toxins to enter the cells, damaging DNA, causing mutations, and further compromising a cell's ability to fight off disease while promoting uncontrolled cell growth.

An acidic pH not only deprives cells of oxygen, it also disables respiratory enzymes that are responsible for utilizing oxygen—a bad combination. Cancer thrives in an acidic environment and does not survive in a normal alkaline environment. An acidic pH reduces the amount of oxygen in body fluids and *reduced oxygen not only turns cancer on, it also drives it.*

Historically, we had little difficulty maintaining normal pH because our diets were rich in alkalizing fresh fruits and vegetables. (Even though some fruits are acidic before you eat them, such as citrus fruits, they have an alkalizing effect in the body.) Today, our diets are very different. Eating the Standard American Diet produces low-grade acidosis, which increases with age. This, along with the accumulation of genetic mutations, is another reason why cancer occurs more often in older people.

Normal cell metabolism produces acids. Problems arise when we add to this burden by consuming acid-forming foods such as sugar, grains, dairy, meat, and highly acidic colas and soft drinks. Overconsumption of animal protein is another big contributor to acidosis. When animal proteins break down in our bodies they metabolize into strong acids. Eating a lot of meat and dairy products, as most Americans do, increases acidosis and your risk of cancer. The American diet is low in minerals, and mineral deficiencies are part of the problem. The body uses minerals to neutralize acids, so when you combine a diet that is already low in minerals with a high animal-protein diet, it causes severe mineral deficiencies. This lowers your pH into highly acidic conditions, creating disease. The bottom line is the majority of the foods most of us eat today have an acidic effect on the body, causing an epidemic of disease and cancer.

Recall that cancer cells ferment sugar to produce energy. One of the metabolic byproducts of fermentation is lactic acid, which makes cells and body fluids even more acidic and less able to deliver oxygen. This has the effect of acidifying normal neighboring cells, inhibiting the transport of oxygen into those cells and helping cancer to spread.

The pH of your cells helps to determine whether or not you get cancer, and if you get cancer, how bad it will be. The more acidic your system becomes, the less oxygenated your cells will be.

The effect of pH on enzymes is important. An acidic environment impairs the body's metabolic machinery and defense mechanisms by causing some enzymes to shut down and others to work when they shouldn't, giving rise to many dysfunctions, including diminished hormone production. For example, the liver's ability to detoxify and to produce hormones is dependent on pH-sensitive enzymes. If your body is too acidic, important hormones will not be produced. When liver detoxification is inadequate, toxins overload the kidneys, and this can produce fatigue, headaches, skin rashes, back and shoulder pain, and a variety of other problems. Too much acid strips the body of critical alkalizing minerals such as zinc, magnesium, and calcium that are necessary to manufacture enzymes. Enzymes are one of the body's best anticancer defense mechanisms; they attack cancer cells and take them apart, and when enzymes are impaired, cancer is encouraged. If the body is too acidic, the stomach produces less acid, thus affecting our ability to properly digest foods and get the nutrition we need. Acidosis causes far-reaching problems affecting many body functions. Viruses thrive in acidic cells, making infection more likely.

Chronic stress creates acidity, and we lead stressful lives. Allergic reactions create acidity, and most of us have allergies and food sensitivities whether we know it or not. Chronic dehydration, chronic infections, most prescription drugs, and many environmental toxins all promote acidity. Cancer itself produces acidity. Too much acid causes cancer, and then cancer cells produce more acid, making matters even worse. This vicious cycle promotes an acid pH, which both switches on and drives cancer.

In Chapter 1, I talked about Paul, a man who had reversed his fully metastasized cancer after being given a 50/50 chance of being alive in six months. When I asked Paul what he thought was the single most important thing he had done to improve his situation, his reply was, "Change my pH." This reply was no surprise because there is a long history in alternative medicine of people like Paul reversing cancer simply by alkalizing their pH. *If you want to prevent or reverse cancer, it is imperative that you normalize your cellular pH. If you are too acidic, you must avoid acid-forming foods, eat an alkalizing diet of fresh fruits and vegetables, and take alkalizing supplements.* Alkalizing supplements include calcium, magnesium, potassium, and zinc.

How do you know what your pH is? There is an indirect, simple, and inexpensive test that provides a reasonable approximation of the pH in your cells when you test your first-morning urine before you have had anything to eat or drink. Your test paper should be graduated from pH 5 to pH 8 with incremental readings (available at www.beyondhealth.com). Wet a small strip of the pH paper with the urine and compare the color against the scale provided. The color will coincide with your pH. As you eat more and more alkaline foods, you should see an improvement in your pH. Below are the pH ranges to look for:

Below 6.0—Dangerous Range
6.0 to 6.5—Unhealthy Range
6.5 to 7.5—Healthy Range
Above 7.5—Dangerous Range

Keep a diary of the foods you eat and also note your first-morning pH measurement. This will allow you to monitor how different foods affect your pH. First-morning pH should consistently run in the acceptable range. Occasional readings outside the acceptable range are okay, but consistent readings below 6.5 are not good, and readings below 6.0 are dangerous. Occasional readings above 7.5 are okay, but consistent readings are not, and a pH of 8.0 is alarming.

Balancing your pH maximizes energy and boosts immunity. Most Americans are too acidic, and most terminal cancer patients have cells that are as much as 1,000 times more acidic than normal. When cells are too acidic, body chemistry changes and cells will no longer properly communicate, self-regulate, and self-repair, which is the essence of disease. Making your cells and body fluids acidic switches cancer on; to keep cancer switched off, keep them alkaline. *You are in control of this very important switch.*

Sugar

Sugar is a leading cause and driver of cancer, and you have control over how much sugar you eat. Sugar is a deadly metabolic poison that harms us in many ways. Sugar not only switches cancer on, it also drives it. Beyond cancer, sugar causes almost every other ailment from the common cold to depression, osteoporosis, and even Alzheimer's. Sugar fuels cancer, and eating sugar is like throwing gasoline on a fire, or flooring the accelerator on the cancer car—the cancer will explode with growth. Sugar is one of the most dangerous substances that most of us are exposed to on a daily basis. With good reason, sugar has been called "death by installment." Recall there is only one disease, caused by deficiency and toxicity; sugar causes both. *Sugar causes disease!*

Sugar is acid-forming in the body, causing cells and tissues to become too acidic. Acidosis impairs oxygen respiration and switches cancer on. Sugar causes the production of saturated fats, because cells turn excess sugar into fat. When these fats are incorporated into cell membranes, they inhibit oxygen transport into the cell. Sugar also causes the production of excess insulin and estrogen. Insulin stimulates cell growth, and estrogen is known to drive prostate, uterine, ovarian, and breast cancers. Unbalancing these hormones upsets all your other hormonal balances, which can result in dire consequences.

Cancer cells ferment sugar in order to create energy and stay alive—this is their food, their fuel. Without sugar, cancer cells will die. Fermenting sugar is a less efficient way to produce energy. Fermentation requires a lot of sugar to obtain the same amount of energy as when combining the sugar with oxygen, which is a more efficient process. This is why people with cancer often crave sugar, and why eating sugar and other simple carbohydrates drives cancer and makes it grow. Cancer patients should not eat sugar, high-glycemic fruits, or any other carbohydrate that is easily converted to sugar such as white flour, white rice, and white potatoes. This means no bread, no pasta, no baked goods, and no breakfast cereals. *It is imperative that cancer patients avoid all sugar and carbohydrate foods.* Eating sugar is like putting gasoline in your cancer car. Sugar

drives cancer by feeding the cancer cells; avoiding sugar is like taking your foot off your cancer accelerator. In short, the car won't
operate without fuel, so stop putting fuel in the cancer tank!

White Flour/Wheat

White flour is deadly, and has almost the same effect as eating sugar. It is lacking in nutrition, and it has a toxic effect on the
body—creating deficiency and toxicity. The digestive system readily
converts white flour into sugar, and the sugar raises the insulin level
of the blood, causing the same devastating problems that eating
sugar does. White flour also has an acidic effect on the body, lowering your pH and causing acidosis. Further, the gluten contained
in the flour is highly allergenic, and the resulting allergic reactions
impair your immunity, produce a flood of pro-inflammatory chemicals, and use up precious nutrients. It has been estimated that up to
half the population is now metabolically reactive to gluten, which
means they suffer, often unknowingly, from gluten's effects.

While white flour is destructive, it appears that wheat itself is a major
health hazard. Modern wheat contains high amounts of compounds
called lectins, which cause systemic inflammation, depress immunity,
and promote disease of all kinds—including cancer. Get wheat out of
your diet. (More on this in Chapter 4, the Nutrition Pathway.)

Alcohol

Alcohol is another cancer switch and driver, and easy to control.
Alcohol has been listed as a known human carcinogen by the U.S.
Department of Health and Human Services, and researchers con-
tinue to find links between even moderate alcohol drinking and an

increased risk of cancer, especially cancers of the breast, liver, rectum, mouth, throat, and esophagus. In fact, some researchers have concluded that there is no minimum level of alcohol consumption that is without risk.

One way alcohol causes cancer is to release free iron in the body. Body iron is usually in the form of proteins such as transferrin and ferritin. Iron becomes dangerous when it is released from these protective proteins, triggering intense inflammation. Alcohol helps to release the iron from its protective proteins, raising the level of free iron. A study in a 2011 *Breast Cancer Research and Treatment* found that iron levels were 5 times higher in the breast fluid of breast cancer patients.

The more alcohol you drink, the greater the risk of developing cancer. Studies show that even social drinkers who consume more than two drinks daily increase their risk of developing cancer. Women are at particular risk. Women who drink as little as one alcoholic beverage a day have an increased cancer risk. N-nitrosamines are potent carcinogens found in alcoholic beverages, especially beer. Alcohol can transport carcinogens into cells and damage DNA, and it also increases blood sugar. It does not directly produce sugar, but it causes the liver to convert glycogen (a sugar-storage carbohydrate) into sugar. Anything that increases blood sugar beyond normal limits helps to feed and drive cancer. Alcohol also increases estrogen in the body by compromising the function of the liver in getting rid of excess estrogen; excess estrogen drives breast cancer.

Alcohol has a profound effect on pH. Alcohol is metabolized by the liver into a compound called acetaldehyde. Acetaldehyde, a potent neurotoxin, is then metabolized into acetic acid, making the body acidic. In order for the liver to detoxify acetaldehyde, critical nutrients such as the amino acid cysteine and the peptide glutathione are required. The more alcohol is consumed, the more these nutrients become depleted, reducing the body's ability to detoxify other toxins. Further, acetaldehyde reacts with polyamines, natural body compounds essential for cell growth, thus triggering a series of reactions that damage DNA, leading to the formation of cancer.

Consuming even one alcoholic drink per day appears to challenge the body with a toxic burden that some people are unable to tolerate. By making carcinogens more bioavailable, damaging DNA, using up critical nutrients, increasing blood sugar levels, and acidifying the body, alcohol is a significant contributor to the cancer process, as it is both a switch and a driver. To prevent cancer, avoid alcohol or use it in moderation—not to exceed one drink per day, with red wine being the best choice. People with cancer should not consume any alcohol.

Dairy/Excess Animal Protein

Milk and the products made from it contain a combination of toxic and carcinogenic chemicals along with growth-promoting hormones. Milk increases blood levels of insulin-like growth factor 1 (IGF-1), a growth hormone that promotes cancer. Milk is also high in casein, a protein that promotes cancer.

Most Americans consume more animal protein than their body can use for its daily needs. This switches cancer on and drives it. Animal protein increases blood levels of IGF-1, which acts as a switch that drives cell growth. Blood levels of IGF-1 are good predictors of cancer—low levels prevent it and high levels promote it. Animal protein is acid producing. As we have already discussed, acidic conditions decrease oxygen metabolism, switching cancer on. Further, the acidic condition caused by excess animal protein suppresses a kidney enzyme, inhibiting the body's production of vitamin D, which is necessary for keeping cancer switched off. A lack of vitamin D enhances the activity of IGF-1, encouraging more cell growth. *Excess animal protein acidifies the body, increases IGF-1, and decreases vitamin D—all of which drive cancer.*

We are constantly exposed to carcinogenic chemicals that must be detoxified before they do us significant harm. A diet high in animal protein not only contains many carcinogenic chemicals, it alters enzyme activity in the liver, which prevents the liver from safely disposing of toxins. This can result in producing chemicals that are more dangerous than the original toxin.

Colin Campbell, in his book *The China Study*, summarized numerous studies indicating that consuming animal protein in excess of the amount needed for growth turns the cancer switch on. Campbell found that when experimental animals predisposed to develop liver cancer were fed carcinogenic aflatoxin, the only animals that got cancer were the ones fed 20 percent animal protein in their diets. No cancer developed in the animals eating only 5 percent animal protein, yet all the animals were equally disposed to getting cancer. Cancer developed only in those animals eating the same kind of high-protein diet that Americans eat. In *The China Study*, Campbell wrote, *"Like flipping a light switch on or off, we could control cancer promotion merely by changing the levels of protein, regardless of the original carcinogen exposure."* This is an enormously significant finding, for it means that you can switch cancer on or off simply by changing the amount of animal protein in your diet. Cutting back on the amount of meat, milk, cheese, yogurt, and eggs in your diet will help to keep cancer's switches and drivers turned off.

Chronic Inflammation

Inflammation is not only an on switch for cancer, it is also a driver of the cancer process. Chronic inflammation is a foundation stone of every chronic disease. It is a major cause of cancer and is necessary for cancer growth and metastasis. This is why it is extremely important that inflammation be minimized. To protect ourselves, we must stop doing the things that we know cause inflammation and switch to a diet and an anti-inflammatory supplement program that suppresses inflammation.

Inflammation promotes cancer in several ways. First, it creates free radicals. The free radicals damage DNA, helping to switch cancer on, and they also damage cell membranes. Damaged membranes impair oxygen transfer into cells, and that helps to switch cancer on. Secondly, inflammation drives cancer by enabling cancer cells to invade adjacent tissues and metastasize.

Most Americans suffer from chronic inflammation due to eating an inflammatory diet of sugar, white flour, processed oils, dairy, and excess animal protein. Our massive overconsumption of pro-inflammatory oils, such as canola, corn, peanut, safflower, soybean, sunflower, most olive oils, and all hydrogenated oils, is one of the major causes, if not the major cause of cancer in our society. We are living in a toxic manmade oxidizing environment filled with ozone, chlorine, herbicides, pesticides, and other environmental chemicals that cause oxidative free-radical damage to our cells and contribute to our inflammation. Making matters worse, we take toxic prescription drugs, live stressful lives, and make ourselves overweight. More than two out of three Americans are overweight, and fat cells produce a constant flood of pro-inflammatory chemicals. In addition, chronic stress dramatically increases the amount of pro-inflammatory chemicals in the body. We are also hoodwinked into accepting health-damaging vaccinations, which result in chronic inflammation. Many people have autoimmune diseases or chronic infections, such as gum infections and yeast infections, which produce a flood of inflammatory chemicals. Wherever there is inflammation, there is massive generation of free radicals that damage DNA, cells, and tissues. Inflammation ages us, literally destroying our bodies, causing people to become sick and frail, not to mention cancerous.

Inflammation is not always bad. It is a natural process that helps the body to heal when injured. Once the healing is done, however, the inflammation is supposed to turn off. When it doesn't turn it off is when we get in trouble. *Chronic* inflammation has a deadly effect on us. In the inflammatory process, chemicals are excreted from immune cells to make tissues more permeable to facilitate the delivery of repair materials to the injured area. Tumors take advantage of inflammation and use the same chemicals to render the natural barriers surrounding them more permeable so the tumor can grow. Cancer cells need inflammation to sustain their growth; that's why inflammation is critical to the cancer process.

The more inflammation people have in their bodies, the more cancer they have and the less likely they are to survive. Studies show that patients who are measured as having the lowest amount of inflammatory chemicals in their blood are twice as likely to survive as those with high levels. The level of inflammation in a cancer patient is a reliable indicator of their chances of survival.

The continuous production of inflammatory chemicals blocks the natural process of apoptosis. *Apoptosis is a process of cell death that is genetically programmed into every cell, preventing the uncontrolled growth of tumors.* By blocking apoptosis, inflammation protects cancer cells from natural cell death.

To prevent and control inflammation, take high-quality anti-inflammatory supplements, such as vitamins A, C, D, E, and carotenes, along with minerals like zinc, selenium, and magnesium, plus other forms of antioxidants like CoQ10, quercetin, alpha lipoic acid, epigallocatechin gallate (EGCG), and curcumin. All of these nutrients need to be of high quality. (More about them in the Supplements chapter—Chapter 10). Numerous nutrients in fresh fruits and vegetables can dramatically reduce inflammation. Toxins must be avoided and stress reduced. Excess weight must be brought under control (read *Never Be Fat Again*).

Sodium and Potassium Imbalance

Excess salt is both an on switch and a driver of cancer. We consume far too much salt (sodium chloride), and this contributes to our cancer epidemic. According to research from the Centers for Disease Control and Prevention (CDC), if you live in the U.S., there is a 90 percent chance that you consume too much sodium. A number of studies, including a 1991 study in the *American Journal of Clinical Nutrition*, have found strong links between excess dietary sodium and cancer. Increasing sodium intake not only increases the incidence of cancer, it also accelerates metastasis.

One of the fundamental changes we have made in our diet is the relative amount of sodium and potassium we consume. Historically, our diets were rich in potassium and low in sodium. Traditional human diets contained about four times as much potassium as sodium. Today, the ratio is reversed, and the average person now consumes four times more sodium than potassium. This is happening because we eat fewer potassium-containing fruits and vegetables and lots of processed foods, which contain enormous amounts of salt. Consuming these salt-filled processed foods has altered the natural balance between sodium and potassium in our bodies. Too much salt damages the body's electrical system and makes our cells too acidic, both leading to dire consequences.

Cells operate best when there is more potassium inside the cell than outside of it and more sodium outside the cell than in it. This difference creates an electrical potential, allowing each cell to function as a little battery, creating the electricity we need to run our body's electrical system. The stronger your batteries, the healthier you are. You can look at the body as an electrically operated device. For example, electricity is used to signal the heart to beat. The voltage of each cell battery affects how cell membranes function. Low voltage presents problems. As we know, the function of the cell membrane is critical to health, and anything that reduces oxygen transfer through the cell membrane contributes to cancer. *Low voltage inhibits oxygen transport into the cell, and cancer cells often measure half the voltage of normal cells.* By eating too much salt and changing the sodium/potassium ratio in our cells, we damage the "battery of life," interfere with the body's self-regulation and repair functions, and create a deficiency of oxygen respiration in our cells.

If your batteries are run down, so are you. In order to function properly, all of your batteries need to be fully charged. Only when fully charged will a cell be able to efficiently bring in all the nutrients it needs, expel its metabolic waste products, and protect itself from infection. A healthy cell maintains a charge of about 90 millivolts, which facilitates delivery of oxygen and other nutrients. A cancer cell is often 45 millivolts and can be as low as 30 millivolts, which blocks oxygen from getting into the cell. The excessive sodium in our processed-food diets forces more sodium into the cell, lowering the voltage and changing the electrical properties of the cell membrane. This is one more argument for not eating nutritionally deprived, toxic, processed foods—they contain too much salt.

In addition to affecting our cell batteries, excess salt also contributes to making our bodies too acidic. Eating a diet with too much salt, not enough potassium-containing foods, and too many acid-forming foods is a recipe for chronic acidosis, which lowers the oxygen-carrying capacity of our body fluids and helps to switch on and drive the cancer process.

Potassium is primarily found in plant foods like fresh fruits and vegetables, while sodium is primarily found in processed foods. To prevent and reverse cancer, restore the normal sodium/potassium balance in your cells. Keep your sodium consumption to less than 1,000 mg per day; one-half teaspoon of salt contains about 1,100 mg of sodium. Read every label carefully—about 70 percent of our salt comes from consuming processed foods. Once again, you are in personal control of an important cancer switch and driver, so get the excess sodium out of your diet. *Eliminate salt-filled processed foods, be careful with the salt shaker, use spices rather than salt, and eat substantially more fresh fruits and vegetables.*

Toxic Chemicals

Many chemicals are known to switch cancer on and/or drive it. Toxins cause cancer via numerous mechanisms. Toxins damage genes, deprive cells of oxygen, interfere with oxygen metabolism inside cells, and disrupt cell-to-cell communications. For example, hemoglobin is a protein in red blood cells that carries oxygen. Hemoglobin has to take on oxygen, carry that oxygen in the bloodstream, and then deliver it to the right place at the right time. Various toxins can interfere with every step of this process, causing oxygen deficiency.

Carbon monoxide is one such toxin, as it reacts with hemoglobin, reducing its ability to carry oxygen. Smokers have high carbon monoxide levels in their blood, which is one way smoking contributes to cancer. People who live and work in the canyons of large cities, such as New York City, have high carbon monoxide levels, owing to the pollution from cars, trucks, and buses. Lead interferes with the manufacture of hemoglobin, and most of us, especially older people, have too much lead in our systems. Then there are the regulatory receptor sites that help to balance the amount of carbon dioxide in the blood. Various toxins can affect the receptors and change how much carbon dioxide is in the blood. This, in turn, can reduce the amount of oxygen available and cause an oxygen deficiency.

Enzymes are molecules that are a critical part of our metabolic machinery. Enzymes break down larger molecules from food into smaller ones, which is necessary for the body to use them. Enzymes then take these smaller molecules and reassemble them into larger ones, such as hormones, neurotransmitters, and antibodies. Respiratory enzymes are responsible for processing oxygen and fuel into a high-energy compound called ATP (adenosine triphosphate). When toxins disable these enzymes, this inhibits oxygen respiration and reduces the amount of energy (ATP) a cell can produce. Without ATP, we would cease to function, and if ATP production is compromised, we will lack energy and get sick. Cigarette smoke contains cyanide. Smokers have elevated cyanide levels in their blood, and cyanide disables an enzyme that helps to produce ATP. Heavy-metal toxicity is another way we disable these enzymes. Enzymes require nutritional minerals such as magnesium, zinc, and selenium in order to function. Toxic metals, such as arsenic, cadmium, lead, and mercury, displace the nutrient minerals in the respiratory enzymes and cause them to stop functioning. This too causes a deficiency of oxygen respiration. Unfortunately, most of us have unhealthy accumulations of heavy metals in our bodies. (For more on how to avoid and get rid of heavy metals see the Toxin Pathway chapter—Chapter 5).

Glutamates

Glutamates are a class of compounds that are used as food additives, the best-known member of which is monosodium glutamate (MSG). Glutamates are cancer drivers. They are added to processed foods to enhance flavor because processing destroys flavor. These chemicals promote cancer and have wide-ranging toxic effects on the body. It is known that some cancer cells have a large number of glutamate receptor sites. Stimulating these receptor sites can drive the cancer process, making cancer grow much faster, become more invasive, and have more deadly consequences.

Glutamates are added to about 80 percent of processed foods, often in high concentrations, and often several forms of glutamates can be found in a single product. The ingredients list is filled with words that sound healthy but are not, such as natural flavors, spices, hydrolyzed vegetable protein, vegetable protein, sodium caseinate, textured protein, soy protein extract, and others. All these contain glutamates. Glutamates are also routinely added to fast foods, like commercial pizzas, but they can also be served in expensive restaurants, especially in soups and the chef's favorite sauces. *This is one more reason why processed foods and fast foods must be avoided by cancer patients.*

Nutrient Deficiencies

Cancer can be caused simply by depriving cells of certain nutrients. An important step in the cancer process is damage to genes.

We know that toxins and radiation damage genes, but here is something else—nutritional deficiencies. Dr. Bruce Ames, a professor of biochemistry and molecular biology at the University of California, Berkeley and a member of the National Academy of Sciences, has observed genetic damage in cells that have been deprived of essential vitamins and minerals that *"rivals and even exceeds the effect of radiation."* Ames, the author of "Micronutrients Prevent Cancer and Delay Aging" said, "What we are seeing is kind of a double whammy. Cells are more likely to sustain genetic damage and are less able to repair the damage." When poor nutrition damages respiratory genes, oxygen respiration in the cell is reduced and cancer is the result. There is much agreement among scientists, including the National Academy of Sciences, that everyone should take at least a multivitamin daily.

Certain nutritional deficiencies vastly increase the risk that cells will sustain cancer-causing genetic damage by promoting damage to DNA and inhibiting DNA repair. These deficiencies include vitamins B6, B12, E, folate, and the minerals magnesium and zinc. When you consider that most Americans are chronically short in at least several essential nutrients, including the above, it is little wonder we have so much cancer.

Beyond damaging genes, vitamin and mineral deficiencies reduce the capacity of respiratory enzymes to combine oxygen with fuel to make energy. Contributing to our cancer epidemic, most Americans are chronically short on essential nutrients that are required for oxygen respiration. Deficiencies of B vitamins, copper, iron, magnesium, manganese, selenium, and zinc contribute to the cancer process.

The shift from a diet of fresh, whole foods to today's standard diet of primarily nutrient-deficient, toxic, processed foods is one of the most fundamental and disastrous changes we have made in human history. In addition, modern chemical-farming methods have depleted our soils of essential minerals, so that even fresh, whole, commercially grown foods are no longer capable of supplying what the body requires for good health.

These changes have substantially reduced the amount of essential nutrients in our diet. These deficiencies depress immunity, damage genes, and reduce oxygen respiration. Even if you get enough oxygen into your cells, if the metabolic machinery to process the oxygen does not operate due to lack of nutrients, the result is like not having the oxygen at all. Oxygen respiration is replaced with sugar fermentation and cancer.

The most important thing you can do to prevent and reverse cancer is consume lots of organically grown, fresh fruits and vegetables and take high-quality supplements. *Nutrients contained in fresh fruits and vegetables are known to interfere with every known step of the cancer process.* This happens with no side effects, only benefits. Nutrients in fruits and vegetables prevent cancer in the first place. If you have been diagnosed with cancer, they turn cancer off by suppressing the switches and drivers that promote the cancer process. You are in control of what you eat.

Platelet Stickiness

Blood clots contribute to the cancer process. When blood platelets stick together, blood forms clots. Large blood clots cause strokes and heart attacks. Small clots, of which we are not even aware, can play a role in the cancer process because they reduce the amount of oxygen available to cells. Blood cells that are sticking together absorb less oxygen and deliver less oxygen. Clumped together, these red blood cells cannot pass through the smaller capillaries so much less oxygen gets delivered to cells served by those capillaries.

Cancer deaths could be sharply reduced if clots were eliminated. Maintaining good blood-flow speed helps to keep tissues well oxygenated. When people die of cancer, 90 percent of the time they are succumbing to metastases, cancer cells that took root in other parts of the body after being shed by a primary tumor. Small clots that restrict the blood flow into capillaries and slow down the blood flow not only deprive cells of needed oxygen, thus helping to switch cancer on, but they also provide an opportunity for cancer cells to stop moving with the flow. Cancer cells that would normally travel through the capillaries are held up and are able to attach themselves to the blood vessel wall and invade neighboring tissues. This helps to drive the cancer process. Fast-moving blood lessens this opportunity.

Platelet stickiness is caused by the same biologically inappropriate supermarket fats and oils that screw up cell membranes. Consuming the correct essential fatty acids reduces platelet stickiness, provides good oxygen transfer and increases blood speed, thus reducing the ability for a cancer cell to attach and invade new tissues. Consuming the correct assortment of essential fatty acids is a must if you want to avoid blood clots. Both fish and flaxseed oils make platelets slippery so they don't stick together as readily; these oils also reduce inflammation. They have been shown in numerous studies to dramatically reduce the risk of clots.

Another source of clots is excess sodium. Excess sodium changes the electrical properties of cells, causing them to become less repellant and, therefore, more likely to stick together.

Sugar causes clots. Eating sugar and refined carbohydrates causes a rapid and dangerous increase in blood sugar. The body responds to this crisis by secreting insulin from the pancreas, causing an insulin spike. Insulin promotes clotting. High insulin levels inhibit the breakdown of fibrin. Fibrin is the principal component of blood clots, and when it can't be readily broken down, clots can be created. Because diabetics have high insulin, they have more blood clots and suffer more heart attacks and strokes. Eating a diet containing sugar, fruit juices, and refined grains increases insulin and promotes blood clotting. Anything that makes your blood insulin levels go up will cause platelet stickiness.

Being overweight promotes blood clots. Fat cells in overweight people produce estrogen, which not only increases the risk of certain cancers, but increases the risk of blood clots as well.

When you increase the amount of sugar in the blood, the sugar reacts with proteins in the blood in a process called *glycation*, which has the effect of thickening your blood and making it flow less freely. Clearly, sugar should be eliminated from your diet, along with other "high-glycemic" foods such as grains, baked goods, sodas, and fruit juices.

Olive oil should play a prominent part in any healthy diet. Its anti-inflammatory and antioxidant effects result in a vascular environment in which platelets are less likely to clump together and form clots. Olive oil is also rich in inhibitors of platelet-activating factor (PAF), which begins the clotting process by causing blood platelets to stick together. However, to get the benefits of olive oil, you have to get real olive oil instead of the usual adulterated oils that masquerade as "extra virgin olive oil" at the supermarket. (Learn more about olive oil in Chapter 4, The Nutrition Pathway.)

Supplementing with anti-fibrin enzymes, such as nattokinase, could also help to reduce clotting and cancer metastasis. Curcumin is especially good at reducing the high fibrinogen levels that promote clotting. Ginkgo biloba is good blood-thinning herb. Like olive oil, it inhibits PAF, decreasing clotting and improving circulation. Ginkgo is also an antioxidant, and it reduces high cholesterol. Vitamin E also helps to prevent clotting, and most Americans are deficient in vitamin E. Magnesium slows clotting speed and stimulates fibrinolysis (the breakdown of fibrin and clots). Garlic also reduces platelet stickiness and clotting. Platelet stickiness drives cancer, but you have control over this process.

Medical X-rays

X-rays are a type of ionizing radiation, and ionizing radiation is one of the best-known and universally recognized causes of cancer. Radiation damages DNA and switches cancer on, yet conventional medicine remains in denial, insisting that diagnostic x-rays are safe, even though it is established fact that ionizing radiation is not safe. In addition to damaging DNA, radiation also damages respiratory enzymes in healthy cells, causing a deficiency of oxygen respiration.

The late Dr. John Gofman, a medical doctor, nuclear physicist, renowned radiation expert, and author of the book *Radiation from Medical Procedures in the Pathogenesis of Cancer and Ischemic Heart Disease,* concluded after decades of research that x-rays are an essential cofactor in more than 60 percent of all cancer. Gofman estimated that more than 80 percent of all breast cancer is caused by chest x-rays, mammograms, and other x-rays for spinal, back, and neck problems. Radiation damage to genes is cumulative over a person's lifetime, and as small exposures accumulate, the risk of developing cancer goes up. In 2005, the National Academy of Sciences announced that each additional radiation exposure, no matter how small, increases the risk of cancer.

CT scans (computed tomography) are particularly dangerous because of their excessive amount of x-ray exposure. A single full-body CT scan exposes a person to a total radiation dose close to the dose linked to cancer in Japanese atomic bomb survivors. Each additional scan adds significantly to a person's total lifetime radiation exposure.

Medical x-rays, including dental x-rays, contribute to our cancer epidemic. Yet, most are unnecessary. Researchers estimate that up to 90 percent of all diagnostic x-rays are of "little or no medical value." Just say "no" to x-rays unless you are convinced they are absolutely necessary. Children are especially vulnerable to radiation and should be protected from x-rays.

Infections

Chronic infections use up immune capacity, making your immune system less able to prevent or fight cancer. In addition, immune reactions use up precious nutrients, create toxins, and produce free radicals that damage genes.

Scientists estimate that about 15 percent of human tumors are linked with viruses. Viral and chronic yeast, fungal, bacterial, and parasitic infections all play a role in the cancer process, even though the roles are not fully understood. Any chronic infection will wear down the immune system. A major waste product of a yeast infection is acetaldehyde, which metabolizes to ethyl alcohol. Ethyl alcohol can disable enzymes needed for energy production, cause free-radial damage to genes and inhibit the absorption of iron. Iron is needed by the blood to carry oxygen. A shortage of iron results in low oxygen levels (remember, cancer is an oxygen-deficiency disease). There are a variety of ways that infections affect us. The immune system responds to infections by producing inflammatory compounds that can damage your tissues and DNA. The hepatitis B virus can switch off as many as 150 genes that are protective against cancer. Human papillomavirus (HPV) is known to inactivate tumor suppressor genes. H. pylori infections induce chronic inflammation. All immune responses use critical nutrients such as zinc, vitamins A, C, and E, and carotenoids, which are often in short supply in the first place, causing deficiencies of these essential nutrients.

Chronic infections are more than just inconveniences. Yeast infections, chronic sinus infections, and tooth infections, such as abscesses in virtually all root-canal treated teeth, need to be addressed and eliminated. Virtually all root-canal teeth are infected, and bacteria trapped in these dead teeth create powerful toxins that poison the entire body and increase your risk for cancer. Some of the toxins from infected root-canal teeth, such as thioethers, are themselves capable of causing cancer in humans. Many alternative cancer specialists recommend that cancer patients remove all teeth that have been treated with root-canal therapy. However, they must be removed safely by dentists very experienced in this procedure. The periodontal ligament and about one millimeter of jawbone should be removed at the same time.

Impaired Apoptosis

Apoptosis prevents cancer, and it switches cancer off. Apoptosis is the body's normal method of disposing of damaged, unwanted, unneeded, or malfunctioning cells, and it is important to preventing and reversing cancer. Sometimes called "cell suicide," apoptosis is a control mechanism that plays a crucial role in maintaining health by eliminating old, unnecessary, and unhealthy cells. In an adult, the number of cells is kept relatively constant through cell death and division. Self-regulation is achieved when the rate of mitosis (cell division) is balanced by cell death. If this equilibrium is disturbed and cells multiply faster than they die, a tumor will develop. A defining characteristic of cancer cells is their ability to prevent normal cell death by producing chemicals that inhibit apoptosis.

Apoptosis is controlled by genes. For apoptosis to happen, cells receive either internal or external signals telling them to die. Any impairment of this process can cause disease. When cells are damaged by free radicals, the apoptosis genes can also be damaged, causing us to lose this protection against cancer. Protecting these genes from harm helps prevent cancer, and repairing and turning apoptosis genes back on helps to reverse it.

The nutrients known to assist with the apoptosis process include curcumin, quercetin, green tea extract, Panax ginseng, resveratrol, vitamin E succinate, and essential fatty acids. Vitamins A, C, E, and D, and the mineral calcium have been shown to help regulate apoptosis. Foods such as blueberries contain a combination of phenols, tannins, flavonols, and anthocyanins that support apoptosis. The anthocyanins in olives are an important benefit of the healthy Mediterranean diet. Foods high in soluble fiber, such as beans, support apoptosis when bacteria in the gut ferment the fiber, thereby creating apoptosis-supporting short-chain fatty acids. Foods such as Brussels sprouts and cabbage contain a compound called sinigrin that is broken down by gut bacteria to form compounds that support apoptosis.

Pectin also supports apoptosis. Pectin refers to a group of complex polysaccharides found in a variety of plant cells. Pectin is used as a thickening agent in the preparation of jams, jellies, and preserves. Apples, grapefruits, oranges, and apricots are known to have high levels of pectin. Generally, 60 to 70 percent of the dietary fiber in citrus fruits is pectin. Other sources include bananas, beets, cabbage, and carrots.

On the other hand, there are things that interfere with apoptosis. Chronic inflammation interferes with apoptosis, allowing cancer to grow. A number of toxic chemicals, including solvents such as benzene and toluene and a class of chemicals called phthalates inhibit apoptosis. Phthalates are used as plasticizers in plastics, primarily in vinyl plastics, to increase their flexibility. They are now widely used in plastic products in the food, construction, home furnishing, and automotive industries. Your new car can give you cancer! That new car smell and the oily coating on the inside of your car's windshield are examples of phthalate contamination. Phthalates are also used extensively in beauty products, perfumes, hairsprays, pesticides, wood finishes, insect repellents, solvents, lubricants, and in the food industry. Everywhere in our environment, they are bioaccumulating in our tissues and having dramatic negative effects on our health.

Inhibiting apoptosis with solvents, phthalates, and chronic inflammation will cause and drive cancer. Enhancing apoptosis with a nutritious diet with lots of fresh fruits and vegetables and high-quality supplements will help to prevent and reverse cancer. It is essential to support this critical biological process.

Angiogenesis

Angiogenesis drives cancer. Angiogenesis is the process by which new blood vessels grow from preexisting vessels. It is a normal process in growth and development, as well as in wound healing. However, this is also a fundamental step in the transition of tumors from a dormant benign state to a growing malignant state. Angiogenesis is essential to the growth of cancer. Without it, tumors cannot grow beyond a small diameter of 1 to 2 millimeters, no bigger than the size of a letter "o" on this page. To prevent or reverse cancer, avoid those things that promote angiogenesis and eat a diet that suppresses angiogenesis.

Tumors promote angiogenesis by secreting various growth factors, which allow the tumor to get bigger by inducing the growth of capillaries into the tumor. This supplies the tumor with required nutrients for growth and takes away toxic waste products. Remember, most of us already have small and relatively harmless clusters of cancer cells in our bodies. The problem begins when these clusters start to grow. Angiogenesis is a necessary and required step for these cancer cells to transition to a growing tumor, and for the tumor to metastasize and spread to other parts of the body.

When cancerous tumor cells release molecules sending signals to surrounding normal tissue, this activates certain genes. These genes make proteins to encourage growth of new blood vessels. The new blood vessels are made from a composite of normal cells and tumor cells. This mixture facilitates the shedding of tumor cells into the blood supply where they can end up in distant locations. The subsequent growth of such metastases also requires a supply of nutrients and more angiogenesis.

Certain chemicals promote angiogenesis, and should be avoided. Angiogenesis is promoted by excess omega-6 fatty acids—the norm in the American diet. This is another reason to avoid all those supermarket oils, such as corn, soy, sunflower, safflower, peanut, and canola oils. These highly processed oils are too rich in omega-6s and should not be consumed. Arsenic promotes angiogenesis. Arsenic is a contaminant in the fluoride chemicals added to tap water—another reason not to drink unpurified tap water.

Bisphenol-A (BPA) also drives angiogenesis. A 2009 study in the *Journal of Pediatric Surgery* found that animals exposed to BPA had over 50 percent higher gross tumor volume, tumor weight, and blood vessel density than those not exposed. BPA is found in numerous plastic products, as well as in the plastic linings of canned-food containers. According to the CDC, more than 90 percent of us are bioaccumulating BPA in our bodies. Avoid water and beverages in plastic bottles, as well as canned foods and beverages.

Diesel exhaust is another promoter of angiogenesis. A 2009 study reported in *Science Daily* found that diesel exhaust activated a chemical signal (vascular endothelial growth factor) that promotes new blood vessel development, which can feed a growing tumor. Diesel exposure also increased levels of a protein (hypoxia-inducible factor 1) that is essential to blood vessel development when oxygen levels are low. Diesel exposure also lowers the activity of an enzyme that has a role in producing substances that can suppress tumor growth. Further, tissues exposed to diesel exhaust develop chronic inflammation, which both causes and drives cancer. As much as possible, avoid diesel exhaust. If you live near a highway, be sure to protect yourself with a high-quality air filter in your home.

Interfering with angiogenesis is a way to stop tumor growth and metastasis. The omega-3 fatty acid DHA is known to suppress angiogenesis. A number of food flavonoids found in vegetables are known to inhibit angiogenesis as well. Anti-angiogenesis nutrients are found in garlic, celery, and green tea. The mineral selenium inhibits angiogenesis—another reason to take a high-quality multivitamin daily. To prevent and reverse cancer, it is important to inhibit angiogenesis by avoiding environmental toxins and by getting good nutrition.

Keeping the Car in the Garage

Recall our analogy between driving your car and driving cancer. To reverse cancer growth, take your foot off the accelerator, apply the brake, turn the ignition switch off, and park the car. But the best strategy of all is to prevent cancer growth. Remember, most of us have microclusters of cancerous cells in our body. Think of these microtumors as cars in a garage. Unless you take a series of actions, the cars will continue to sit there, going nowhere. So here is something else you can do: Keep the car in the garage! Locking cancer in the garage is a lot easier than trying to stop the cancer once it is out of the garage, going at high speed, and doing physical damage to your body.

These microclusters of cancer cells in our body are just waiting for an invitation to grow. But these cells are surrounded with connective tissue made of collagen and elastin, acting like a garage. Encapsulated in this confining environment, a tumor cannot grow. To break out of the garage and grow, cancer cells produce *collagen-digesting enzymes,* which dissolve the surrounding connective tissue and allow the cancer cells to get out of the garage and move through the tissue. Collagen-dissolving enzymes play a major role in the spread of cancer, and the more enzymes a cancer cell can produce and the more susceptible the collagen is to the enzymes, the faster the cancer will grow and metastasize.

Collagen dissolving is a natural process. Immune cells use this mechanism to cut through tissue in order to get access to damaged or infected tissue and do their jobs. This is a useful process, and it is normally carefully controlled. However, when out of control, serious infections, chronic inflammation, and cancer occur.

Mother Nature knows how to control the collagen-dissolving

process and protect us from infections, inflammation, and cancer, but our poor diets do not support nature's control system. Strong, healthy collagen is dependent on adequate amounts of vitamin C, which most of us don't have. Poorly constructed collagen fibers are more susceptible to damage. One especially critical nutrient is the amino acid lysine, and most of us don't get enough lysine. Lysine is not only used to make collagen, it also attaches to the sites on the collagen molecules where collagen-dissolving enzymes attach to attack the collagen. If you start with healthy collagen, when lysine attaches to these sites, it blocks the availability of collagen-dissolving enzymes and collagen dissolving is inhibited. Lysine is effectively the lock on the garage door. Lysine not only inhibits infections and chronic inflammation, but prevents cancer from happening and works to prevent the spread of existing cancer.

Nutrients including vitamin C, quercetin, proline, and lysine are essential to build strong collagen. If you have cancer, supplementation with these nutrients is a must.

You Control the Off Switch

In this chapter, we have explored what cancer is and how it happens. We have determined that a deficiency of oxygen respiration in your cells is the prime cause of cancer. We have focused on the cancer process and the biological switches that turn it on and the drivers that allow it to grow and spread.

Of all the switches and drivers described in this chapter, not all of them are necessarily operating in every case. However, by paying attention to all of them, you will have your best shot at preventing and reversing cancer.

Cancer is a biological process, and in order for cancer to happen, you have to turn that process on. If you can turn the process on, you can turn it off. To solve any problem, you have to remove the causes. The good news is that by knowing the causes, you can have control over the process, so you can turn cancer off and keep it off.

Most Americans, especially those over age fifty, now have numerous microclusters of cancerous cells in their bodies. *Our only real option is to keep those microtumors from growing.* Even if you have microtumors that are already growing, they take years to develop to the stage where they can be diagnosed. This means that you have time to change your lifestyle and make them go away before they become a problem. Start now by avoiding processed oils, sugar, salt, wheat, milk products, and excess animal protein. As much as possible, avoid toxins in the food you eat and in your environment. These are all critical to exercising your control over the cancer process. Eating well is not rocket science—avoid processed foods. Eat more fresh vegetables and get on a high-quality supplement program. Let us now have a more detailed look at how the Six Pathways to health or disease can help to further your control over the cancer process.

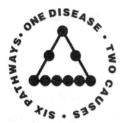

4

THE NUTRITION PATHWAY

What we humans consume for food has undergone
more profound change in the last century than in the previous
one hundred thousand years . . . what we put into our bodies
has sown the seeds for our current epidemics of illness and disease.

—*Randall Fitzgerald, author of* The Hundred-Year Lie

Food is the breakthrough drug of the twenty-first century.

—*Jean Carper, author of* Food: Your Miracle Medicine

Trying to beat cancer while eating a diet that constantly raises
blood glucose is like trying to put out a forest fire while
someone nearby is throwing gasoline on the trees.

—*Patrick Quillin, author of* Beating Cancer with Nutrition

N utritional deficiency is the single most important cause of *all* disease—not only chronic illnesses like heart disease and cancer, but infectious diseases, including colds and flu. Remember from previous chapters, there is only one disease—malfunctioning cells—and only two causes of disease—deficiency and toxicity. There is no such thing as a "disease" as we have been indoctrinated to understand this term. The medical profession has given different names to thousands of conditions, calling them diseases and imbuing them with almost magical powers to wreak havoc on hapless victims who are powerless to avoid being stricken. This model disempowers the individual. All these so-called diseases are symptoms of one condition: malfunctioning cells. Unless cells malfunction, disease cannot happen. A cell is either functioning normally or it isn't—one or the other. When cells malfunction, they can produce thousands of different symptoms, not thousands of different diseases. Disease is the malfunction in the cells, not the symptoms we observe. Cells malfunction when they don't get all the nutrients they need to perform their complex life-giving tasks.

Nutrition Is the Key to Good Health

To get sick, all you have to do is eat the Standard American Diet (SAD). The SAD has been depleted of essential nutrients and is loaded with toxic chemicals. When immigrants move to the United States and adopt the SAD, their cancer risk increases. This is why a 2009 study in *Cancer Epidemiology, Biomarkers and Prevention* found that Hispanics living in Florida have a 40 percent higher risk of cancer than those who live in their native countries. A cancer-causing diet creates an internal environment that supports cancer. To reverse cancer, you must eat a diet that creates an environment that does *not* support cancer. *You must be willing to shift to an anti-cancer diet.* For most people this will require a fundamental change from their normal cancer-causing diet, but don't let that stop you.

The very worst thing you can do is nothing! For those who are eating the cancer-causing SAD, the changes in your diet will be substantial. Take it one step at a time, and keep improving. Start with getting the sugar out of your life and eating more salads with dressings made of healthy oils. Get on a good supplement program. When it comes to food choices, most people are doing the wrong things most of the time. Turn that around and do things right most of the time—the results will be dramatic. You don't have to be a fanatic, and you don't have to be perfect. Each additional step you take will bring you closer to achieving a cancer-free life.

Good Diets Work

Simply eating a diet of predominantly fruits and vegetables can cut your cancer risk by 50 percent and in some cases by 75 percent! Nutrient deficiencies will cause all your new cells to be improperly constructed and will also create chemical imbalances in those cells. The result will be cellular malfunction and disease. For example, a deficiency of an essential nutrient such as vitamin D or an excess of omega-6 fatty acids will suppress immunity and promote exactly the environment needed for cancer to grow.

You are what you eat. Every cell in your body is made from what you eat and drink. The problem is there are vast differences between the historically wholesome and nutritious diet of our ancestors and the processed and chemical-based foods we eat today. If you don't eat the right things, it is not possible to build or operate your cells properly.

According to DNA analysis, humans have changed very little in the past 40,000 years, while our diet has changed dramatically. Our genes are still those of our hunter-gatherer ancestors and require the same nutrition as they did then. We are not getting that nutrition, and the result is our catastrophic epidemic of chronic disease—and cancer. Modern diets are overloaded with biologically inappropriate sugar, grains, dairy, and processed foods. The data clearly shows that countries that consume more fresh vegetables have less cancer.

The single most important thing anyone can do to maintain health, stay biologically young, and prevent or reverse disease is—eat a good diet. Yet, the single largest impediment to improving health is that most people think they are already eating a good diet. Because of this colossal delusion, few people see the need for change, especially if the change is more than minimal. The Standard American Diet will *not* sustain healthy life. Even the strictest adherence to a diet will not be helpful if you are misinformed about which foods are really healthy. In fact, according to a 1998 report by the National Academy of Sciences, *even if you eat a good diet*, it is no longer possible to get all the nutrition you need and supplementation is now a necessity.

Major changes in diet are now needed to provide what our bodies require, plus supplementation with high-quality vitamins, minerals, and other nutrients.

More than two thousand years ago, Hippocrates, the father of modern medicine, said, "Let food be thy medicine." Hippocrates was right then, and he is still right. Tragically, modern physicians ignore Hippocrates and choose prescription drugs for their medicine. Cells are not made of drugs, they are made of nutrients. If something has gone wrong, you can bet that a lack of nutrients is part, if not all, of the problem. So when doctors prescribe drugs, the nutrient deficiency is not being addressed. Meanwhile, these highly toxic chemicals poison your cells, create nutritional deficiencies, make you even sicker, and keep you sick. Nutrients prevent and reverse disease while drugs are toxins that cause disease. If you want to prevent or reverse disease, your cells need nutrients—once your poor diet makes you sick, drugs are not going to solve your problem. *Every food choice you make, every bite you eat will affect your health for better or for worse.* You make that choice at every meal.

Your cells have critical jobs to do. They cannot do those jobs unless they obtain all of the essential nutrients they need on a regular basis. Without these nutrients, they *will* malfunction, and you *will* get sick. A chronic deficiency of even *one* essential nutrient will make you sick. All nutrients act together as a team, and a chronic shortage of even one will undermine the whole system and your health. The average American is chronically deficient in several essential nutrients. According to the U.S. Department of Agriculture's (USDA) 1996 Continuing Survey of Food Intakes for Individuals, more than 70 percent of Americans do not consume the recommended daily allowance (RDA) for zinc. Eighty percent do not get the RDA for vitamin B6, and 75 percent do not get sufficient magnesium—and these are only three nutrients. Furthermore, the RDA is only the minimum amount required to prevent overt deficiency disease. The RDA is *not* sufficient to maintain optimal health. The amount needed for good health is often several times the RDA—almost all of us are not getting what we need.

Medical researchers estimate that our ancestors consumed four times more nutrients than we do today, and for certain nutrients that number is twenty or even fifty times higher. Yet the changes in our environment and lifestyle make our need for nutrients the highest ever. Our intake of nutrients is down, while the need is up. Most

people are unaware of the unprecedented burden that our exposure to environmental toxins is placing on our bodies, dramatically
increasing our need for nutrients. Meanwhile, the concept of eating
for nutrition and health is not the norm in our society; for many,
the idea comes as a shock. Most people make food choices based
on what tastes good, or what is convenient. Making matters worse,
physicians often tell cancer patients they can eat anything they want.

Cancer can be switched on or off with nutrition. Certain "foods"
promote disease, while others support health. You need to learn
which do what. We now know that a chronic deficiency of even
a single nutrient will make you sick and can cause cancer. Many
people have cured their cancers by doing nothing more than significantly changing their diet. In fact, if you are a cancer patient and
you are not dramatically changing your diet, you will sabotage any
other cancer treatment you choose.

Most of us are still eating the diet we grew up with. But the American diet can best be described as bizarre. No one in history has ever
consumed such a diet. Historically unprecedented, modern diets are
biologically incapable of supporting healthy life. Modern diets are
so bad that medical pioneer and author of the breakthrough book
Mental and Elemental Nutrients, Dr. Carl Pfeiffer, concluded: "The
average human diet, nutritionally unfit for rats, must be equally
unsatisfactory or even more so in meeting human needs." The diet
most of us eat will not support healthy life in rats, yet we feed this
diet to our children! Our children are in such poor health, they are
projected to be the first generation in 200 years to die younger than
their parents. Diabetes, asthma, allergies, and cognitive/behavioral
problems are epidemic, and after accidents, cancer is now the leading cause of death for children.

If you have metastasized cancer, the choice is this: change your

diet or die. Your doctor cannot save you. Only *you* can save you—
if you give your immune system a chance to go to work. Start by
changing your diet.

Once you make the change and become accustomed to your new
and improved diet, your tastes will change. You won't miss the old
diet, and you will feel better than you have ever felt. You'll think of
food in an entirely new way; as either health-destroying or health
sustaining. Remember this: *Nothing tastes as good as health feels!*

Most people are aware that genetic mutations cause cancer. The
single most important cause of genetic mutations is malnutrition. A
deficiency of even a few nutrients will result in genetic damage that
is equal to, or greater than, the damage caused by radiation. Once
damaged, DNA needs to be repaired, and this is why the body has
a DNA repair system. Our poor nutrition not only damages DNA,
but then we lack the nutrients required to operate the repair system,
compounding the problem.

What you eat affects whether or not you get cancer and whether
you will die or recover from it. Even a slight amount of malnutrition can have a substantial effect on your DNA and your immune
system, making you susceptible to infections and cancer. Every cell
is dependent on a supply of essential nutrients daily to perform all
of its required functions, including the regulation of cancer's on/
off switches. Whether or not you supply these nutrients is a critical
determinant of your health.

What you eat also affects your moods and behavior and your
ability to learn, think, and remember. Bad nutritional choices have
an impact on the ability to enjoy life to the fullest, and, for some
people, even contribute to a descent into depression, violence, suicide, or criminal activities.

Your diet can make the difference between getting sick and not getting sick—between having colds and the flu and not having them—between rapid aging and slow aging—between having cancer and not having cancer. We shop at the supermarket, come out with carts loaded with factory-produced boxes, jars, bottles, and packages and call it food. It's garbage! Food supports health—garbage damages health and is unfit to eat. It's almost hard to believe that ninety cents out of every American food dollar is spent to purchase garbage—processed foods that are low in nutrition and high in toxins. This is devastating to our health, and it's why the health of our people is in a long-term decline.

Americans think of themselves as the best-fed people in the world. We are not. According to the WHO, there are about 1 billion people in the world who are starving to death because they are unable to obtain enough food. These folks can't even get enough calories—an enormous tragedy. But here is the really shocking news and perhaps an even worse tragedy—there is another group of 1 billion people who are also *starving to death*—not because they cannot obtain food—*but because they choose to eat the wrong foods.* The 300 million Americans are part of that second group. *Most Americans are starving to death!* As a consequence of our poor food choices, our cells are malfunctioning on a massive scale, and we are experiencing an unprecedented epidemic of cancer and other chronic illnesses. We need to make better food choices.

How Our Poor Food Choices Began

It all started with the Industrial Revolution in the latter part of the 1700s. Coal-fueled steam engines introduced machine-based manufacturing and changed life forever as people moved off the farms and into cities to work in factories. This influx of people into the cities and reduction in the number of farmers producing readily available fresh foods created a need to process foods in ways that gave them shelf life in order to store foods for long periods. This began a period of drastic changes in our diet that are still ongoing. Most of our calories today come from "foods" that did not even exist only a few hundred years ago. Processed foods like white flour, refined sugar, and white rice were considered "perfect" solutions. Their shelf life is pretty much forever. They supply calories, produce energy, and take away your hunger—*but*—they lack essential nutrients. Soon, other methods of processing for long shelf life, such as canning, freezing, and irradiating were developed.

Processing is the ultimate robber of nutrition. You get shelf life and convenience, but you lose nutrients, and, in some cases, almost all of the nutrition is lost. Not only are nutrients lost, but toxins are generated as well as added, creating both deficiency and toxicity— the two causes of all disease. Toxins are added to processed foods in the form of preservatives to give shelf life, artificial colors to make food appealing, artificial flavors to replace lost flavor, flavor enhancers to increase flavor, salt to mask bad flavors and improve color, chemicals to help retain moisture, and processing aids to make the manufacturing process go more smoothly. Ninety cents out of every food dollar is spent on these toxic, nutritionally deficient, disease-causing, processed foods. Some people eat little else. What you are buying is disease!

It is depressing to go to a supermarket (I call it the disease store) and watch people pay good money for grocery carts loaded with every imaginable disease, including cancer. Often, there will be no real food whatsoever in the cart. It will be filled with processed foods in the form of bread, cookies, baked goods, and breakfast cereals; canned goods; frozen pizzas; milk, cheese, and dairy products; fruit drinks and sodas; fruits and vegetables sprayed with toxic chemicals; foods too old to retain much nutrition; refined sugar in many forms; processed oils; hydrogenated fats; artificial colors, flavors, and preservatives; farmed fish and feedlot-raised meat. The cart will be loaded with diabetes, heart disease, arthritis, Alzheimer's, osteoporosis, accelerated aging, and cancer. Then after decades of spending a lot of money to buy cancer, somehow it is still a surprise when people get what they paid for, and the cancer finally arrives.

A key aspect of healthy eating is choosing foods that have not been adulterated. Eating foods that are as close as possible to their natural state is the only way to get the maximum amount of the nutrients that are found in fresh, raw foods. Today's food supply is enormously compromised. The combination of modern chemical farming, harvesting before ripening, processing, pasteurizing, irradiating, storing, and shipping have all conspired to reduce the nutritional quality of our food to below that required for healthy life. Farming with artificial fertilizers does not replace minerals in the soil. Our soils are now stripped of essential minerals, and if the minerals are not in the soil, they do not get into the plant, and when you eat the plant, you don't get what you need. Harvesting produce before it is ripe helps to get the food to you before it rots, but it reduces the nutritional content by up to 80 percent because a lot of the nutrition is developed in the last day or two of ripening.

Then there is the problem of distribution. Food is meant to be harvested when ripe and consumed shortly thereafter. Most people don't know that *with each passing hour after harvesting*, nutrition is lost. It is significant that the average age of produce in the supermarket is two weeks, and some items are a year or more old. "Fresh" apples average about ten months old and can easily be over a year old. They may still look like apples, but they have little nutritional value. Studies on "fresh" oranges have found that many contain no vitamin C whatsoever. These so-called "fresh" oranges are harvested green, stored in warehouses, artificially colored, and sold as fresh. In fact, the uniform color of non-organic oranges is often due to the injection of an artificial dye into the skins—one reason to eat only organic oranges. Food is remarkably hardy, but nutrients are not. Nutrients are easily lost or destroyed. For example, spinach loses 60 percent of its folic acid in three days. Vegetables such as asparagus, broccoli, and green beans lose 50 percent of their vitamin C before they reach the produce section. Cooking these vegetables results in even more losses, including another 25 percent of the vitamin C, 70 percent of vitamin B1, and 50 percent of B2.

Over the past twenty-five years, the incidence of esophageal adenocarcinoma has increased 350 percent, faster than any other cancer in the western world. Research has shown that this type of esophageal cancer is increasing 5 to 10 percent per year in developed countries. A 2002 German study, reported in the *Journal of Cancer Research and Clinical Oncology*, said vitamin C, vitamin E, beta-carotene and folic acid supplements significantly reduce the risk of all esophageal cancers. This cancer is increasing because these nutrients are lacking in our modern diets. Supplementing with vitamin C was associated with a 66 percent reduction, and supplemental vitamin E reduced esophageal cancer risk by an astonishing 87 percent—*two simple and inexpensive ways to keep cancer turned off.*

Mineral deficiencies are also a critical problem. Nobel Prize winner Dr. Linus Pauling once said, "You can trace every sickness, every disease and every ailment to a mineral deficiency." Yet according to the 1992 Earth Summit report, 99 percent of Americans are mineral deficient. No wonder more than three out of four Americans have a diagnosable chronic disease. You may have no symptoms, but if you consume foods that have little nutritional value or are toxic, you are more than likely to be in the early stages of disease.

The nutritional content of every vegetable grown in the United States has undergone huge declines. A 2001 study in the *Nutrition Practitioner* looked at calcium levels in food over the period 1940 to 1991. On average, in the space of fifty years, the calcium content of vegetables dropped by 46 percent. It is even lower today, and calcium helps to prevent cancer. *For example, in order to get the same nutrition you got in one carrot a half century ago, you now have to eat two carrots to get the same amount of calcium, four carrots to get the same magnesium, and up to twenty carrots to get the same amount of zinc.* How many people are eating all those extra vegetables? All bodily processes depend on the action and interaction of minerals. A shortage of even one mineral can throw the entire body out of balance.

Unfortunately, conventional physicians have almost no training in nutrition and biochemistry and give patients advice that makes matters worse. Most oncologists will tell their patients that cancer has nothing to do with nutrition and that it doesn't matter what they eat. Typical is the case of Stacy, a forty-eight-year-old cancer patient who was suffering a recurrence of metastasized melanoma. Stacy questioned her physicians about diet. She was told she could eat whatever she wanted. One doctor told her that nutrition had absolutely nothing to do with cancer. He told her to eat whatever made her happy, and he jokingly said he would write her a prescription for ice cream. Like most doctors, he was simply unaware of the critical role nutrition plays in causing disease. Stacy's oncologist actually served candy to the cancer patients in his waiting room, oblivious to the fact that sugar drives cancer like gasoline drives fire.

Stacy's recurrence of melanoma was diagnosed as a "significant metastasis to the lower ilium." She was advised to undergo immediate surgery—she refused. Her oncologist was adamant. He followed her out of the office into the hall saying, "Schedule the surgery now! Schedule the surgery now!" Stacy was sufficiently well informed to know that her metastasized melanoma was a death sentence. Given the grim statistics on that type of cancer, she knew that conventional medicine could not save her. If she wanted to live, Stacy would have to take charge of her own health.

Stacy purchased organic vegetables, juiced them, and took vitamin supplements. Three months after the "significant metastasis" diagnosis, all testing showed her to be cancer free. After her radiologist called her with the good news of her test results, she told him what she had done to rid herself of the cancer. He simply stated, "Well, whatever it is you are doing, keep doing it." He didn't ask her any questions and was not curious about how she had accomplished this incredible feat. Seven years later, with no medical treatment, she is still in robust health and now grows her own organic vegetables—*cancer can be switched on or off through nutrition.*

Since Stacy's original melanoma diagnosis in 2003, four family friends were diagnosed with melanoma. Despite pleading with them to take a more natural approach to healing, just as my brother pleaded with his five friends, they all chose conventional treatment with surgery, chemo, and radiation—they are all dead.

I asked Stacy if she would write something for inclusion in this book. Here is what she wrote:

> *It is crucially important to give our cells what they need to be successful in fighting disease and building the immune system. We also need to take away all the toxic ingredients; this includes any negativity. I believe very strongly that our cells are eaves-*

dropping on our thoughts. We need to look at anything in our recent past that was traumatic or upsetting to us, and face it. I was incredibly fortunate to find the book Never Be Sick Again, *one of the first books I came across in my search for answers. This book provided a basic, fundamental message that made the difference between surviving my disease or dying from it. Importantly, it also gave me an understanding of the "why" behind making these necessary changes. We cannot allow others to decide our outcome. So a doctor who expresses a poor prognosis for us cannot be allowed to dictate how or if our disease will progress—this is entirely up to the patient.*

The cancer process is enormously complex, involving hundreds of genes and many biochemical processes in the body, but Mother Nature has provided natural healing for us. As complex as the cancer process is, *there are chemicals in fruits and vegetables that interfere in every known step of the cancer process.* In fact, there are chemicals in fruits and vegetables that have been observed to kill cancer cells and even restore cancer cells to normal. *Fruits and vegetables will not only prevent cancer, they can cure cancer!* Fruits and vegetables address the two causes of disease, deficiency and toxicity, helping to restore cancer cells to normal. Standard cancer treatments cause deficiency and toxicity. They cannot and do not restore cells to normal, which is why they don't work. Good nutrition is the key to good health. Your first commitment must be to your diet. You will not get well by continuing to eat the same diet that made you sick in the first place.

Nutrition Regulates
Cancer's On and Off Switches

Curing cancer is about shutting down the cancer process; it is *not* about shrinking or removing tumors. To shut the cancer process down, certain biochemical processes need to be supported and others need to be inhibited. Three critical processes involved in turning cancer on or off are *inflammation, apoptosis*, and *angiogenesis*. Inflammation is a foundation stone of every chronic disease—including cancer. Inflammation both causes and drives cancer, and it is essential to the cancer process. Most Americans are in a chronic inflammatory state. Inflammation damages DNA, damages cell membranes, impairs oxygen transport into cells, and it makes the natural barriers surrounding cells more permeable so tumors can grow. Cancer cells need inflammation to sustain their growth—shutting down inflammation is essential to reversing cancer. *Apoptosis* is the process by which cells die when they become sufficiently abnormal. Apoptosis protects us from cancer. *Helping to maintain healthy apoptosis or to restore apoptosis is essential for preventing and reversing cancer. Angiogenesis* is the process by which new blood vessels are stimulated to grow and feed a growing tumor—something you want to inhibit.

In 2005, five studies were presented at the American Association for Cancer Research's 4th Annual International Conference on Frontiers in Cancer Prevention Research. These particular studies demonstrated that adding certain vegetables and herbs, such as broccoli sprouts, cabbage, ginkgo biloba, and garlic, can prevent and, in some cases, even stop the growth of cancer.

There are an enormous number of chemical interactions between compounds found in foods and the body's cells and DNA. These chemicals can change cell signaling and instructions given to genes, thus reducing inflammation, enhancing apoptosis, and inhibiting angiogenesis. Adding fresh fruits and vegetables to your diet can reap healthy benefits at any stage of life. Studies and long-term observation have shown that broccoli can reverse breast cancer. Carrots can reverse lung cancer. Ginger, onions, and garlic shrink tumors throughout the body. There is even new data on walnuts. Research presented at the March 2010 annual meeting of the American Chemical Society and published in *Science Daily* found that walnut consumption slows the growth of prostate cancer in mice and has beneficial effects on multiple genes related to the control of tumor growth and metabolism. Researcher Paul Davis of the UC Davis Cancer Center said, "This study shows that when mice with prostate tumors consume an amount of walnuts that could easily be eaten by a man, tumor growth is controlled. This leaves me very hopeful that it could be beneficial in patients." Study after study has proven that real food, whether it is walnuts, onions, or carrots, protects against disease and cancer, and that processed food causes disease and cancer.

Many of the things that we know cause and promote cancer are the very things that cause and promote inflammation. People with more inflammation have more cancer, and people with cancer who have more inflammation have more aggressive cancer that is more likely to spread and kill. Controlling inflammation is essential. Fruits and vegetables contain anti-inflammatory chemicals that help to prevent and control chronic inflammation. By combining these healthy foods with antioxidant supplements and adequate omega-3 oils, plus eating a diet that does not contain hydrogenated oils or excessive omega-6 oils, you are creating a healthy internal environment that will not support cancer.

People who eat a diet high in fresh fruits and vegetables have a lower incidence of cancer. Among the nutrients contained in fruits and vegetables is a class of about 5,000 compounds called flavonoids; hundreds of these compounds can be found in a single fruit or vegetable, and they all work together as a team. It is important to eat a variety of fruits and vegetables to get all the different flavonoids working together. Flavonoids support apoptosis and inhibit angiogenesis. Flavonoids are antioxidants that help to control inflammation, but they also perform numerous other functions. They are known to suppress and even kill cancer cells. One of the functions of flavonoids is to help to control a cell-signaling molecule called NFkB. This compound is normally found in every cell; it gives instructions to genes telling them to produce inflammatory chemicals and encouraging cells to grow—not something you want if your concern is cancer. In the absence of sufficient flavonoids to control NFkB's signaling activity, cells grow and inflammatory chemicals are produced. When flavonoids are present, the signaling effect of NFkB is controlled, inflammation is diminished, and tumors stop growing—in some cases, they even disappear. Flavonoids such as quercetin, curcumin, and ellagic acid are found in common fruits and vegetables, including cauliflower, broccoli, and Brussels sprouts. They are known to inhibit a large number of cell-signaling molecules that are essential for switching cancer on and driving it to grow and metastasize. Flavonoids inhibit the enzymes that make it possible for tumors to invade surrounding tissue. Consuming a diet rich in flavonoids is a must, as is taking flavonoid supplements. Flavonoids, minerals and vitamins strengthen the immune system, helping it attack cancer cells.

In 1993, a study in the *Journal of Cellular Biochemistry* found that beta-carotene, an antioxidant found in carrots and other vegetables, was a powerful cancer inhibitor. Beta-carotene could restore precancerous cells to normal, thereby preventing cancer from happening. In a six-month test, four-out-of-five cancer patients experienced dramatic reductions in the size of their tumors by taking a beta-carotene supplement daily. Another carotene is lycopene, a bright red carotenoid, found in red fruits and vegetables such as tomatoes and watermelons. Men with the highest levels of lycopene in their blood have the lowest risk of prostate cancer.

One problem with getting the nutrients we need is that most people cook their foods. Cooking food is another major change we have made in our diets. Cooking common vegetables, such as carrots, can cause losses of 75 percent of the vitamin C, 70 percent of the vitamin B1, 50 percent of the vitamin B2, and 60 percent of vitamin B3. *The higher the heat and the longer the cooking time, the more nutrients are lost.* Cooking reduces the availability of many of the precious nutrients and phytochemicals. Produce such as apples, beets, cabbage, and cauliflower lose most of their anticancer activity when they are cooked. *As much as possible, foods need to be eaten raw.* Vegetables such as broccoli and spinach may be lightly steamed or quickly stir-fried if necessary.

Although the human body is capable of making its own enzymes, we also get enzymes directly from our food. Cooking food deactivates its health-sustaining enzymes. This puts stress on the body, which must manufacture extra enzymes in order to compensate for the enzymes lost in cooking. Obtaining enzymes is one reason why eating raw foods is so important, and why cooked foods contribute to our epidemic of chronic disease.

Within my lifetime, the consumption of raw food has decreased. According to USDA statistics, over the last century, average consumption of fresh apples declined by more than three-fourths, fresh cabbage by more than two-thirds, and fresh fruit by more than one-third. During that same period, consumption of processed vegetables went up hundreds of percent and consumption of processed fruits went up by 1,000 percent. If you must eat cooked foods, it is best to eat something raw first, such as a salad before the main course. Cooked food appears to be so alien to the human system that it provokes an immune response, as if you are being exposed to a virus. Scientist Udo Erasmus, author of *Fats and Oils*, wrote, "When cooked (or dead) food is eaten, a defense reaction occurs in the tissues of the stomach and digestive tract. This reaction is similar to the reaction we find in infections and around tumors and involves the accumulation of white blood cells, swelling, and a fever-like increase in temperature of the stomach and intestinal tissues." This reaction does not occur if raw food is consumed prior to eating the cooked food.

How you cook makes a difference. Cooking food at high temperatures, such as in grilling, frying, and barbecuing, not only destroys nutrients, but poisons the food by producing enormously powerful carcinogens. The high heat of grilling causes reactions with the proteins in red meat, poultry, and fish, producing carcinogenic chemicals called heterocyclic amines. Another class of cancer-causing agents, polycyclic aromatic hydrocarbons, forms when the juices from meats drip and hit the heat source, rising in the smoke and contaminating the meat. This delivers two classes of powerful carcinogens at the same time. Meat that has been blackened is the worst of all—never eat blackened meat. Even well done meat is highly contaminated, and numerous studies have shown that people who eat meat cooked at higher temperatures get more cancer. Anytime you cook meat at high temperatures, whether by barbecuing, frying, or broiling, carcinogens are created. A 1990 study in *Cancer Research* found that children born to mothers who eat a lot of these carcinogens have a high risk of developing cancer—and childhood cancer is epidemic. Microwave ovens are found in almost every kitchen, and microwaved food is very dangerous, causing deficiencies and toxicities that drive cancer. Microwaving not only destroys most of the nutrition in the food, it also produces dangerous toxins and carcinogens that poison the body. Eating microwaved food damages cell-to-cell communication, stresses the immune system, and lowers the oxygen-carrying capacity of the blood—*all of which cause and drive the cancer process.*

Research reported in the April/May 1995 *Nexus* by Dr. Hans Hertel and Dr. Bernard Blanc of the Swiss Federal Institute of Technology found pathological changes in the blood of volunteers who ate microwaved food. Blood samples from test subjects demonstrated impaired immunity due to decreased lymphocytes (white blood cells) and decreased hemoglobin. Decreased hemoglobin lowers the oxygen carrying capacity of the blood, making less oxygen available to cells. The combination of less oxygen, impaired immunity, and microwave cooking's production of carcinogenic compounds causes cancer.

Microwaving food destroys nutrients. A 2003 study in the *Journal of the Science of Food and Agriculture* reported that broccoli lost 97 percent of its antioxidants when cooked in a microwave. By contrast, only 11 percent was lost when steamed. Foods today are already nutrient deficient; why make them worse by cooking them in a microwave? If you must cook, steaming is generally the least damaging way to cook.

Research over decades has clearly demonstrated that a number of readily available foods such as cruciferous vegetables (cabbage, broccoli, kale, Brussels sprouts, turnips, cauliflower, radishes, bok choy, and watercress) have a major impact on cancer prevention and reversal. Cancer-fighting foods all contain large amounts of phytochemicals. These chemicals are nature's way of protecting plants against disease and environmental stress. Phytochemicals give fruits and vegetables their brilliant colors, and they are primarily responsible for the cancer-prevention capabilities of these healthy foods. By choosing a variety of fresh fruits and vegetables, you can provide your body with thousands of different phytochemicals, offering enormous protection against disease.

As previously stated, flavonoids, such as quercetin, support apoptosis. Curcumin, vitamin E succinate, green tea extract, and resveratrol also support apoptosis. Omega-3 fats inhibit angiogenesis, while nicotine promotes angiogenesis, which is one more reason why smoking supports cancer and is unhealthy. The prescription is simple. Eat more fresh fruits and vegetables and correct your ratio of omega-6 to omega-3 fats by supplementing with more omega-3s. And of course, don't smoke!

Certain foods are known to promote tumor growth and spread. Sugar, excess omega-6 oils, hydrogenated oils, excess animal protein, and milk products all promote cancer. *Cancer cells differ from normal cells in that they are totally dependent on sugar to produce energy.* To feed a growing tumor, you need to eat lots of sugar. One approach to shutting down the cancer process is to starve the cancer cells by not feeding them the food they need to multiply. Raising the sugar content of the blood feeds cancer cells and helps them grow. In addition, sugar increases blood insulin, which is a powerful promoter of tumor spread and growth. Eating carbohydrates, such as sugar, fruit juices, and grains, increases insulin. Normalizing your insulin levels is one of the most important things you can do to lower your risk of cancer.

Oils high in omega-6s, such as corn, safflower, sunflower, peanut, soybean, and canola oils, are known to support cancer progression. Never eat these oils, or any of the thousands of products made with them, including baked goods and salad dressings.

Excess animal protein, especially dairy protein, drives cancer. Data in *The China Study* shows that animal protein beyond what can be used for growth and daily repairs, promotes cancer, and the average American eats ten times more than the rural Chinese people in the study (70 grams per day vs. 7.1 grams). Excess animal protein is able to turn cancer on in experimental animals 100 percent of the time. A high animal-protein diet increases estrogen, and excess estrogen is known to promote a number of cancers, including breast and prostate cancer. Excess animal protein acidifies the body, and cancer thrives in an acid environment. Animal protein also contains large amounts of the amino acid methionine. Excess methionine is a known cancer promoter.

What Not to Eat—The Big Four and Others

What I call the Big Four are "foods" you should definitely not eat. These four foods are: sugar, wheat, processed oils, and dairy/excess animal protein. These foods are primary causes of disease, and they switch on and drive cancer.

Sugar

Sugar is a major culprit in the cancer process; those who consume the highest amount of sugar have the most cancer. One of the single largest changes we have made in our diet over the last century is the enormous amount of refined sugar we eat. Our genes are still those of our hunter/gatherer ancestors, and we are not biologically designed to handle this load of refined sugars. Because of our biology, sugar is a deadly metabolic poison that switches on and drives the cancer process. It is killing us.

Once you have cancer, sugar feeds the cancer cells, so the more sugar you eat, the faster your cancer will grow. Eating sugar produces a flood of inflammatory free radicals that damage DNA. Sugar makes cells oxygen deficient and causes oxygen-deprived cells to become cancer cells. Sugar accelerates the aging process. Even a modest increase in blood sugar generates free radicals and causes inflammation. Sugar is a deadly metabolic poison that may even be the largest single contributor to our epidemic of chronic and degenerative disease. According to chemist and twice Nobel Laureate Dr. Linus Pauling, "Sugar is the most hazardous foodstuff in the American diet."

The fact is the sugary foods we were given as rewards and treats as children, and that have become so much a part of our normal diet, cause biochemical chaos in our bodies. At best, these foods are dangerous, and at worst, they are deadly.

On average, Americans now get about 20 percent of their calories from sugar, and many of our young people get twice that. Sugar creates massive and continuing disruption to our normal biochemistry. Even two teaspoons of sugar (one can of soda contains ten to thirteen teaspoons) causes a wide range of deficiencies and toxicities, resulting in massive cellular malfunction lasting for a period of six to eight hours. Sugar disrupts hormone, fat, carbohydrate, protein, and mineral metabolism. All this affects immunity, the digestive process, the cardiovascular system, the nervous system, and hormone and enzyme production. Eating sugar several times a day puts your body into continuous biochemical chaos, which throws the body out of balance so it no longer properly communicates, self-regulates, or self-repairs—*this is disease!*

Eating sugar is worse than eating nothing! In *A History of Nutrition,* Elmer McCollum cited experiments in which animals fed water alone lived substantially longer than those fed sugar and water. When you eat sugar, the body requires certain nutrients for it to be metabolized. These include B vitamins, calcium, magnesium, chromium, and zinc. Sugar does not contain these nutrients, so your bones, teeth, and other tissues are robbed of these essential vitamins and minerals in order to process the sugar you are eating. This depletes your reserves, creates deficiencies, and throws the body out of balance, making you susceptible to disease. The purpose of food is to nourish our bodies. Sugar does the opposite. Nutritionist and best-selling author of *Fit for Life,* Harvey Diamond, calls processed and refined sugar "a deadly, virulent poison."

Since cancer cells ferment sugar to produce their energy, eating sugar or anything that quickly metabolizes into sugar such as white flour and white potatoes, will feed your cancer and make it worse. Cancer cells require several times more sugar than normal cells, so when you raise the sugar content of the blood, you make sugar more available to the cancer cells. Sugar feeds the cancer, and you cannot expect to put out the fire while feeding the flames.

In the body, sugar is acid forming. When consumed every day, it produces a continuously over-acid condition, which both causes and drives cancer. Sugar is rapidly absorbed into the bloodstream and quickly distributed to body cells. This happens so fast that there is insufficient oxygen available to effectively burn and metabolize the sugar. The result is incomplete burning and formation of a toxic acid called pyruvic acid. Pyruvic acid accumulates in the brain and nervous system and damages these tissues, causing neurological diseases. When eaten daily, sugar causes the body to become too acidic, and precious minerals such as calcium and magnesium are lost from the bones and teeth as the body tries to neutralize the acid and rectify the imbalance. This acidic condition alone fundamentally changes your body chemistry, causing numerous chronic diseases including cancer.

Sugar interferes with vitamin C metabolism and depresses immunity. Sugar and vitamin C have a similar chemical structure and compete with one another to enter cells. When a lot of sugar is present, it wins, creating an artificial shortage of vitamin C inside the cell. Immune cells need a lot of vitamin C to function normally. In fact, white blood cells, to fight infections, require fifty times as much vitamin C as do other cells. *Even a small amount of refined sugar can suppress your immune system*, making you susceptible to colds, flu, and all types of infections as well as *cancer*.

Refined sugar is absorbed so rapidly that it increases the sugar content of the blood beyond normal limits, creating a crisis. The body responds to this crisis by secreting insulin from the pancreas. Insulin signals cells to lower blood sugar by absorbing the sugar into the cells where it is either burned for energy or stored as fat. Once this excess insulin is produced, your blood insulin level will remain abnormally high for hours. Unfortunately, high insulin creates a cascade of negative effects. It is a powerful stimulator of inflammation and cancer growth and metastasis.

One of the most damaging things you can do to your body is increase your blood insulin, and this happens every time you eat sugar. Insulin is a switch that turns cancer on. If you eat sugar several times a day, insulin will be high all day, every day. Some researchers believe that insulin may be the single largest cause of chronic disease. Dr. David Katz, director of the Prevention Research Center at Yale Medical School and author of *Nutrition in Clinical Practice* had this to say: "Is insulin *the* master control of all disease? I don't know, but it's certainly a candidate for that role." People who live the healthiest and longest eat the least sugar and have the lowest insulin.

Insulin not only switches cancer on, it also drives it. Cancer cells have six to ten times the number of insulin receptors as normal cells. Insulin stimulates cell growth, signaling cancer cells to grow. Excess insulin also suppresses production of IGFBP-3 (insulin-like growth factor binding protein-3). IGFBP-3 inhibits the spread of cancer cells and supports apoptosis, triggering the death of cancer cells. You don't want to suppress something so useful, but this is what happens when you eat sugar.

Whenever insulin is increased, so is another hormone called insulin-like growth factor (IGF), which also stimulates inflammation, cancer growth, and metastasis. IGF's job is to stimulate cell growth, making cancer cells grow faster. IGF also promotes the production of inflammatory factors, and inflammation is necessary for the growth and metastasis of cancer.

Most Americans, both men and women, are suffering from hormonal imbalances. Sugar causes hormonal imbalances, leading to a host of health problems—including cancer. Sugar elevates insulin, and excess insulin increases estrogen, and these imbalances throw your entire hormone system out of balance. Adding to this problem, sugar makes you fat, and fat cells produce estrogen, adding to the excess you already have. Excess estrogen causes enlarged prostates and drives both prostate and breast cancers. Excess estrogen causes cancer by displacing iron from its protective proteins and increasing the level of free iron in the body, which is highly inflammatory. To make matters worse, we are already unwittingly absorbing a lot of estrogen-like chemicals from commercially raised cattle and poultry and from the pesticides on nonorganic foods. The estrogen-like chemical bisphenol-A leaches from plastic food and drink containers, such as the resin lining of most food and beverage cans, plastic water bottles, and polycarbonate containers.

As if all these problems were not enough, metabolizing sugar is responsible for yet another cell-damaging disaster. AGEs (advanced glycation end-products) are formed when a sugar molecule reacts with an amino acid, either in food before we eat it or in the body after we eat it. AGEs form in foods during the cooking process, particularly as food browns. Foods likely to supply AGEs include bacon, hot dogs, cured and smoked meats, and baked beans. AGEs also form inside the body. When you increase the sugar in the blood, it reacts with proteins, fats, enzymes, and even the DNA in your cells. A breakfast of eggs and orange juice puts both sugar and protein into the blood at the same time, forming AGEs. *Any protein meal followed by a sugary dessert will create AGEs.*

Once critical molecules in the body have reacted to form AGEs, they become much more susceptible to damage from free radicals. AGEs damage DNA, as well as the enzymes that are needed to repair DNA. Disabled enzymes also shut down critical functions inside cells including oxygen respiration and energy production. AGEs also are absorbed into various body tissues where they remain for long periods of time and initiate long-term chronic inflammation. Immune cells try to get rid of AGEs. However, if you eat a lot of sugar and create a lot of AGEs, the immune system becomes exhausted, making you more susceptible to infections and cancer. All of the above contribute to switching cancer on and driving it. Get the sugar out of your life, and you won't have to worry about AGEs.

Americans devour an incredible 160 pounds of sugar per person each year—almost a half-pound per person per day! By contrast, the average person eats only 8.5 pounds of broccoli per year. Think about that—160 pounds of a nutritionally worthless, empty-calorie poison that switches on and drives cancer versus only 8.5 pounds of a healthy food that prevents and reverses cancer. Clearly, we have our priorities wrong.

Getting sugar out of your diet is a simple choice that you can make, but you may be surprised to learn how many processed foods contain sugar. Getting sugar out of your eating regimen means much more than eliminating desserts.

Learn to be a label reader. When you read the labels, look for more than the word sugar in the list of ingredients. Below is a list (far from complete) of some of the names that will tell you sugar is in a product.

Sugar	Corn syrup	Maltose
Beet sugar	Dextrose	Evaporated cane
Brown sugar	Fruit juices	juice
Cane sugar	Fruit juice concen-	Honey
Confectioner's sugar	trate	Maltodextrin
Organic sugar	High-fructose corn	Malt syrup
Raw sugar	syrup	Maple syrup
Sugar cane syrup	Fructose	Molasses
Barley malt	Glucose	Turbinado sugar
Brown rice syrup	Lactose	

If you are going to eat something containing sugar, at least limit the amount you eat by checking the number of grams of sugar you may be consuming. *If there are more than 4 grams in the amount you intend to eat, reject the item.* Consider a can of baked beans, which is a processed food that should be avoided anyway. A typical can may read: white beans, water, molasses, sugar, fructose, brown sugar—this product is loaded with four different kinds of sugar. A typical can may contain 20 grams of sugar. A typical bottle of salad dressing is often loaded with sugar, not to mention sugar-loaded spaghetti sauce, pancake syrup, cured meats, yogurt, and ketchup. To be safe, get the sugar out of your life, and get all the processed foods out of your life. If you don't eat processed foods, you don't need to worry about added sugar. Sugar improves the shelf life and flavor of processed foods and therefore is added to most of them. Fresh broccoli, sunflower sprouts, Brazil nuts, and brown rice don't need ingredient lists and have no added sugars. Fresh, whole foods make life simple and healthier.

As you avoid all the sweeteners listed as sugars, you can use a little pure stevia extract when sweetness is necessary. Stevia is a calorie-free herb that is naturally sweet. In fact, it is 100 times sweeter than sugar. It does not cause a rise in blood sugar or insulin.

Artificial synthetic sweeteners are *not* an option. They all have toxic effects on the body. Aspartame, used in most diet sodas, is known to be particularly toxic. One of the breakdown products of this molecule is formaldehyde. Formaldehyde accumulates in our cells where it damages DNA and causes cancer. Drinking even one can of diet soda can cause DNA damage that leads to cancer. Your risk increases with each can consumed. Aspartame is an excitotoxin. It can penetrate the blood-brain barrier and damage the brain and nervous system. Aspartame also increases your risk of strokes and heart attacks. Splenda is a newer artificial sweetener, and it may not penetrate the brain as aspartame does, but it can adversely affect the body in several ways because it is an unnatural, manmade chemical. The side effects of Splenda include skin rashes/flushing, panic-like agitation, dizziness and numbness, diarrhea, swelling, muscle aches, headaches, bladder issues, and severe gastrointestinal problems. Animal studies show that Splenda reduces the amount of good bacteria in the intestines by 50 percent, increases the pH level in the intestines, and contributes to increases in body weight.

Wheat

Most people are aware that white flour is deficient in nutrients and not good for them. To make white flour, the whole grain has been seriously depleted of over twenty essential nutrients, including 72 percent of its zinc and 85 percent of its vitamin B6. When a handful of these nutrients are added back, the flour is called "enriched." White flour is mostly starch, and quickly metabolizes into sugar, causing all the same problems that sugar creates. Eating white flour is almost the same as eating sugar.

Like sugar, white flour causes an increase in blood sugar, insulin, and estrogen, and produces a flood of pro-inflammatory chemicals and free radicals. All of these work to switch cancer on and drive it. The average American consumes about 200 pounds of this toxic garbage every year.

When I ask people if they eat white flour, many claim they don't. When I point out that white flour is a major ingredient in many of their favorite foods, they are shocked to discover how much of it they do eat. Most people don't realize they are consuming white flour when they are eating breakfast cereal, bread, a dinner roll, a bagel, a pretzel, a cookie, a pancake, pasta, pizza, or a piece of pie. It's all white flour, and it's all inflammatory and enormously damaging to human health, disrupting vitamin and mineral metabolism and hormone balance. Even something labeled as "whole wheat" bread or "whole grain" cereal is usually mostly white flour.

While the problems with white flour are well known, most people are unaware that grains themselves may be a problem, and that wheat is the worst grain of all. The wheat we eat today differs from what our ancestors consumed. Modern wheat has been hybridized to achieve higher protein content. Some of that increased protein is in the form of *gluten*, and some is in the form of a class of proteins called *lectins*. Gluten is a type of protein that is found in certain grains, such as wheat, rye, oats, and barley. It is highly allergenic to humans. By increasing the protein content of the wheat, we have created wheat that is high in gluten and, therefore, highly allergenic. Researchers have estimated that as much as half the population may now be metabolically reactive (allergic) to gluten, but most people are unaware of their sensitivity. Nonetheless, they suffer a wide range of health problems including the common cold, depression, eczema, and irritable bowel syndrome, completely unaware that gluten is the problem. Immune reactions to gluten produce free radicals, inflammation, and acids that make the body more acidic. An overworked immune system, free-radical damage, inflammation, and acidosis help to switch on and drive cancer. Gluten sensitivity is causing an epidemic of chronic disease.

Grains were a very minor part of the human diet until about 10,000 years ago. Now grains represent about half of all the food consumed. All plants contain natural toxins to protect the plant from viruses, bacteria, fungi, and predators. Our genes are well adapted to handle the toxins in fruits and vegetables, but not so for the relatively recent addition of the special toxins in grains. Anthropological evidence indicates that when we started eating grains, our health declined. Infant mortality increased, lifespan shortened, infectious diseases increased, and bone disorders and dental decay appeared.

Grains contain nutrients, but cooking is usually necessary to make them edible. Cooking significantly diminishes the nutritional value. Baked goods that contain yeast present a special problem, and should never be consumed by cancer patients. Many studies have linked bread and other bakery products with cancer. This is due to the carcinogenic mycotoxins they contain, which are metabolic waste products of the yeast used to make the bread. In addition, grains contain anti-nutrients called phytates. Phytates react with calcium, making calcium unavailable to you, possibly resulting in calcium deficiency.

Grains also contain a class of proteins called *lectins*, which can damage gut tissue and decrease absorption of nutrients. Research presented in a 2008 *FASEB Journal,* a 2000 *Gut,* a 1999 *Lancet,* a 1995 *Pediatric Allergy and Immunology*, a 1993 *British Journal of Nutrition*, and numerous other sources indicate that lectins may be the biggest grain problem of all. Lectins are a class of defensive glycoprotein compounds that plants use to protect themselves from insects—they are powerful natural insecticides. Lectins are found in legumes and nightshades, such as tomatoes and potatoes, but are exceptionally high in seeds of the grass family such as wheat, spelt, rye, and rice. Lectins are part of the protein content of these foods. However, lectins are especially high in modern hybridized wheat.

Over centuries, selective breeding of wheat has increased its protein content, and the lectin concentration has increased proportionately. While higher protein may have been desirable from a nutritional standpoint, higher amounts of lectins are not desirable from a health standpoint because of their toxicity.

Lectins are highly stable molecules that are resistant to degradation through a wide range of pH and temperatures. They survive cooking, sprouting, fermentation, and digestion. Being very stable and resistant to breaking down in the body, lectins tend to accumulate and become incorporated into tissues, where they interfere with normal biological processes. We are now consuming a lot of high-lectin wheat, and it is accumulating in our tissues, putting a continuous toxic load on us. Ironically, whole wheat contains more lectins than white flour, and in this regard, may be an even bigger threat to health than white flour.

Lectins are designed to attach to receptor sites on the cell membrane of bacteria and fungi and disrupt their function. This does a marvelous job of protecting wheat from infection by bacteria and fungi, but humans have exactly the same receptor sites! Consuming wheat appears to be having a devastating effect on human health, including switching on and driving cancer. In fact, lectins can do direct damage to the majority of tissues in the human body, and this helps to explain why chronic inflammatory diseases are more common in wheat-consuming populations. The inflammation created by lectins damages DNA, switches cancer on, and drives it.

When we eat wheat, the lectins damage our gastrointestinal tract, causing injury to the gut tissue and creating holes in the tissue that make it more permeable to larger molecules. This is called a leaky gut. Once the gut is leaky, undigested molecules, including gluten, enter into the bloodstream. The immune system sees these molecules as invaders and attacks them, creating inflammation. Increased intestinal permeability is now recognized as causing a wide variety of problems that result in chronic inflammatory and autoimmune syndromes, including inflammatory bowel diseases, celiac diseases, multiple sclerosis, eczema, and several others. Lectins not only damage gut tissue, they pass through the gut and stimulate the production of pro-inflammatory chemicals throughout the body. All the above result in chronic systemic inflammation, which both switches on and drives cancer and compromises immune defenses, the body's first line of defense against cancer. In addition, these immune responses increase the body's acid load, creating the acidic environment that switches on and drives cancer.

Lectins, even in small quantities, have profoundly adverse effects on the entire body. At exceedingly small concentrations lectins stimulate the production of pro-inflammatory chemicals such as interleukins 1, 6, and 8 in intestinal and immune cells.

Lectins damage the thymus gland, which is essential to immunity, and also directly damage immune cells in the blood. They damage the thyroid gland. Antibodies created in response to the lectins have been found to cross-react with other body proteins, thereby causing autoimmune diseases, including the thyroid disease Hashimoto's thyroiditis. Autoimmune diseases depress immune function and are inflammatory, thus contributing to cancer. Lectins have been found to play a direct role in the development of celiac disease that is entirely independent of gluten's effects. Lectins have the ability to pass through the blood-brain barrier and directly damage brain cells, as well as attaching to, and thus damaging, the myelin sheath coating on nerves. Lectins also exhibit insulin-like properties, which can cause insulin resistance (diabetes) and weight gain. They signal genes, causing production of chemical compounds such as epidermal growth factor, which, when elevated, increase the risk of cancer. Lectins stimulate platelet stickiness and blood clots. In short, lectins help to turn cancer on and facilitate its spread throughout the body.

Most people think of wheat as a good food. However, there is sufficient evidence that it is instead a toxin and a major cause of disease. *Anyone with a chronic illness, especially cancer patients, must avoid all products containing wheat.* Further, cancer patients should eliminate, or at least minimize, the consumption of grains in general.

Processed Oils

Cancer can be switched on *by eating the wrong oils and switched* off *by eating the right oils.* The improper construction of cell membranes with inappropriate oils is probably the single most important cause of oxygen deficiency and cancer.

Virtually any oil you buy at the supermarket is the wrong oil, including *all hydrogenated oils, canola, corn, cottonseed, peanut, safflower, soybean, sunflower,* and *most olive oils.* When a cell membrane (the wall separating the interior of the cell from the rest of the world) is constructed out of processed supermarket oils, this inhibits oxygen transport across the membrane into the cell, causing oxygen deficiency and both switching on and driving cancer. To prevent or reverse cancer, these products must *not* be consumed.

When a cell in the body is worn out, a new one is made. Our cell membranes are constructed mostly of oils, and to keep ourselves in good repair, we build millions of new cells every second of every day. Cell membranes have the exacting task of regulating what goes in and out of a cell. Keeping the wrong things out, letting the right things in, delivering essential nutrients, removing metabolic wastes, and doing it all correctly is a complex task. However, cell membranes do it all extremely well—*if* you construct them properly in the first place. To do that, you need the correct oils in the correct ratios to each other, and these oils must be available when the cell is being created. The good oils include unprocessed, high-quality coconut, fish, flaxseed, and olive oils. Unless you are consuming the correct oils and in the correct ratios, the membranes will not be properly constructed.

Once again, remember that oxygen deficiency (a lack of oxygen respiration) is the prime cause of cancer. Even if you have sufficient oxygen in your blood, your cells will not be able to use this oxygen if it is unable get through the membrane and into the cell. Improper construction of the cell membrane with the wrong oils not only inhibits oxygen transport into the cell, it also inhibits the transport of other essential nutrients as well as the transport of metabolic wastes out of cells. This causes deficiency and toxicity in your cells and results in cellular malfunction and diseases of every description.

Humans have a need for specific oils called *essential fatty acids* (EFAs). There are two categories of EFAs: omega-3 and omega-6. We need both types, but it is important that these oils be consumed in the proper ratio to each other. Researchers estimate that the proper ratio of 6s to 3s is ideally about 1:1, and these must be available to the body as needed when new cells are constructed.

Due to consumption of the usual supermarket oils, most Americans consume far too much omega-6 and too little omega-3 fatty acids. Historically, we consumed about an equal amount of each. The current ratio in our diet is about 20:1, and for some people as bad as 50:1. In short, we get far too much omega-6 and not near enough omega-3 oils. It's so bad that about 90 percent of the U.S. population is deficient in omega-3 fatty acids, and a 1991 study in the *World Review of Nutrition and Dietetics* showed that 20 percent of us have so little omega-3 in our blood that it cannot be measured by standard tests. Biologically speaking, this is a disaster and an invitation to cancer. Numerous studies have shown that *excess omega-6 oils suppress the immune system and drive cancer—power-*

fully promoting cancer growth and metastasis. In addition, excess omega-6s increase insulin levels, and elevated insulin drives cancer, increases inflammation, and suppresses immunity. On the other hand, omega-3s inhibit all of these and have been shown to inhibit the growth of tumors.

These same fats and oils you buy at the supermarket are also used in processed foods, fast foods, and restaurant foods. They are not only chemically imbalanced, supplying too much omega-6 and too little omega-3, but they are also highly processed. Commercial processing subjects them to heat, chemicals, and oxidation, which result in significantly changing their molecular structure and making them toxic to the body. Most supermarket oils undergo processing to make them crystal clear and to extend shelf life. This bleaching and deodorizing process usually takes place at about 500 degrees Fahrenheit, far above 320 degrees, at which massive *trans fat* formation occurs. Above 392 degrees, powerful toxins called *lipid peroxides* are formed. *There is no safe level of lipid peroxides or trans fats.* Processed oils precipitate a chain of oxidative events in the body that can severely damage cells. Yet another problem is that about 40 percent of edible oils, especially soy and corn oils, contain solvent residues from their manufacture, and solvents are known to inhibit apoptosis.

Another problem with these processed oils is that most cells prefer to use oil as a fuel. To create energy, the fuel has to be processed by metabolic machinery (enzymes) to combine it with oxygen. Enzymes are designed to fit and interact with very specific molecules. The processed oils that most of us consume have had their molecular structure altered through exposure to heat, oxygen, and hydrogenation. So even if you have enough oxygen in the cell, you may still be unable to make the energy you need because the misshaped oil molecule will not fit the appropriate enzyme and cannot be processed into energy. You are supplying the wrong fuel—not having the correct fuel inhibits oxygen respiration.

When the correct cellular building materials are not available, your body will make your new cells out of what is available. Think of building a house out of cardboard instead of high-quality plywood because the plywood is unavailable, but the cardboard is. Good oils, the essential fatty acids, are important building blocks of life. They are essential for building healthy cell membranes and as raw materials for building essential body chemicals. Incorrect molecules from the wrong oils compromise the structure and function of cells throughout the body. This interferes with critical cell-to-cell communications that are necessary for keeping the body in balance. Wrong oils interfere with the transport of nutrients into cells, and of toxic wastes out of cells. They also compromise the electrical properties of cells.

Because processed oils have been deprived of their natural antioxidants, toxic preservatives and other additives have been added to the oil, and these also interfere with oxygen transport. Almost all the processed food products we eat, such as salad dressings, baked goods, chips, breakfast cereals, and restaurant foods, are made with biologically incorrect oils, which contain toxins.

The fats we call *hydrogenated oils* pose a special problem. Hydrogenated oils are uniquely dangerous, and they are found in everything from baked goods to breakfast cereals to peanut butter. They are manmade fats containing a variety of unnatural molecules, including trans fats, all of which are toxic to your body. Some products are now being labeled as trans-fat free. This can be deceptive. Trans fats only have to be disclosed on the label if the food contains more than 0.5 grams per serving. Even that amount is toxic, but to avoid listing trans fats, or to claim "trans-fat free" on their label, food manufacturers simply adjust the serving size until the trans fat content falls under 0.5 grams per serving. Thus modern food labels often have serving sizes that are much smaller than the amount you would normally consume. So be sure to read food labels carefully. Never consume anything containing hydrogenated oils, which are sometimes listed as "margarine" or "vegetable shortening."

The imbalance of omega-6 and omega-3 oils in our diet will both initiate and perpetuate inflammation. This is highly significant because inflammation is a common denominator of all chronic disease and is essential to the cancer process. Both classes of EFAs produce body chemicals called prostaglandins. Inflammatory prostaglandins are produced from omega-6 fatty acids, and they suppress the immune system and increase inflammation, heart disease, and cancer. However, when sufficient omega-3 oils are present, anti-inflammatory prostaglandins are produced, and these offset and balance those from the omega-6s. Anti-inflammatory prostaglandins from omega-3s suppress inflammation, tumor development, blood pressure, water retention, blood platelet stickiness, and cholesterol levels. Excess omega-6s dramatically lower the amount of vitamin E in the body, which increases free-radical damage to DNA and tissues, promoting the growth and metastasis of tumors. Too many 6s also suppress the immune system, which can activate hidden and undeveloped cancers. In addition, essential fatty acid imbalance causes the clumping of red blood cells, which slows down blood flow, restricts blood flow to the smaller capillaries and results in poor oxygen delivery to cells.

While the primary reason for this enormous imbalance of 6s and 3s is the excessive consumption of the supermarket oils used in our homes and in processed foods, a secondary reason for this imbalance is the decrease in the consumption of "real" fish, meat, and eggs. For example, most of the salmon and a lot of other fish available today have been farmed in artificial environments. Farmed fish are grain fed, as opposed to the normal diet they would consume in their natural environment of oceans and rivers, and they contain the wrong fatty-acid ratios. The same holds true for beef and chicken, which are fed grains that change their fatty-acid ratios.

Consider that a real egg (produced organically from hens fed a natural diet) contains about 300 milligrams of the omega-3 fatty acid DHA (docosahexaenoic acid). The standard, grain-fed, make-believe egg from the supermarket averages only 18 mg, while being high in omega-6s. How important is this? DHA has been found to inhibit genes associated with tumor growth and to increase the activity of tumor-suppressor genes and genes associated with apoptosis (tumor cell death)—all of which work to *turn off* the cancer process. Not surprisingly, a study reported in the March 25, 2009 *Science Daily* found that omega-3 fatty acids were even protective against advanced prostate cancer. *This is why DHA-rich, high-quality fish oil should be part of an anticancer diet,* and why these make-believe foods, which are deficient in omega-3s, are doing so much damage to our health.

Nearly all cattle are shipped to feedlots prior to slaughter to "fatten them up." If you eat this grain-fed beef, as most Americans do, you worsen your omega-3 to -6 fatty acid ratio. Natural beef is rich in omega-3s, but grain-fed beef is rich in omega-6s. *If you choose to eat beef, eat grass-fed, organic beef.* It is available online and at health food stores. Just eating organic meats is not good enough. That just means the animals were fed organic grains. The meat contains fewer pesticides, but it still has the wrong fatty-acid ratio.

Essential fatty acids are found in almost all natural foods. What differs is the amount and the ratios of 6s to 3s. Flaxseed oil is one of nature's richest sources of EFAs. Other rich sources include fish, green leafy vegetables, nuts, and seeds. Flaxseeds freshly ground in a small coffee grinder make an excellent addition to fresh salads. To eat a proper balance of EFAs, avoid processed oils and foods. Instead, fill your grocery cart with fresh organic vegetables, fruits, raw nuts, and organic fish and meats. Use high-quality olive oil for cooking and for salad dressings (most olive oil is adulterated with toxic oils). Flaxseed oil is also excellent for salads. Use a mixture of both olive and flax oil for good health.

To get as much oxygen as possible into the cells, the cells must be constructed with the proper oils. Avoid supermarket oils, all hydrogenated oils, and all food products containing these oils. Avoid grain-fed animals, eggs, and fish—they are too rich in omega-6s. Studies show that decreasing the amount of omega-6s stops the growth of tumors. *Conversely, increasing omega-6s will "rescue" dying tumors and bring them back to life.*

Anticancer oils include olive, coconut, flaxseed, and fish oils, but these must be unprocessed, high-quality oils and most brands do not measure up. Be sure to supplement with high-quality flaxseed and fish oils to help give your body the oils it needs to transport oxygen into your cells. Importantly, unless you build a cell membrane out of the correct oils, you will impair oxygen transport into the cell. *If you want to prevent or reverse cancer, you need to change your oil!*

Dairy/Excess Animal Protein

Dairy and excess animal protein both switch on and drive the cancer process. High-animal-protein diets promote cancer, and low-animal-protein diets dramatically inhibit cancer. Americans have been terribly misled into consuming dairy and far too much animal protein. Americans are among the world's highest consumers of milk products, and we also consume about ten times too much animal protein. Protein is required to construct essential molecules such as hormones and enzymes as well as structural tissue, and all these molecules constantly need replacement. Protein is an essential nutrient, and without it, life cannot be sustained. However, animal protein, in excess of the amount needed for growth, promotes cancer.

Dairy

Consuming milk is both unnatural and unhealthy. This may be the first time you are hearing that, but nowhere in nature does one species drink the milk of another or drink milk after weaning. Only humans do these things, and we suffer the consequences with heart disease, osteoporosis, diabetes, infections, arthritis, allergies, and cancer. Most Americans have been brainwashed when it comes to dairy products. I certainly was. I grew up believing that milk, cheese, and yogurt were vital parts of a healthy diet. The first time someone suggested that dairy products were not healthy, I thought he was crazy. We've already looked at the damaging effects of eating sugar and elevating insulin levels in your body. Milk also increases insulin levels, promoting cancer. No one should be drinking milk or consuming products containing milk.

People who consume the most milk have more cancer. Television commercials tell us that milk "does a body good," but modern milk is a toxic soup. It is loaded with fifty-nine biologically active hormones, dozens of allergens, up to fifty-two powerful antibiotics, pesticides, herbicides, PCBs, dioxins (up to 200 times the safe levels), blood, pus, feces, solvents, viruses, excessive bacteria, and even radioactive compounds.

Of those fifty-nine biologically active hormones contained in your milk, one is the powerful growth hormone IGF-1 (insulin-like growth factor 1). IGF-1 instructs cells to grow. Instructing cells to grow may be fine for the infant, for whom milk is intended, but in adults, it promotes cancer. IGF-1 is a switch that turns cancer on, and people with the highest levels of IGF-1 experience the most cancer. IGF-1 is known to be a factor in the rapid growth and proliferation of breast, colon, and prostate cancers, and most likely plays a role in all cancers.

Many studies have shown powerful connections between milk and fatal prostate cancer. Not only does milk contain IGF-1, it also contains a number of other growth-promoting factors (polypeptides that stimulate cell proliferation). Adding to all the previous studies, a 2010 study in the journal *Prostate* found a more than 200 percent increase in the risk of prostate cancer associated with an increased intake of dairy products.

Cows treated with synthetic growth hormones such as rBGH produce milk especially high in IGF-1. Drinking only one glass will double the amount of IGF-1 in your body. Most of the milk used to make ice cream comes from rBGH-treated cows and one serving of ice cream gives you twelve times as much of this powerful cancer accelerator as you would get in one serving of milk, because IGF-1 gets concentrated in the cream. IGF-1 is rocket fuel for cancer. Most ice cream is also loaded with sugar and other toxic chemicals including artificial colors, flavors, and processing aids. Most ice cream also contains carrageenan, which is used as a thickening, emulsifying, and stabilizing agent. Carrageenan has an inflammatory and immunosuppressive effect on the body, and degraded carrageenan is a known carcinogen. While most, but not all foods, use undegraded carrageenan, there is evidence it degrades in the digestive system. Carrageenan is also used in yogurt, custards, jellies, cream cheese, cottage cheese, and other dairy products, as well as chocolate products, pie fillings, salad dressings, soups, soy-milk, as a fat substitute in processed meats, and in toothpaste.

Virtually all milk is pasteurized and homogenized. This process-ing substantially changes the chemical and physical properties of the milk and, for many reasons, makes it less nutritious, more toxic, and more carcinogenic. Millions of us have paid a very high price for the misguided advice put out by the dairy industry. News stories tell us to drink milk to ensure proper calcium intake, yet countries with the highest milk consumption have the most osteoporosis.

Milk and dairy products are not part of a healthy diet. Even back when most of us were farmers, traditional milk from one's own cow was not a healthy food choice, but it wasn't a disaster either. Mod-ern milk on, the other hand, is a highly processed and allergenic make-believe food that is a threat to anyone's health. Americans are among the biggest milk consumers in the world. And, like other countries that have high consumption of dairy products, we have among the world's highest rates of osteoporosis, diabetes, heart attack, allergy, and cancer.

Consider the case of Jane Plant, a geology professor who wrote the book *Your Life in Your Hands*. Dr. Plant cured herself of breast cancer by changing her diet and getting the milk out of her life. Plant was first diagnosed with cancer at age forty-two. Over a five-year period, her cancer recurred four times "despite a radical mastec-tomy, three further operations, 35 radiotherapy treatments, several chemotherapy treatments, and irradiation of my ovaries to induce the menopause." Having experienced firsthand how conventional cancer treatments fail, her message now is that breast cancer can be treated, and even prevented, by simple changes in diet. Plant points out that milk, in particular, contains growth factors and hormones that promote cancer. She offers a clear explanation of the mechanism whereby high levels of growth factors cause the promotion and proliferation of cancer cells. Her diet now consists of foods that have been shown to protect against cancer. Plant notes that even in Hiroshima, the chances of contracting breast cancer are half that of Western nations. Only when Chinese and Japanese women move to milk-consuming Europe or the United States does their chance of contracting breast cancer dramatically increase.

Beyond the problem of growth factors and growth hormones, is the problem of milk protein. The largest and most comprehensive nutrition study done to date was "The China Study," conducted by world-renowned nutrition researcher Dr. Colin Campbell, who wrote a book with that same title. Campbell found that the most powerful cancer driver of all was milk protein. Casein, the predominant protein in cow's milk, promotes cancer at every stage in the cancer process.

Casein in cow's milk is difficult for humans to digest. Because undigested casein molecules are highly allergenic, an estimated half our population is allergic to milk. Dairy allergies present a serious health problem, leading to numerous disorders. Continual immune reactions to dairy protein will put the body in a state of chronic inflammation, which promotes cancer. Casein turns cancer on in experimental animals 100 percent of the time. As if all that isn't bad enough, cow's milk contains viruses that promote cancer, especially leukemia and lymphoma. More than half the dairy herds in America are infected with these viruses, and people living in areas near the infected herds suffer significantly more leukemia.

Pasteurized milk is an acidic food. Most Americans are eating too many acidic foods already, and milk throws their systems further out of balance. In *Fit for Life: A New Beginning*, author and nutritionist Harvey Diamond asserts:

> *It is a well-established fact that the high protein content of meat and dairy products turns the blood acidic, which draws calcium out of the bones. This causes the body to lose or excrete more calcium than it takes in. The deficit must be made up from the body's calcium reserve, which is primarily the bones.*

Think about this: milk causes calcium losses and osteoporosis, yet people with osteoporosis are instructed to consume more milk! Calcium is indeed needed, but drinking milk causes you to lose calcium. Vitamin D is critical for calcium metabolism, which is why most milk is "fortified" with vitamin D. However, a study in a 2001 *American Journal of Clinical Nutrition* found that those who consumed the most milk actually have the lowest vitamin D levels. Calcium and vitamin D are both needed to prevent cancer, but industrial milk is not a good source of either.

When I tell people not to drink milk, they often ask, "Where will I get my calcium?" I inform them that 70 percent of the world's people do not drink milk. Where do they get their calcium? They get it from plant foods. Green vegetables, such as kale, broccoli, and collard greens, are loaded with calcium.

Paul Nison, author of *The Raw Life,* has stated that "dairy is the cause of most disease in the world today." When a prominent Washington, D.C., pediatrician was asked in an interview what single change to the American diet could provide the greatest health benefits, Dr. Russell Bunai replied, "The elimination of milk products."

Excess Animal Protein

The recommended daily allowance (RDA) for total protein is 50 to 60 grams per day. Many Americans get twice this amount. Our average consumption of animal protein alone is about 70 grams per day. Americans average more animal protein than the RDA for total protein. By contrast, most rural Chinese, who are far healthier than we are, average one-tenth of that, 7 grams of animal protein per day (about the amount contained in one egg). Excess animal protein promotes cancer, obesity, heart disease, diabetes, osteoporosis, and kidney, eye, brain, and autoimmune diseases. A high-animal-protein diet changes the ratio of estrogens in the body, shifting the balance to those that stimulate cancer. People who are on high-protein diets to lose weight need to be aware of this danger. Animal protein is also rich in a fat called arachidonic acid, and studies have linked arachidonic acid to promoting tumor growth and metastasis. Averaging 7 grams or less per day of animal protein is a worthy goal—approximately one egg or a piece of fish or meat the size of the palm of your hand. The remainder of the RDA should be plant protein.

Meat, especially red meat, contains iron. While iron is an essential nutrient and is needed for oxygen transport in the blood, excess iron accelerates cancer growth and metastasis. Cancer is dependent on iron for its growth, and in addition, iron is a free-radical generator and can damage DNA. The lung cancer rate is 300 percent higher in red meat eaters. The way to measure your iron levels is with a blood test for ferritin. Any doctor can order this test. If your ferritin is high, you have a problem and need to reduce your iron level.

Animal protein can be safely and beneficially consumed in small quantities, but the fish you eat should not be farmed, and the eggs and meat should be organic. A good rule is to use animal protein as a condiment, not as a main course. You do not need to consume animal protein at every meal or even every day. Most of your protein should come from plant-based foods. Most people have been so conditioned to think of meat and dairy as their source of protein, they don't even think about the protein in plant foods. Consider this: Calorie-for-calorie, spinach has as much protein as beef.

Here are some of Dr. Colin Campbell's conclusions from *The China Study*:

- High animal-protein intake, in excess of the amount needed for growth, promotes cancer.
- Low-animal-protein diets inhibit cancer.
- Children who eat the highest protein diets are the most likely to get cancer.
- Once you have cancer, low-protein diets dramatically block subsequent cancer growth.
- People who eat the most animal-based foods get the most chronic disease.
- Cow's milk protein is an exceptionally potent cancer promoter, and casein (a protein in milk) may be one of the most cancer-causing food substances that we consume.

Much to the surprise of everyone, including Dr. Campbell himself, the shocking conclusion of his study was that excess animal protein is one of the most powerful disease promoters ever discovered. Animal protein beyond what is needed for growth and daily repairs is able to turn cancer on in experimental animals 100 percent of the time. You can switch cancer *on* by feeding animal protein to the test animals, and switch it *off* when you stop.

Excess animal protein appears to be an important factor in chronic disease. Dr. Campbell's research linked the intake of animal protein with obesity, Alzheimer's, osteoporosis, diabetes, heart disease, and kidney and eye disorders, among other ailments. Plant protein does *not* have a cancer-promoting effect, and large amounts can be safely consumed. Here are some ways to cut down on animal protein:

- Begin to introduce more primarily vegetarian meals.
- Build meals around fresh, raw healthy salads as the main course, rather than meats. A small amount of high-quality animal protein or protein-rich sprouts can be added to your main-course salad.
- Avocados contain good essential fats and can be used to replace meat in meals.
- Nuts and seeds (raw and soaked/sprouted) are a good source of protein and healthy fat, which can be satisfying.
- Lentils can be easily adapted to replace ground beef in Mexican recipes, shepherd's pies, meatballs, and stuffed peppers.
- If you do eat meat, make sure it is not grilled, charred, or browned in any way. When fat drips into an open flame, dangerous carcinogens called polycyclic aromatic hydrocarbons are formed. Cooking meat at high temperatures produces carcinogens called heterocyclic aromatic amines. All proteins cooked at high temperatures contain several chemicals that have been proven to cause cancer in laboratory animals. Barbecuing is the worst way to prepare meat because of both the open flame and higher temperatures.
- When you cook meat, it is best to slow cook it at a low temperature using a crockpot; cooking on low overnight is ideal.

To summarize, *cancer can be switched off by changing the level of animal protein in the diet.* To prevent cancer, limit animal protein to occasional small amounts. To reverse cancer, avoid all milk and dairy products, and almost all animal protein. At least 90 percent of our protein should be derived from plant foods such as vegetables, whole grains, legumes, lentils, seeds, nuts, and sprouts. Fish and seafood are the healthiest forms of animal protein; they most closely resemble the diet of primitive man. An occasional small portion of fresh fish would be the safest animal protein to consume. Farmed or canned fish are not options. Farmed fish contain toxins and the wrong fatty acid ratios. Canning causes numerous problems; nutrition is destroyed and toxins are introduced. You can limit your exposure to mercury by selecting fish species from less polluted geographical areas such as the Pacific Ocean and Alaska or by choosing brands that have tested low for mercury content.

Salt

Salt is another health-damaging substance people commonly consume. Unknown to most people, common table salt is a leading cause of disease, and as you learned in Chapter 3, excess sodium increases the incidence of cancer and accelerates metastasis. Eating too much salt results in an excess of sodium and a relative deficiency of potassium. This upsets the ratio of sodium to potassium inside our cells, causing cellular malfunction and disease. The average American male consumes more than 10,000 milligrams of salt per day. Consider that number in light of a January 2010 study in the *New England Journal of Medicine,* which estimated that cutting salt intake by just 3,000 mg per day would prevent enough heart attacks and strokes to save $24 billion from the national healthcare tab.

We need sodium to help our nerves function properly, to aid nutrient absorption, and for maintaining the right balance of water and minerals in our bodies. The human body requires about 220 mg of sodium per day. One teaspoon of refined salt contains about 2,300 mg of sodium—about ten times what we need. Try to keep sodium intake to less than 1,000 mg per day or *less than a half teaspoon*. (In special circumstances, such as excessive sweating or chronic diarrhea, higher levels may be necessary.) Even the government is concerned about excess sodium consumption and is now recommending that most adults in the United States eat no more two-thirds of a teaspoon of salt each day, but only about 5 percent of us are actually doing that.

Natural foods, which are rich in potassium and low in sodium, are what we were designed to eat. Unfortunately, we have changed to a sodium-rich diet of processed foods, and it is making us sick. Even eating at a "healthy" salad restaurant can be a *big* health hazard. Consider this: if you have a bowl of the split-pea soup, you will consume 1,430 mg of sodium. A serving of their "healthy" non-fat Italian salad dressing adds another 1,350 mg. Two "healthy" low-fat muffins add another 1,400 mg. A serving of their mushroom marinara sauce on your hot pasta adds another 318 mg. Choosing a couple of the salad offerings adds another 400 mg, and chocolate pudding for dessert adds another 177 mg. This adds up to a whopping 5,075 mg of sodium—*at just one meal*—and the body needs only 220 mg per day.

One of our biggest sources of sodium is in products made from grains such as bread, pasta, and pizza crust. The tomato sauce and cheese add even more sodium. One slice of whole-wheat bread typically contains about 100 mg. Another source is not only the lunch-meat and sausage you'd expect, but prepared chicken dinners and other prepared and packaged meats. There are 709 mg in two ounces of turkey breast lunchmeat. Still more can be found in processed vegetables including vegetable-based soups and sauces and canned vegetables, not to mention potato products such as chips and fries. There are 390 mg of sodium in a half-cup serving of canned peas and 780 mg in one cup of canned vegetable beef soup. One cup of low-fat milk contains 107 mg of sodium, and one ounce of cheddar cheese contains 180 mg. There are 200 mg in one cup of cornflakes. Many people don't realize these foods contain any sodium at all!

When your sodium intake is too high, you get weak bones. For every 2,000 mg of salt you eat, you will lose about 23 mg of calcium in your urine. Calcium is necessary to prevent cancer. Unless you replace these calcium losses, and most people don't eat enough bioavailable calcium to fully replace them all, then eating an average of 5,000 mg of sodium per day could result in calcium losses as high as 2.5 percent of your skeleton annually. In only ten years, you will lose 25 percent of your bone structure! Since this loss is progressive, older people tend to have weak bones, and today even young people suffer from weak bones. Excess sodium also increases the risk of high blood pressure, which is a major cause of heart disease and stroke. In fact, people who consume more than 4,000 mg per day double their risk of stroke compared to those consuming less than 1,500 mg. Other ramifications of excess sodium include chronic fatigue, neurological disorders, premature aging, weight gain, impaired immune function, and cancer—*excess sodium drives cancer and accelerates cancer metastasis.*

Mother Nature tells us the balance of sodium and potassium we need. Human milk contains three times as much potassium as sodium. Yet we are consuming four times as much sodium as potassium! Fast foods are loaded with salt. About 75 percent of our salt

intake comes from eating processed foods. It takes a lot of awareness to eat a low-salt diet, but you can do it. In restaurants, soups
often contain a lot of salt—avoid them. Many restaurants use too
much salt—request less. Read labels carefully. Your body will thank
you with the gift of better health. To increase potassium, eat a diet
of *fresh* fruits, vegetables, nuts, seeds, and grains. Foods that are
high in potassium include: bananas, oranges, avocados, tomatoes,
broccoli, lima beans, melons, cucumber, papayas, mangos, kiwi, and
spinach. These same foods contain lots of other nutrients that our
bodies need to be healthy.

Glutamates

Glutamates are a class of compounds known as excitotoxins that
are used by the processed-food, fast-food, and restaurant industries
to enhance the flavor of their foods. The best-known glutamate is
monosodium glutamate (MSG). Glutamates are especially dangerous for people with brain cancer, where they have been shown
to dramatically increase the growth and aggressiveness of these
tumors.

Glutamates produce enormous amounts of free radicals in the
body, and free-radical damage is known to cause cancer. By consuming foods on a daily basis that are high in glutamates, you will
do a lot of free-radical damage to cells, tissues, and DNA. Constant
damage to DNA will switch cancer on. The resulting inflammation
will promote tumor growth as well as invasiveness and metastasis, a
special danger to the cancer patient.

People are exposed to glutamates daily because they are in about
80 percent of all processed foods. Glutamates are cleverly disguised
on food labels with words such as natural flavors, spices, hydrolyzed

vegetable protein, vegetable protein, sodium caseinate, textured protein, soy protein extract, and others. Even baby formula can contain glutamate in the form of caseinate. When you start to look for it, you may be shocked at how often you will find glutamate. It's everywhere. Commercial pizza and most fast foods are known to have a lot. Glutamates damage the brain and nervous system. They are also known to damage DNA and to cause diabetes, obesity, and heart attacks. Avoid this stuff!

Genetically Modified Food

An entirely new threat to our health is genetically modified (GM) foods. GM foods have been modified in the laboratory to enhance desired traits such as increased resistance to herbicides or improved nutritional content. Genetic modifications are created by inserting genetic material from one organism into the permanent genetic code of another. Biotechnologists have engineered numerous novel creations, such as potatoes with genes from bacteria, pigs with human genes, fish with cattle genes, tomatoes with fish genes, and thousands of other plant, animal, and insect combinations. At an alarming rate, these creations are now being patented and released into the environment.

This is potentially one of the most dangerous experiments ever done. Absolutely no one has *any* idea of what the long-term effects of these experiments will be, yet millions of people are unwittingly eating these foods daily. They have the potential for altering all the life on the planet, yet they are constantly being released into the environment with little or no consideration for the dire consequences to come. Congress has yet to pass a single law to regulate them, and no one is responsible for investigating whether they are safe. They are not safe!

The Center for Food Safety estimates that 70 percent of all the processed foods on supermarket shelves contain genetically engineered ingredients. The main genetically engineered foods already on the market are: white potatoes, tomatoes, soybeans, corn, canola, and papayas grown in Hawaii. Corn, canola, and soybeans are used in many processed food products. Packaged foods in a supermarket, in the form of cereals, baby food and formula, salad dressing, chips, cookies, and bread, contain either some GM canola oil, soy oil, soy flour, soy lecithin, soy protein, corn oil, corn starch, or corn syrup. That's the reality. Yet only 40 percent of Americans know that most of the foods they are buying are GM. Almost 25 percent of consumers believe that GM foods are not even being sold in America. If you needed another reason to avoid all processed foods, this is a big one.

More than 90 percent of soy and over 70 percent of all corn grown in the United States is now GM, and up to half of the organic corn and soy is GM contaminated. If you are concerned about eating GM foods, then corn and soy are no longer food choices you can make in America. Even organic corn and soy products are contaminated because the pollen from GM farms blows in the wind, seeds get commingled in the seed distribution process, and sometimes the same farm machinery is used on different farms. This contamination is already enormous, and labels saying GM-free cannot be trusted.

What does this have to do with cancer? Cancer rates have soared since the introduction of GM foods, and there is reason to believe that GM foods are contributing to this increase. In 1994, the Food and Drug Administration (FDA) approved the sale of genetically engineered bovine growth hormone (rBGH). This product is injected into dairy cows to force them to give more milk. However, this causes a 500 percent increase of IGF-1 in the milk of these cows. As mentioned earlier, people with elevated levels of IGF-1 are much more likely to get cancer. Due to these concerns, the European Union has banned the use of rBGH since 1994, and Canada banned it in 1999. In fact, rBGH is banned in every industrialized country, with the exception of the United States. Now that you are aware of this, do you want to continue to feed this cancer-causing milk to your children?

One of Scotland's leading experts in tissue diseases, Dr. Stanley Ewen, a gut pathologist at Aberdeen Royal Infirmary, has warned that GM food can give you cancer. Ewen is concerned about the use of the cauliflower mosaic virus as a promoter in GM foods, with unpredictable health effects. The virus is used like a tiny engine to drive implanted genes to express themselves. Ewen pointed out that the virus is infectious, and when we eat these foods, they could act as a growth factor in our stomach or colon, encouraging the growth of polyps. The faster and bigger polyps grow, the more likely they are to be cancerous. Animal feeding studies of GM foods have already observed what appears to be precancerous cell growth.

Our immune systems are our first line of defense against cancer. Between 1995 and 1998, studies on genetically-modified potatoes by researcher Dr. Arpad Pusztai at the Rowett Research Institute in Scotland found that rats fed genetically modified potatoes experienced intestinal damage and harm to their immune systems. These effects were not observed in rats fed natural potatoes. After making his data public, Dr. Pusztai was immediately fired from his job. The folks who supply GM seeds want to keep this kind of knowledge from getting out to the public—and they are succeeding. As you might expect, and as was intended, other scientists are not rushing to continue Dr. Pusztai's research.

The bacteria in our gut play a prominent role in our immune defense against disease. Today, health has been compromised in most people because the natural balance of those bacteria has been altered due to our poor diets, drinking chlorinated water, getting vaccinations, and especially by taking antibiotics. Alarmingly, eating even one serving of GM food has been found to change the genetic structure of our healthy bacteria. Evidence from the only human GM feeding trial ever published, a 2004 study in *Nature Biotechnology*, showed that GM foods may be inserting genes into our healthy bacteria and causing them to produce concentrated pesticides in our guts for the rest of our lives—and eating only *one* serving can do this. Some researchers believe that this may be the reason that bees living near and pollinating GM crops have died in large numbers. Autopsies of the bees showed that they died from something that looked like colon cancer. We may already be in the midst of catastrophic damage to our health.

Even the limited number of studies that have been done over the past decade have revealed that GM foods can pose serious risks to humans, domesticated animals, wildlife, and the environment. Human health effects can include higher risks of toxicity, antibiotic resistance, immune suppression, allergenicity, and cancer. Jeffrey Smith, author of *Seeds of Deception* and *Genetic Roulette: The Documented Health Risks of Genetically Engineered Foods,* provides overwhelming evidence that GM foods are unsafe and should never have been introduced. Rats fed GM corn died within three weeks, while mice developed liver and pancreatic problems. A study sponsored by the Austrian government found that cattle, pigs, and sheep became sterile after being fed GM corn. Sheep have died after grazing in GM cotton fields. Allergies are already a problem, considering allergies to soy have skyrocketed by 50 percent in the United Kingdom, coinciding with the introduction of GM soy imports from the United States. Soy may be our fastest-growing allergy.

As for environmental impacts, the use of genetic engineering in agriculture could lead to uncontrolled biological pollution, threatening numerous microbial, plant, and animal species with extinction, and the potential contamination of all life on the planet with novel and possibly hazardous genetic material. Don't eat this stuff—most of it is contained in processed foods. Processed foods are garbage; unfit for human consumption, they destroy your health and make you sick.

Food Combining

How you eat is important. If you eat the wrong combination of foods at a meal, the food may not be properly digested. If the food isn't properly digested, you can't get the full nutritional value. Further, undigested food promotes the creation of dangerous toxins that poison the body. The resulting deficiency and toxicity contribute to the cancer process.

Proper food combining means eating those foods together that require the same chemical environment for their digestion. Each type of food requires a different combination of digestive juices to be properly digested. Starchy foods, such as grains in any form (bread, pasta, rice, etc.), need an alkaline environment for the body to break down and use the nutrients they contain. Proteins, on the other hand, require a highly acidic environment. If you eat both a starch and a protein at the same time, expect problems. As your body pours alkaline components into the digestive system in order to break down starches, it also releases acid to digest proteins. The acids and alkalis neutralize each other so that nothing gets digested properly. Your valuable digestive enzymes are wasted as more and more are poured into the system to break down this combination.

Your body is working so hard that you may feel sluggish. Starches require less time in the stomach before moving on to the intestinal tract, where much of their digestion occurs. When starches enter the stomach with proteins, which require a longer time there, they get held up. The starch begins to ferment, creating toxins and causing gas, bloating, abdominal discomfort, acid indigestion, poor nutrient absorption, and many other problems. Since most people in our society eat protein along with starch (the meat-and-potatoes diet), indigestion has become normal. Americans spend more than 2 billion dollars a year on antacids!

Fruit inherently contains all of the enzymes necessary for its digestion, so it can and should pass through the system in much less time than either starch or protein. Some fruits, such as melons, are only in the stomach for fifteen to twenty minutes, while others are there slightly longer, but none as long as starch, let alone protein. When you eat a big meal and then have fruit for dessert, your stomach is already full and mixing in enzymes as it churns the meal. Along comes fruit, which is designed to pass right through, but now it cannot. It is stuck behind the meal. When fruit is forced to remain in the stomach with a starch, the mixture ferments and creates toxins that spread throughout the body. If the fruit remains in the stomach with a protein meal, digestion is again impaired, and the protein putrefies, similarly resulting in powerful toxins being released into your body. With impaired digestion, you cannot reap the nourishment from the food consumed, so you may be hungry again soon because your body is malnourished. You eat more to satisfy your hunger, but you are actually toxifying your body even more.

Our digestive systems were not designed to eat what has become the "normal" dict in our nation. Many of these foods may still be enjoyed, but learning a new way to eat them will maximize the benefit you receive from them. If you eat three meals a day, have one fruit meal, one starch meal, and one protein meal (not necessarily animal protein). Fruit is a wonderful morning food (as long as you don't have a blood sugar problem). Since the stomach is empty, fruit can pass right through, and the body can easily absorb and incorporate all of its life-giving vitamins, minerals, trace minerals, and enzymes to make us flourish. Eating fruit in the morning also extends the time the body has to "rest" since active digestion is not required. Lunch can be a starch and vegetable meal for which the body readily provides an alkaline environment *or* a protein and vegetable meal, prompting the system to make an acid environment. Either way, your body will be able to extract all of the goodness and put it to use to replenish and repair your cells. You won't feel so sleepy after lunch because digesting the meal will not take all the energy from your body. You'll feel better because your body is not struggling with an impossible task. You will feel energized as your body is able to actually use the nutrients, which have been broken down and can be absorbed. In addition, you will not be poisoned by the fermentation byproducts. For dinner, you can eat a meal of either starch *or* protein with vegetables. This makes for optimal digestion.

The common eating habits of our culture constantly create bad combinations for digestion. Americans love a hearty meat sandwich or a meat-and-potatoes meal. Most popular foods today are based upon poor food combinations—spaghetti and meatballs, chicken stir-fry over rice, pizza, hamburgers, tacos, almost all types of sandwiches, and trail mixes which combine protein nuts, starchy grains, and dried fruit. You can make better choices by following these four guidelines:

• Eat starches (grains, starchy vegetables such as potatoes, sweet potato, corn, legumes and beans, pasta or bread) with vegetables, but *not* with protein or fruit.

- Eat protein (nuts, seeds, or the small amount of meat or fish you may choose to consume) with non-starchy vegetables, and *not* with starches.
- Eat fruit alone. (Acid fruits, such as citrus fruits, apples, mango, all berries, cherries, pears, apricots, and peaches may be eaten with raw nuts.)
- Melons should be eaten alone. Sweet fruits should ideally be eaten after acid fruits.

The Anticancer Diet

The most important thing anyone can do to prevent and reverse cancer is to eat a good diet. Almost all Americans are suffering from malnutrition, and malnutrition leads to a vicious cycle of genetic damage, immune dysfunction, and disease. If choosing what you eat is not about providing your cells all the nutrition they need, then you are choosing cellular malfunction, disease, and cancer. While certain so-called "foods" contribute to cancer, real foods are protective. You need to know which is which. The Standard American Diet is a cancer-causing diet. An anticancer diet will both prevent and even cure most cancer.

To beat cancer, you have to first get off your bad *cancer-causing* diet and then get on a good *anticancer* diet. In this chapter, you have just learned about the Big Four and other foods to avoid. To prevent and reverse cancer, it is *mandatory* to stay away from the Big Four (sugar, wheat, processed oils, and dairy/excess animal protein), which are contained in most processed foods. They are the foundation of a bad diet, and they support the initiation, growth, and metastasis of cancer.

The Right Foods

Cutting bad foods out of your life is one step; putting good foods in is another. A diet consisting primarily of fresh plant foods is an anticancer diet.

There are well-known mechanisms for interfering with tumor growth and inducing apoptosis (cancer-cell death), and plant foods contain all the chemicals necessary to interfere with the cancer process at every level. The biochemistry of cancer is extremely complex, requiring the successful navigation of numerous biochemical pathways, and it is possible to interfere with each of these. Existing clusters of cancer cells can be kept small and harmless. For those who already have diagnosable cancer, taking positive action can simply make the cancer disappear—*surgery, chemotherapy, and radiation are not required.* In fact, standard cancer treatments damage the body, making survival less likely. Improving nutrition is a much better approach. *Only one out of ten Americans is even meeting the current USDA guidelines for consumption of fruits and vegetables.* In fact, cancer may be considered as a vegetable-deficiency disease.

Raw, fresh vegetables along with fruits, nuts, seeds, and beans must be the foundation of your diet. Hundreds of studies show that eating more fruits and vegetables reduces the risk of all types of cancers because plant foods contain nutrients and phytochemicals that interfere with the cancer process. Eighty percent of your diet should consist of raw fruits and vegetables—remember that cooking food destroys critical nutrients.

Eating more fruits and vegetables actually decreases your appetite for fatty foods, which themselves increase the risk of cancer. Fruits and vegetables contain natural agents that block carcinogens. Vegetables that are most important to reducing the risk of cancer are the cruciferous vegetables: broccoli, cabbage, Brussels sprouts, mustard greens, kale, and cauliflower. Other good vegetables include carrots, onions, beets, and spinach. Good fruits include avocados, cherries, blackberries, blueberries, pineapples, watermelon, kiwis, mangos, plums, and honeydew melons. In general, cancer patients should consume fruits in moderation because of their sugar content. Fruit juices should be completely avoided, even by healthy people, because they rapidly increase blood sugar and insulin.

The critical anticancer nutrients in vegetables can be made even more bioavailable by juicing or "blenderizing." Using a juicer or powerful blender to mechanically break the tough cell walls of the plant releases more nutrition. In fact, you can get three times the nutrition from the same food than if you chewed it. For the cancer patient, getting this extra nutrition is critical. Normal chewing makes only a fraction of the nutrition available, and most people don't chew well anyway. A combination of juicing and blenderizing is best. Juicing allows you to consume more vegetables and get more nutrients because the juice lacks the fiber and is less filling. Blenderizing retains the fiber. Ideally, juices should be drunk immediately after they are prepared. *If you want to prevent cancer or stop cancer dead in its tracks, juicing and blenderizing vegetables are two of the most important things you can do.*

There are a variety of suitable juicers and blenders on the market. Choose a variety of vegetables and drink as much as possible every day. A healthy combination includes carrots, celery, tomatoes, kale, turnip greens, spinach, broccoli, and beets. An apple or a slice of lemon adds good flavor.

Fiber helps to prevent cancer by producing fuel for the cells lining the gut and by supporting friendly bacteria that metabolize estrogen in the colon, protecting against estrogen-driven cancers such as breast and prostate cancers. Although fiber is very important, it is lacking in our diets because we eat so much processed food and not enough fresh fruits and vegetables. A 2007 study in the *International Journal of Epidemiology* found that a fiber-rich diet cut the risk of breast cancer in half. The researchers recommended at least 30 grams of fiber per day. Many experts recommend 35 to 45 grams per day. The average American gets about 15 grams.

Fiber helps to normalize the body's insulin and estrogen levels. High insulin drives cancer; high estrogen drives breast and prostate cancer. In addition, fresh foods that are high in fiber are also high in nutrition, including the flavonoids and antioxidants that we know to be helpful in preventing and reversing cancer. Good fiber sources include: kidney beans, garbanzo beans, navy beans, whole grains, legumes, and raw vegetables. Get used to looking at the package label to find the fiber content of foods. In addition to the fiber, the above foods are excellent sources of protein. As you work to reduce the amount of animal protein in your diet, increase the amount of these excellent sources of plant protein.

As a general rule, as much as possible, fruits and vegetables *should* be organic—animal protein *must* be organic. Vegetables, including sprouts, *must* be the foundation of an anticancer diet. The fiber, enzymes, chlorophyll, minerals, and many other nutrients they contain are essential. Consuming an anticancer diet is not just something nice to do; it is a necessity.

Dozens of anticancer compounds have been identified in plants. Plant flavonoids, including quercetin, interfere with the effects of estrogen in stimulating breast and prostate cancer. In fact, plant flavonoids will act to prevent cells from becoming cancerous, even when exposed to powerful carcinogens. In addition, they inhibit the growth of cancer cells and stimulate cancer-cell death. Olive oil helps to protect DNA from oxidative damage, which can make a cell turn cancerous. Both green and black teas inhibit DNA damage and can prevent cancer cells from dividing, thus inhibiting cancer growth. Herbs such as silymarin and ginkgo biloba also contain powerful anticancer compounds. Numerous plant chemicals are known to inhibit and suppress cancer growth mechanisms. Many fruits and vegetables contain carotenes. Animal experiments and human experience have shown that high amounts of dietary carotenes stop cancer from growing.

As much as possible, have organic salads, vegetables, vegetable juices, and sprouts for breakfast, lunch, and dinner. Leafy dark-green vegetables such as kale, spinach, and Swiss chard are high in nutritional content, and a combination of dark-green leaves, mushrooms, and onions is known to have powerful anticancer effects. A 2009 study in the *International Journal of Cancer* found that women who consumed the most mushrooms were 64 percent less likely to get breast cancer. Since all vegetables have different kinds and amounts of nutrients, it is best to eat a variety. Following is a list to include in your anticancer diet:

arugula	cauliflower	lettuce	radishes
asparagus	celery	mustard	scallions
beets	collards	greens	sea vegetables
broccoli	cucumbers	okra	spinach
Brussels	eggplant	onion	squash
sprouts	garlic	parsley	Swiss chard
cabbage	green beans	peas	turnips
carrots	kale	peppers	watercress

The foods listed are highly protective against cancer and are even curative. You want a diet high in fresh, organic fruits and vegetables and high in omega-3 fatty acids. Occasional non-gluten grains such as buckwheat, millet, brown rice, quinoa, and amaranth are okay in moderation. Legumes and lentils are good sources of plant protein. Occasional small portions of high-quality fish and organic eggs can be added. Sprouts are an excellent food choice and highly recommended on an anticancer diet. However, store-bought sprouts are too often contaminated with dangerous bacteria and mold. Growing your own sprouts is simple to do and the best choice; it's an inexpensive way to produce your own high-quality food. There are entire books on this subject, so people can learn to do sprouting in their own kitchens.

Nuts are a good food choice. They can be a small part of an anticancer diet, but many nuts, such as cashews and peanuts (which are not really nuts), are too contaminated with mold to be safe. The molds produce carcinogenic aflatoxins that enter the liver and block a very important tumor-suppressor gene, which is why people who consume lots of aflatoxins often develop liver cancer. Nuts should be organic, whole, and unprocessed. The best choices are almonds, macadamias, Brazil nuts, and walnuts. According to research at the UC Davis Cancer Center, which was presented at a 2010 annual meeting of the American Chemical Society, walnuts affect several genes that control tumor growth and metabolism—interfering with the cancer process, cutting cancer risk, and also slowing the growth of tumors. In this animal study, the human equivalent of just two handfuls of walnuts a day was found to cut breast cancer risk in half.

Drinking an adequate amount of water is also essential. Studies show that most people are chronically dehydrated, especially those over age fifty. Even a small amount of dehydration will affect all the chemistry in your body. Water helps to hydrate the body and to remove toxins. Most experts recommend drinking at least eight glasses per day. However, the water has to be pure. Tap water is not appropriate. I recommend a reverse osmosis system for drinking water.

A wealth of scientific research shows that regular tea drinking, especially green and white tea, inhibits colon, breast, prostate, lung, melanoma, ovarian, and bladder cancer. The phytochemicals in tea suppress signaling molecules needed for cancer cell reproduction and block enzymes needed for tumor invasion—inhibiting the cancer process. Green tea extract (EGCG) has been shown to inhibit hormone-sensitive cancers, such as breast and prostate cancers. It also has been demonstrated to inhibit hematological cancers, like leukemia and multiple myeloma. In addition, it inhibits the development of ovarian cancer and lung cancer and reduces the growth of lung cancers should they develop. It also curbs the invasion of bladder cancer. Daily consumption of high-quality tea is recommended for an anticancer diet. High-quality tea is necessary because a lot of the tea imported today contains excessive amounts of pesticides and fluoride. Tea consumption does not need to be excessive. Some studies in the above research used the equivalent of drinking two to three cups of white tea per day.

A 2005 study in the *Archives of Internal Medicine* found that only 3 percent of American adults practice what is considered a healthy lifestyle. Only 23 percent of us are eating as much as five servings of fruits and vegetables per day. Federal guidelines recommend nine servings. Since we know there are nutrients in fresh fruits and vegetables that interfere with every known step of the cancer process, it should be obvious that an anticancer diet must include lots of fresh produce. Preferably, the produce should be organically grown, as fresh as possible, and consumed raw. Studies show that people who eat organic foods have virtually no pesticides in their urine, while those eating nonorganic foods often exceed safety levels.

There are many ways in which nutrients help to prevent and reverse cancer. In order for the body to self-regulate and remain in homeostasis, cell-to-cell communications must be maintained. Such communications help to regulate cell growth and prevent cancer from happening. Certain chemicals in foods are known to facilitate your communications network by increasing chemical messengers. Flavonoids found in celery and parsley and carotenes found in carrots, tomatoes, watermelons, and pink grapefruit are known to be effective.

The Bottom Line

While we may call the above an anticancer diet, in reality it is the diet humans are intended to eat. To recap, if you have cancer, here is a list of important changes you need to make in your diet:

- Avoid all processed foods
- Avoid restaurant foods, unless organic and raw
- Eat organically produced foods
- Eat a primarily plant-based diet
- Get on a high-quality supplement program
- Avoid processed, supermarket fats and oils
- Consume a balance of healthy omega-6 and omega-3 oils
- Include high-quality flaxseed and olive oils in your diet
- Avoid sugar and wheat, and minimize grains
- Avoid all dairy products
- Avoid alcohol and coffee

• Avoid foods high in mold such as peanuts, corn, and
  dried fruits
• Avoid barbecued and microwaved foods
• Minimize animal protein, and it must be organic
• Juice or blenderize fresh vegetables every day

Every disease is either caused by or greatly influenced by what you eat. Human nutrition is extremely complex, but the choice that we need to make is simple. Either we continue to think of foods as entertainment and eat foods that make us sick, or we realize that food supplies essential raw materials for our cells and eat foods we need to make us healthy. Cells are chemical factories. More than 100,000 chemical reactions take place in each cell every second. Every moment of every day, thousands and thousands of chemicals that you need to stay alive and function are being produced. The raw materials for these chemical reactions come from the food you eat.

Because a chronic shortage of even one essential nutrient will affect the entire system and cause disease, we need to be mindful of everything we put in our mouth. Every mouthful should supply the maximum amount of nutrition, and we have to train ourselves to think about this. To get the nutrition we need, we have to eat real food. Real food is what nature provides, and it is loaded with nutrition. Unfortunately, real food is now in short supply—some people eat almost no real food at all. What they eat is garbage. Garbage is something that is not fit to eat and will make you sick, but we don't call it garbage. We call it food. There are only two causes of disease—deficiency and toxicity. Modern processed foods cause both. This is why the Standard American Diet will not support healthy life—even in rats.

Ninety cents out of every American food dollar is spent to

purchase processed foods that cause disease. Then we wonder why cancer is an out-of-control epidemic. We are getting what we pay for!

Foods that switch on and drive cancer include sugar, wheat, processed oils, dairy, and excess animal protein. Contributing are non-foods like aspartame, glutamates, alcohol, fluoride, chlorine, and coffee.

What nature provides is food; what man provides is garbage. If it comes out of a factory, it is low in nutrition and high in toxins and will make you sick. Here is a short list of what comes out of factories: bread and other baked goods, milk, breakfast cereal, ice cream, cookies, sodas, canned foods, frozen entrees, candy, vegetable shortening, margarine, and salad oils. Contrast this to freshly harvested organic produce, and you get the picture. Foods that inhibit and even kill cancer cells include broccoli, cabbage, Brussels sprouts, mustard greens, kale, cauliflower, purple grapes, red raspberries, strawberries, carrots, pineapples, almonds, and walnuts.

If you have cancer, it is a given that you are suffering from multiple nutritional deficiencies. To overcome these deficiencies, changing your diet and taking high-quality supplements is essential. Until we start eating for nutrition and stop eating garbage, our epidemic of chronic disease will continue, and cancer will soon be affecting more than half our population. Health is a choice—the challenge is to choose it.

Nothing tastes as good as health feels.

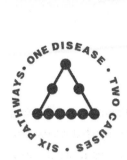

5

THE TOXIN
PATHWAY

We are now one of the most polluted species on the face of this planet . . .
Indeed, we are all so contaminated that if we were cannibals
our meat would be banned from human consumption.

—*Paula Baillie-Hamilton, M.D., author of* Toxic Overload

We are not all exposed to a single agent, a single radiation
or a single type of radiation, and we're not exposed
at a single point in time. It's a cumulative effect.

—*William Suk, National Institute of Environmental Health Sciences*

Toxicity is one of the two causes of all disease, and today
we are living in a chemically based society where almost all
Americans are in toxic overload. Never before in history has

171

the human organism been exposed to so many toxins. Our bodies are not designed to protect themselves from such an overwhelming onslaught of manmade chemicals, and these chemicals are bioaccumulating inside us. This overload, along with our poor diets, is directly responsible for our epidemic of chronic disease and cancer as well as the many mystery illnesses, such as chemical sensitivity syndrome, that are products of the late twentieth century.

For the last century, mankind has been unwittingly involved in a vast and complex chemistry experiment. We live in a sea of toxins, and we now know that this experiment in chemical living is having a catastrophic effect on our health, interfering with vital biologic processes, and causing our cells and systems to malfunction. Yet the experiment is not only continuing; it is expanding. Each year, more and more toxic chemicals are put into our environment. We are bioaccumulating hundreds of these toxins, which are being passed on to unborn babies, damaging their future health. We get sicker as we get older because we progressively become more toxic. We are now one of the most polluted species on the planet. These chemicals are scrambling our biochemistry, causing massive cellular malfunction, disease, and cancer.

By retirement age, our accumulated toxic loads are more than sufficient to cause cancer. To make matters worse, the detoxification capacity of our kidneys and liver diminishes with age, further challenging older people, who have the highest concentrations of toxic chemicals. Contributing even more to this toxic overload, most older people are on prescription drugs, adding substantially to their toxic burden, causing fatigue, poor memory, and disorientation. Resistance to disease plummets as toxins build up in our bodies.

The threat to our health comes not only from individual chemicals, but also from the total chemical load we are sustaining and the interactions of the hundreds of chemicals stored in our tissues. Certain chemicals in combination become thousands of times more toxic than any one acting alone. Certain food additives, which alone do not harm test animals, will kill them when fed to them in combination. Babies are being born loaded with toxins acquired from their mothers, causing an epidemic of birth defects, hyperactivity disorders, learning disabilities, *and childhood cancer*. It's scary that almost nothing is known about the toxicity of the millions of possible combinations of these various chemicals and their carcinogenicity under various circumstances.

Toxins compromise immunity, and the result is a body that is not capable of destroying the excessive numbers of cancerous cells that are being produced. Sooner or later, some of these cells survive and multiply, and then you have cancer.

The body is able to cope with toxins to a certain point; then you get sick! Some researchers believe we have already crossed the line and may have compromised all future life on the planet. As bad as things are, there are actions each of us can take to reduce the impact of toxins on our health. We can:

- reduce our daily exposure to toxins,
- nutritionally support our detoxification systems, and
- remove stored toxins from our bodies.

If you do these three things, your body will thank you with the gift of better health.

Health is created when all the exquisitely complex metabolic machinery inside your cells is operating normally. While this is happening, you cannot be sick. We get sick by failing to supply the nutrients our cells need and by introducing toxins into the system.

A toxin is any substance that interferes with normal cellular function, causing cells to malfunction—even water can be toxic if too much gets into a cell. Toxins can affect us in numerous ways. Some toxins, such as heavy metals like lead and mercury, shut down enzymes making them unable to produce all the critical molecules we need every moment of every day. Some toxins mimic hormones and give false signals to cells and genes, increasing the risk of hormone-dependent cancers. Others inhibit cell-to-cell communications, interfering with the body's ability to self-regulate. Disrupted communications damage the body's feedback mechanisms and the ability to balance cell growth may be lost. Some toxins directly damage DNA, causing mutations, while others react with DNA and change how genes express—both of these reprogram the cell's control system. Programming errors can lead to uncontrolled cell multiplication. Some toxins interfere with oxygen transport, while others damage immunity. All of the above contribute to the cancer process. The resulting malfunctions throw our chemistry out of balance and our bodies cease to effectively communicate, self-regulate, and self-repair. Once this happens, this is the one disease—no matter what you name it or how many names you give it!

Today almost every American is in toxic overload, and toxicity is a major cause of disease and cancer. Given the magnitude of the problem, it may surprise you to learn that, according to the 2008-2009 President's Cancer Panel, less than 10 percent of the nearly 80,000 chemicals used in commerce today have been tested for their capacity to cause cancer or do other damage to your health. Several thousand of these chemicals are already known to be carcinogenic. We are told that our daily exposure to each is very small, and in general, this is true. However, we are being exposed to small amounts of thousands of toxins daily, and when you add up all the small amounts, the exposure is significant. According to scientists at the United Nations Educational, Scientific and Cultural Organization (UNESCO), the total toxicity to which we are being exposed can be as much as seventy-five times the dose considered toxic in animals. When you consider that these chemicals accumulate in your tissues and build up year after year, you begin to understand why you must protect yourself as much as you can. Comparisons of cancer tissues with healthy tissues show that cancer tissues have a much higher concentration of toxic chemicals.

In 2009, the CDC published its Fourth National Report on Human Exposure to Environmental Chemicals. This is an ongoing survey that tests blood and urine samples in the United States pop-ulation every two years. In this report, 75 new chemicals were added to the list for a total of 212 chemicals tested. All 212 were found to be in the blood and urine of most Americans. Six chemicals were found in virtually every person. The six were:

- polybrominated diphenyl ethers (PDEs)
- bisphenol-A (BPA)
- perfluorooctanoic acid (PFOA)
- acrylamide
- mercury
- methyl tert-butyl ether (MTBE)

Each of these is known to be highly dangerous and a threat to your health. PDEs are used as flame retardants. These chemicals are added to a large variety of consumer products, including furniture, mattresses, carpeting, and computers, to decrease fire risk. They are known to build up in human fat tissue, causing damage to the nervous system, liver, and kidneys. PDEs have also been linked to sexual dysfunction, thyroid problems, brain disorders, and *cancer*. PDEs have contaminated our homes and our food supply. American women's breast milk has the highest PDE levels in the world. We are feeding high levels of these dangerous chemicals to our babies! Before purchasing carpets, mattresses, and upholstered furniture, check to see if they have been treated with flame retardants—most of them have.

BPA is found in a variety of plastic products including water bottles and can linings. BPA leaches out of polycarbonates and epoxies and can be found in almost all food and beverage cans. About 85 percent of all the food cans sold in the United States have plastic linings, which will leach out BPA. Researchers have found cans of corn and other foods to contain BPA levels far in excess of what causes cancer cells to proliferate. BPA is toxic even at *exceedingly low* concentrations. More than 90 percent of those tested in the CDC study were found to have biologically active levels of BPA in their bodies. Bisphenol-A is an endocrine disruptor, which can mimic the body's own hormones and unbalance the entire hormone system. Growing scientific evidence has linked BPA to a host of problems, including heart disease, diabetes, sexual dysfunction, immune dysfunction, behavioral problems, asthma, obesity, liver damage, DNA damage, and *cancer*. There is particular concern about BPA's effect on the development of fetuses, infants, and young children. BPA is capable of altering the expression of genes, changing the way the genes work, and this change can be passed on to the next generation. It is scary to think that even if we ban a toxic chemical like BPA, the problems may remain as they are passed down to the next generation. This can make the next generation more susceptible to cancer, even if they themselves have not been exposed to the chemical. The cumulative effects of toxins such as BPA over several generations may help to explain the dramatic increases in breast and prostate cancers and why cancer is epidemic in our children. Avoid using plastic water bottles and do not consume canned foods or beverages.

PFOA is used in nonstick cookware, stain-resistant clothing, certain food packaging, and heat-resistant products. Studies verify that PFOA contributes to liver and immune system dysfunction as well as infertility, other reproductive problems, and *cancer*.

Acrylamide is a chemical formed when frying, roasting, grilling, or baking carbohydrate-rich foods at temperatures above 120 degrees centigrade (248 degrees Fahrenheit). Acrylamide is found in a number of foods, such as fried chicken, bread, chips, French fries, and even coffee. Tobacco smoking also generates substantial amounts of acrylamide. Acrylamide is known to cause *cancer*.

Mercury both causes and drives cancer. Mercury is one of the most toxic metals known. Yet it is found in virtually every American, accumulating in our bodies, causing harm even in extremely small amounts. The principle sources are silver dental fillings, vaccinations, and fish. Mercury drives cancer by inhibiting apoptosis. It creates DNA-damaging oxidative stress, and it disables enzymes needed for oxygen respiration. Mercury cuts the oxygen-carrying capacity of the blood in half, damages immunity and lowers T-cell counts. Studies have shown that removing mercury fillings from your mouth can result in 50 to 300 percent increases in T-cell counts. In fact, white cell abnormalities, such as those observed in leukemia, have normalized when mercury amalgam fillings were removed. Elevated levels of mercury and other toxic metals, such as lead, cadmium, and arsenic, disrupt essential body chemistry. They *must* be measured and removed when fighting cancer.

MTBE is a gasoline additive that is not used today. However, it is still being detected in water supplies as well as in most Americans' bodies. MTBE causes neurological and reproductive problems and is thought to be a potential human carcinogen at high doses. Cigarette smoke contains MTBE.

With each additional exposure, many types of toxins gradually build up in our bodies to levels where they can do major damage. Even worse, toxins start accumulating before we are born. Testifying on October 26, 2010 before the U.S. Senate Subcommittee on Superfund, Toxins, and Environmental Health, Ken Cook, president of the Environmental Working Group said, "We've measured hundreds and hundreds of toxic chemicals in the blood of babies that are still in the womb." An average of 232 chemicals in the cord blood of newborn babies has been reported. These chemicals are known to cause birth defects, abnormal development, damage to the brain and nervous system, and cancer. Is it any wonder our children are so sick and have so much cancer? Research shows that children born with the highest amounts of chemicals in their bodies have lower IQs, more behavioral problems, and suffer more cancer both as children and as adults, when compared to children who have fewer chemicals in their bodies. This is why it is essential that women who are planning to have children avoid toxins and engage in proactive detoxification activities.

Toxins even cause deficiency. Most people are unaware of the unprecedented burden that our exposure to toxins is placing on our bodies. Every molecule that you put into the body has to be metabolized in some way. Some molecules are beneficial to the body, while others place a burden on it. Processing toxic molecules dramatically increases our need for nutrients, particularly antioxidants. Our need for antioxidants more than *tripled* in the twenty-year period from 1970 to 1990, and it is undoubtedly even higher today. Meanwhile, in the same period, the antioxidant level available in foods was *cut to less than half!* When you consider that the need in 1970 was already greatly elevated over historical levels, you can begin to understand that the declining nutritional content of our foods combined with our increased nutritional needs is a prescription for an epidemic of chronic disease. Supplementation has become essential.

We don't realize how many toxins bombard us every day because we can't see them. The buildup of toxins in the body reduces cell oxygenation and damages DNA, causing cell mutation. Even very small amounts of toxins can be devastating to your health. Yet we now live in a sea of chemicals to which we are exposed every moment of every day. We can't escape them. They are in the air we breathe, the water we drink, and the food we eat. They are in our toothpaste, shampoo, cosmetics, cars, clothes, newspapers, magazines, furniture, and the prescription and over-the-counter drugs we take. These chemicals affect every cell in the body. More than 3,000 chemicals are added to our food. More than 700 chemicals can be found in city drinking water. One billion pounds of pesticides are used in the United States every year, and a percentage of that ends up in our bodies. The oceans are so contaminated that it is now unsafe to eat more than a small quantity of fish. Many of these chemicals act as switches that turn cancer on and others act as drivers that speed the cancer process.

Because so many of us have taken antibiotics, which destroy the normal gut bacteria and allow yeast and fungi to grow, yeast infections can be a major source of toxicity and cancer. Yeast produces acetaldehyde, which produces ethyl alcohol. The alcohol destroys enzymes needed for cell energy and releases DNA-damaging free radicals. This causes fatigue and impairs oxygen respiration. It also inhibits the absorption of iron, which is needed to transport oxygen in the blood, further impairing oxygen respiration. Cancer patients need to test for and eliminate yeast infections. Supplements and changes in diet are essential to eliminate yeast. Sugar and all refined grains must be dropped from the diet.

Constant exposure to tens of thousands of chemicals, from before birth onward, leads to the creation of excessive free radicals that damage genes and create excessive numbers of cancer cells. High-stress lifestyles, immune systems weakened by a diet of sugar and processed food, exposure to health-damaging prescription drugs and vaccinations, plus excessive cancer cells caused by damaged genes are the norm for most Americans. This leaves us less able to protect ourselves from cancer. Only you have the power to change this by choosing to eat a good diet and by lowering your toxic load. Our toxic overload combined with our nutrient deficiencies creates a devastating synergy.

Reduce Daily Exposure

Hundreds of toxic chemicals are bioaccumulating in our bodies. Toxins from pesticides and industrial waste store in our fatty tissues and do genetic damage to cells. A woman's breast tissue is about one-third fat, which helps to explain the epidemic of breast cancer. To get well and stay well, one of the things you must learn is how to reduce your daily exposure to toxins. While the body has the ability to detoxify harmful chemicals, that capacity is being overloaded. You need to determine where your toxic exposures are coming from and avoid them as best you can. About 80 percent of your toxic exposure *is* under your personal control to avoid. By exercising this control, you can reduce your toxic load to manageable levels. All you have to do is learn how to make better choices regarding the foods you eat, the air you breathe, the water you drink, and the products you purchase. By making different choices and lowering the amount of toxins you are taking in, you will substantially reduce your toxic burden, give your body the opportunity to safely detoxify the remainder, and help to keep yourself healthy and free of disease.

The Food You Eat

To reduce your toxic load, start with the foods you eat. Unfortunately, almost the entire food supply has been poisoned to one degree or another—there is little available at a supermarket that is not toxic. As much as possible, avoid processed foods and eat only fresh, organically produced foods.

Many people do not have a reliable supply of high-quality organic foods. You must select from among the least toxic options and minimize the amount of toxins you are consuming. For example, bisphenol-A is found in plastic water bottles, so eliminate your consumption of water packaged in plastic bottles—use glass bottles. Bisphenol-A is also found in almost all canned foods and beverages, and consumption of sodas has been linked to higher BPA levels in teenagers. Avoid canned foods and beverages.

Meat, dairy products, and large fish are contaminated with insecticides, fungicides, weed killers, hormones, antibiotics, prescription drugs, industrial chemicals, PCBs, dioxins, flame retardants, and heavy metals. About 90 percent of human exposure to many of these toxic contaminants comes from eating these foods. Eat only organic meat, in small quantities, and cut out dairy entirely. Some pesticides are known carcinogens, yet the United States is the world's largest user of pesticides. People with high exposures to pesticides, such as farmers, pesticide applicators, manufacturers, and crop dusters have high rates of all kinds of cancer. By eating only organic eggs and meat and avoiding dairy products, you can substantially reduce your exposure to these toxic chemicals by about 80 percent.

As you can see, what may have appeared to you as an impossible task is actually quite doable, when you can achieve an 80 percent reduction so easily. Studies in both the United States and Europe show that by eating less meat you can cut cancer risk in half. For people who travel, avoiding these toxins can be a problem, but you make the best choices you can under the circumstances. When you travel, eat fruit plates for breakfast and salads for other meals. Dinner can be fresh-caught wild fish with a side of vegetables and a salad.

According to the USDA, more than 70 percent of fruits and vegetables contain pesticide residues, which begin to accumulate in us at an early age, reaching concentrations that cause major cellular malfunction and disease. It is a fact that people who eat organic foods have substantially less pesticide residue in their tissues. The question you need to ask yourself is how much "gunk" can you put in your cells before they get really screwed up and make you sick? The answer in some cases is it doesn't take much. The combined effects of multiple pesticides acting together can greatly magnify the effects of any of them acting alone. If you eliminate dairy and nonorganic meats and choose organic fruits and vegetables, you can reduce most of your pesticide exposure. Do not use pesticides in your home or garden. There are many safe alternatives. If you must use a pesticide around your home, garden, or office, use a safe natural product like Orange Guard.

When forced to purchase nonorganic produce, it is good to know which are the safest. For a variety of reasons, certain produce is less heavily sprayed with pesticides than others. Following is a list of produce that is generally the *least contaminated*:

Asparagus	Grapefruit	Peas
Avocados	Kiwi	Pineapple
Bananas	Mangoes	Plums
Blueberries	Melons	Radishes
Broccoli	Mushrooms	Tangerines
Cabbage	Onions	Tomatoes
Cauliflower	Oranges	Watermelons
Eggplant	Papaya	

On the other hand, here is a list of produce that *needs to be organic* because of heavy pesticide contamination:

Apples	Lettuce	Pumpkin
Celery	Nectarines	Raspberries
Cherries	Peaches	Spinach
Cucumbers	Pears	Squash
Grapes	Peppers	Strawberries
Green beans	Potatoes	

Does it really make a difference if you eat organic? A 2003 study in *Environmental Health Perspectives* fed one group of children a diet that was 75 percent organic foods while another group was fed 75 percent conventional foods. The children's urine was measured for pesticides. The children eating conventional foods measured four times higher than the official safety limit. Yet, after only a few days, the children in the organic group measured only one-sixth as much as the conventional group and within the safety limit. Eating organic does make a huge difference.

It is best to eliminate all processed foods. Not only are they deficient in nutrition, but they are virtually all contaminated with toxins. Flame retardants are found in dairy products, meat products, and farmed salmon. Milk is a toxic soup filled with pesticides, antibiotics, dioxins, hormones, sulfa drugs, tranquilizers, and other contaminants. Bread is often contaminated with potassium bromate, used as a dough conditioner. Bromate competes with iodine in the thyroid, causing thyroid malfunction. Commercial peanut butter is loaded with toxic chemical residues. According to the 1982–1986 Total Diet Study, conducted by the FDA, peanut butter had a whopping 183 residues, including highly carcinogenic aflatoxin, produced by a mold that grows on peanuts, as well as on grains such as corn, wheat, and barley. Aflatoxin is one of the most carcinogenic chemicals on earth. Frozen French fries contained seventy different pesticide residues. Frozen pizzas had sixty-seven industrial chemical and pesticide residues. Frozen chocolate cake contained sixty-one toxic residues, and milk chocolate had ninety-three. All these toxins accumulate in your body, exaggerate each other's impact, and systematically destroy your health. You are spending a lot of money to make yourself sick, and if you keep doing it, you will succeed. Advertisers never mention this when they write those catchy jingles for processed foods.

Of special concern are processed meats. In 2007, the World Cancer Research Fund and the American Institute for Cancer Research reviewed more than 7,000 clinical studies examining the connection between diet and cancer, coming to this conclusion: No amount of processed meat is safe, and no one should eat processed meats.

The Fund's *Food, Nutrition, Physical Activity and the Prevention of Cancer: a Global Perspective* study concluded:

> *There is strong evidence that . . . processed meats are causes of bowel cancer, and that there is no amount of processed meat that can be confidently shown not to increase risk. . . . Try to*

avoid processed meats such as bacon, ham, salami, corned beef,
and some sausages.

Prior studies have found that processed meats increase the risk of bladder cancer by 59 percent and pancreatic cancer by 67 percent.

Processed meats such as bacon, ham, hot dogs, pastrami, pepperoni, salami, and some sausages and hamburgers are preserved by salting, smoking, or adding chemical preservatives. Smoking creates carcinogenic polycyclic aromatic hydrocarbons, which contaminate the meat. Preservatives in the form of chemicals called nitrites are added to these meats to prevent bacterial growth and to help maintain color. Unfortunately, nitrates can be converted by heat or the presence of stomach acids into compounds called nitrosamines, which are known carcinogens.

The toxins in packaging materials (such as plastic wrap, plastic bottles, milk containers, juice boxes, Styrofoam, and epoxy can linings) can leach toxins into our foods before we eat them. Portions of the polymers, plasticizers, stabilizers, fillers, and even colorants in plastic wrap can dissolve into the food. Avoid foods packaged in plastic. Choose foods packaged in more appropriate materials, such as paper and glass. Even the wax paper used to package breakfast cereals has been found to leach toxic chemicals into the cereal. Ironically, people sometimes spend extra money to buy organic foods when those foods may be wrapped in toxic packaging. Why purchase organic meat in a Styrofoam tray topped with plastic shrink-wrap or organic canned goods in an epoxy-lined can? As much as possible, you have to know about every aspect of the foods you eat, including the safety of their packaging.

The Water

According to a December 2009 analysis by the *New York Times*, during the prior five years, more than 20 percent of the water treatment systems in the United States had violated the safety standards in the Safe Drinking Water Act. The *Times* found that about 50 million Americans have been drinking water with unsafe levels of toxic chemicals like arsenic (a carcinogen), tetrachloroethylene (a carcinogen), radioactive substances like uranium (carcinogens), prescription drugs, and dangerous bacteria found in sewage. Meanwhile, studies in the *American Journal of Epidemiology* indicate that negative health effects from these chemicals occur at concentrations even lower than the existing standards. The *Times* said, "Studies indicate that drinking water contaminants are linked to millions of instances of illness within the United Stated each year."

Half of all groundwater wells contain pesticide residues. Ninety percent of the fluoride used to fluoridate American water systems is a toxic waste that comes from the pollution-scrubbing devices of the phosphate fertilizer industry. Most fluoridated water contains arsenic because the arsenic is a contaminant in the fluoride product added to the water. In 2001, the National Research Council warned "Even very low concentrations of arsenic in drinking water appear to be associated with a higher incidence of cancer." Phosphate fertilizers themselves are a problem. Phosphate fertilizers are often contaminated with cadmium. The cadmium gets into the groundwater and into the food, and people with high cadmium levels have high cancer rates. Phosphate fertilizers also accelerate the leaching of carcinogenic arsenic from soils into groundwater and plants. For example, phosphate-treated soil increases arsenic accumulation in wheat. Another problem is nitrates, primarily from applying nitrogen fertilizers, which end up in the drinking water. In the body, they are metabolized into N-nitroso compounds that have been shown to cause tumors at multiple organ sites in every animal species tested. Humans with high nitrate exposure have higher cancer rates.

A 2010 study by the Environmental Working Group found hexavalent chromium in the tap water of thirty-one out of thirty-five cities sampled. Of these cities, twenty-five had levels that exceeded the goal level proposed in California, which has been trying to reduce the chemical in its water supply. Hexavalent chromium is used in industrial operations such as chrome plating and the manufacturing of plastics and dyes, and it is well known to cause lung cancer when inhaled. New evidence shows it causes cancer in laboratory animals when ingested. It has been linked to liver and kidney damage in animals as well as to leukemia, stomach cancer, and other cancers. Sadly, even if your water is not contaminated with any of these substances, it may still be unsafe to drink.

Even if your water starts out pure, *most tap water in the United States contains chlorine and fluoride and is unfit to drink*. Chlorine, added to kill bacteria (which are single cell organisms), kills and injures your cells as well. While toxic, chlorine at least does something of value. Fluoride, on the other hand is a dangerous toxin that does only harm. Fluoride is lacking in any benefits, while having catastrophic effects on both physical and mental health. These health-destroying toxins *must* be removed from your water. In a more rational society, they would not be there in the first place. Currently, the best solution is to use a high-quality reverse osmosis system to filter your drinking water.

Chlorine

Chlorine is added to our drinking water to protect us from pathogens, and to this end has been effective. But chlorine and the compounds it forms in the water are dangerous to your health. If you drink, bathe, shower, or swim in chlorinated water you are inhaling and absorbing chlorine into your body, which can damage genes and cells. Chlorine itself is dangerous, but when it reacts with organic compounds in the water it forms cancer-causing *organochlorine compounds*. These chlorinated chemicals do not break down easily and are very stable in the environment. They are easily absorbed into our bodies and accumulate over time. The average American is accumulating over 175 of these organochlorine compounds! Numerous studies, including one in a 1996 *Cancer Causes and Control* have all found that the risk of cancer increases with both duration and amount of exposure to the chlorination byproducts in tap water, and that chlorination byproducts represent an important risk factor for cancer. Hot water, used to shower, vaporizes the chlorine and other chlorinated chemicals in the water, damaging the lungs through inhalation. These organochlorine compounds are also absorbed through the skin. Exposure to vaporized chlorine is 100 times more damaging than drinking chlorinated water.

Swimming in chlorinated water is especially dangerous and causes aggravated respiratory conditions such as asthma, plus dry and brittle hair, dry skin, rashes, and eye irritations. However, most important is what is happening at the cellular level. Chlorine penetrates the skin, readily passing through cell walls and oxidizing the fatty acids in the cells. This damages DNA and disrupts life-sustaining functions. Beyond the chlorine itself, swimming pools and hot tubs often have high levels of these extremely toxic organochlorine compounds, and again, these can be absorbed through the skin or inhaled from the fumes near the surface of the pool or the tub. Numerous studies have found that chlorinated swimming pools are detrimental to health. One study in a 2010 *European*

Respiratory Journal found that young children who swim in chlorinated pools suffer permanent lung damage, increasing their lifelong
risk of respiratory infections, allergies, and asthma. Children who
had spent twenty or more hours by age two in chlorinated outdoor
pools were twice as likely to suffer from lung infections compared to
children who had not been to chlorinated pools at all. Children who
had been to indoor pools were three-and-one-half times as likely to
have a history of lung infections.

One of the chemicals formed in chlorinated water is chloroform.
A 2003 report by the U.S. Environmental Protection Agency (EPA)
said, "Showering is suspected as the primary cause of elevated levels
of chloroform in nearly every home because of chlorine in the water."
The chloroform can enter your body through the lungs or the skin and
be carried in your bloodstream to all parts of the body. Chloroform
is known to cause cancer in animals. Higher levels of chlorine compounds have been found in breast tissue of women with breast cancer.
High-quality water filters are essential for almost every household.

Fluoride

Fluoride both switches on and drives cancer. Federal health offi-
cials continue to call fluoridation one of the ten great public-health
achievements of the twentieth century, while it has long been
known as one of our greatest public-health blunders. The scientific
evidence that fluoride causes cancer is overwhelming, and this has
been known for decades, despite attempts to obscure it. For example, recorded in the *Congressional Record* of 21 July 1976, the chief
chemist of the National Cancer Institute, Dr. Dean Burke, stated
before Congress, "In point of fact, fluoride causes more cancer
death, and causes it faster than any other chemical."

Fluoride is a general cellular poison, doing catastrophic biological damage that is beyond the scope of this chapter to describe, yet many of us are now ingesting daily amounts that far exceed even the government's inadequate safety standards. Hundreds of studies have found a connection between fluoride and cancer; cities that fluoridate their water have significantly more cancer deaths than cities that do not fluoridate. Fluoride causes cancer by reacting with enzymes, changing their shape and disabling them. Nevertheless, two-thirds of Americans drink fluoridated tap water.

We get this deadly toxin not only from our water, but also from toothpaste and from processed foods made with fluoridated water, including sodas, fruit juices, beer, and breakfast cereals. Many commercial fruit juices have been found to contain large amounts of fluoride. Crops watered with fluoridated water concentrate the fluoride and pass it on to you when you eat those foods. Tea leaves accumulate more fluoride than any other edible plant, and the fluoride content in tea has risen dramatically over the last twenty years. Some teas contain alarming levels of fluoride due to the use of fluoride-containing fertilizers and pesticides. Then people compound this problem by brewing their tea with fluoridated water. The average American is getting a daily toxic dose of fluoride that far exceeds even the EPA's inadequate safety standards.

According to the National Academy of Sciences, fluoride levels found in tap water inhibit over 100 enzymes in the body, including critical DNA repair enzymes. Numerous studies have shown that fluoride can result in genetic damage at concentrations as low as 1 part per million (ppm), the amount commonly found in fluoridated drinking water and mistakenly considered safe by the government. Further, the damage increases as the fluoride concentration goes up. One reason why older people have more cancer is because of a decline in their ability to repair damaged DNA—as little as 1 ppm of fluoride can disrupt DNA repair enzymes by 50 percent.

In 1982, at a meeting of the Japanese Association for Cancer Research, data was presented proving that even 1 ppm of fluoride is capable of transforming normal cells into cancer cells. Research in *Cell Biology and Toxicology* reported that a fluoride concentration of 1 ppm drives cancer, increasing tumor growth rates by 25 percent. This is why cancer death rates are higher in fluoridated communities. Doctor P. D. Cohn, in a 1992 New Jersey Department of Health study, found that bone cancer in young men was six times higher where the water was fluoridated. Fluoride switches on and drives cancer by poisoning respiratory enzymes, creating a deficiency of oxygen respiration and disrupting apoptosis and other cancer-protective mechanisms.

The reduction of tooth decay is the supposed justification for putting fluoride in tap water. However, numerous studies show fluoride does nothing to protect teeth. In fact, cities that fluoridate often have higher cavity rates. Fluoride damages your bones and teeth by binding to minerals such as calcium and magnesium, creating deficiencies of these minerals at the cellular level. In a 1992 interview with Andrew W. Saul of the editorial board of the *Journal of Orthomolecular Medicine,* Robert Carton, Ph.D., a former EPA scientist said, "Fluoridation is the greatest case of scientific fraud of this century." He added, "EPA has more than enough evidence to shut down fluoridation right now," and, "Fluoridation constitutes unlawful medical research. It is banned in most of Europe; European Union human rights legislation makes it illegal."

Most people are unaware that the FDA has *never* approved adding fluoride to drinking water. We have been adding this extremely toxic poison to drinking water and giving people cancer for over a

half century without FDA approval. Fluoride falls through a loop-
hole in the law! To be approved by the FDA, a substance must be
safe and effective—fluoride is neither.

Why don't we admit we have made a mistake and stop fluoridating
water? If we admit how toxic this stuff is, how much damage it has
done, how many people have been given cancer, weak bones, and bad
teeth, then the American Dental Association, dentists, water depart-
ments, toothpaste manufacturers, and the companies who sell these
toxic chemicals would all be sued out of existence—it's almost unthink-
able. So the charade that fluoride is safe and beneficial continues. To
avoid fluoride, use a reverse osmosis system to purify your drinking
water, do not use fluoride toothpaste, and avoid processed foods. Only
you can control the care and maintenance of your own body.

Bottled Water

Is bottled water safe? If you can get bottled water from a high-
quality source in glass bottles, the answer is yes. The quality of bottled water varies widely, and many brands have been found to be
no better than, and in some cases worse than, ordinary tap water.
In addition, toxins from the plastic bottles, such as carcinogenic
BPA, will leach into the water. A 2009 report by the Environmental Working Group on ten popular bottled water brands found an
average of eight chemical contaminants in each brand and half the
brands contained bacterial contamination. In some cases, the chemicals even exceeded the legal limits for bottled water contaminants.
A high-quality reverse osmosis system removes chlorine and toxic
chlorinated compounds; it also removes prescription drugs, arsenic,
aluminum, fluoride, and other toxins from the water. This is the
water you want to put in a glass bottle and carry with you.

The Air

Air pollution has been long recognized as causing ailments from allergies to *cancer*. Inhaling particles is known to disrupt the heart's beat-to-beat variations, and reduced heart rate variability has been associated with increased risk for mortality from all causes. It is estimated that 64,000 Americans die prematurely each year from heart and lung disease caused by particulate pollution. However, you don't have to live downwind of a power plant or drive behind a truck to be poisoned by air pollution. While you may think of your home as your castle, it may be more like a toxic waste dump. Toxicity from indoor air pollution affects the health of most Americans, producing a wide variety of symptoms, including anxiety, depression, fatigue, headaches, poor concentration, and poor mental acuity, as well as bodily aches and pains. When people complain of these symptoms, however, their physicians *almost never* suggest indoor pollutants as a probable (or even possible) cause.

Home Pollutants

Indoor air is a health risk due to the combined effects of multiple toxic sources concentrated in a confined space. Some of the most polluted air you can breathe is found right in your own home. The EPA has found that most indoor air is two to five times more polluted than that found outdoors, and it can easily be a hundred times more polluted. The combination of indoor pollution and the fact that most Americans spend 90 percent of their time indoors creates a serious health challenge that must be addressed.

There are multiple sources of indoor pollutants, including polluted outside air with all its particles and chemicals coming into our homes, but also the building materials, furnishings, mattresses, gas appliances, furnaces, cleaning and consumer products, tobacco smoke, incense, deodorants, carpets, paint, household cleansers, copy machines, printers, electronic equipment, dry-cleaning, newspapers, and magazines. Anything you can smell that is not a natural smell is almost certainly toxic. The longer you breathe it, and the more concentrated it is, the more damage it inflicts, putting another burden on our already overstressed bodies.

Building Materials

Building materials themselves, such as plywood, particleboard, and paints outgas formaldehyde, putting this common indoor pollutant and carcinogen into the air of your home. Formaldehyde causes serious damage to DNA, and the damage is cumulative as exposure continues. It is known to cause cancer. Houses and furniture made of particleboard will greatly increase the amount of formaldehyde and other chemicals you breathe in your home. While the industry will tell you that safer particleboards have been available since the 1980s, they outgas other toxic chemicals and are still far from being safe enough.

Carpets

Carpets made of synthetic fibers will outgas copious amounts of toxic chemicals, some of them for decades. New carpets are especially toxic. Synthetic-fiber carpets can contain as many as 200 toxic chemicals, which will outgas from the fibers, dyes, adhesives, backing, fire retardants, fungicides, antistatic and stain-resistant treatments, and the padding. Researchers at Anderson Laboratories, an independent materials testing laboratory, measured the effects of carpet toxicity on 110 families and found that 82 percent developed diverse health problems within three months of installation, including irregular heartbeat, fatigue, rashes, memory loss, muscle pain, blurred vision, and tremors. A 1995 study in the *Journal of Nutritional and Environmental Medicine* found that mice exposed to fumes from new carpets died in a matter of hours, while carpets up to twelve years old caused neurological problems. You can be certain that many of the chemicals outgassing from synthetic-fiber carpets will be cancer causing. Install only natural fiber carpets, tile, or hardwood floors with area rugs.

Appliances

Dangerous gases and particles are generated by household appliances such as gas stoves, water heaters, furnaces, space heaters, and fireplaces. These can release toxins such as nitrogen dioxide, carbon monoxide, methane, and other gases, along with fine particles, into the indoor air. Furnaces and gas water heaters should be kept outside the living space, such as in a shed or unattached garage. If this is not possible consider switching to an electric water heater. Gas stoves should be used only with good ventilation; an electric stove is preferable. Use fireplaces sparingly and never use artificial logs as they put a heavy hydrocarbon load into the living space.

Hot water used in dishwashers, clothes washers, bathtubs, and showers vaporizes the chlorine and other chemicals in the tap water, as well as the bleaches or detergents being used. Exposure by breathing these chemicals exceeds exposure from drinking the water because the inhaled gases go directly into the bloodstream. In fact, about two-thirds of our exposure to chlorine results from inhalation of vapors and skin absorption when showering. Good ventilation is essential, as is using a water filter for showering.

Paradichlorobenzene, found in mothballs and deodorizers, is another common indoor pollutant and also a carcinogen. Cedar chips are a more benign alternative to mothballs.

Cars

New cars are particularly dangerous. The chemicals contained in a new car's plastics, adhesives, and seating materials pollute the interior air of the car with known endocrine disrupters and carcinogens. One class of these chemicals is called phthalates, which disrupt normal hormone function by mimicking estrogen. Phthalates are also found in plastic bottles, food packaging, hoses, shower curtains, vinyl wall coverings, toys, cosmetics, hair conditioners, and fragrances. Phthalates cause sexual development abnormalities in children and contribute to cancer. During the first few months, try to leave a new car parked in the hot sun with the windows up to bake out the toxins. Air it out regularly, and be sure to air it out before you drive and keep it well ventilated while driving.

Attached garages are another problem. Exhaust fumes as well as hydrocarbon vapors coming from the engine can enter the living space. Whenever possible, leave the garage door open, so as to ventilate that space, especially after returning from a trip where the engine and oil are hot.

Never use pesticides in or around the home. If such is necessary, use a safe alternative. A 2006 study in the journal *Occupational and Environmental Medicine* found that the risk of developing leukemia was twice as likely in children whose mothers had used insecticides in the home before birth and long after birth. The use of insecticidal shampoos for head lice also doubled the risk of leukemia. Tobacco smoke, perfume, cosmetics, cleaning products, aerosol products, and all manner of scented products are toxic and should be avoided. There are safe alternatives for virtually all of these.

Airborne Particles

The average American breathes in about two heaping tablespoons of airborne particles each day. The smallest of these particles are capable of lodging deep in the lungs where they remain and cause serious problems. In 2004, Canadian researchers reported in the journal *Science* that fine airborne particles can cause *genetic mutations* that are passed on to future generations. Such damage is fundamental in the development of cancer. Most of these fine particles emanate from industrial plants, power plants, incinerators, and diesel-burning vehicles. In the MATES II report, a study of Los Angeles air completed in 1999, concluded that 71 percent of the cancer risk from air contaminants came from diesel emissions. The negative health effects of air pollution may be felt immediately, years later, or as has now been discovered, even in the next generation. Immediate effects can be felt after a single exposure, but most effects are subtler, causing damage to health without your knowledge. Even colds, flu, and asthma can result from the damage to immunity caused by breathing polluted air.

All Americans need to reduce their toxic load and to be aware of the health risks posed by air pollution. To protect ourselves, we must begin with our personal environment and stop introducing pollutants. Be aware of the problems with carpets, paints, cleaning materials, deodorizers, mattresses, gas appliances, fragrances, dry-cleaning chemicals, and so forth.

Work on reducing the amount of pollutants you introduce into your environment. Toward this end, filters are needed: shower, drinking water, and air filters. Genetic damage caused by fine particles is preventable by filtering the air with a HEPA (high efficiency particulate air) filter. Due to the unprecedented levels of air pollution we are now exposed to, air filters have become a virtual necessity, especially if you live in an urban environment or are near a heavily traveled highway with diesel emissions.

Other Sources

Besides the more well-known sources of toxic exposure mentioned so far, there are also other sources that may surprise you.

The Bathroom

Look in your bathrooms. Likely there are enough toxic chemicals there to make anybody sick. In addition to the toxic chlorinated water coming out of the tap, toxic bathroom products include toilet bowl cleaners, hair spray, and deodorizers. Toilet deodorizers are made from paradichlorobenzene, the same carcinogenic chemical found in mothballs. All of these products can be replaced with safer, simpler yet effective items available in health food stores.

The Laundry Room

Detergents, bleach, spot removers, and fabric softeners all contain chemicals that are toxic to you and to the environment. Manufacturers have lulled us into complacency with the term "biodegradable" detergents. This fact has little to do with the eventual health and environmental impact of these synthetic chemicals. "Biodegradable" only means that at some point the detergent will lose its foaming properties. Purchase unscented products. Detergents can be replaced with soap-based products, while bleach can be replaced with safer oxygen bleaches such as sodium percarbonate and hydrogen peroxide.

Furniture

Today furniture often is made with toxic synthetic materials (polyester, polyurethane, polystyrene, and polyvinyl chloride), which outgas toxic vapors and present significant health risks. Some types of furniture are made of particleboard, which as already mentioned will outgas formaldehyde, and then are covered with a wood or plastic veneer. Alarmingly, most *children's* furniture is made with toxic particleboard. Research shows that bringing particleboard furniture into an empty house triples the formaldehyde levels in the air. Most homes today are made with particleboard, but this problem can be particularly acute in mobile homes where *everything* may be made from particleboard. Buy furniture made from natural materials, such as solid wood or metal. Another less expensive option is used furniture made of these materials.

Clothing

Even the clothes you wear can be toxic. Have you ever gone into a clothing store and noticed the chemical-laden atmosphere? That unhealthy air results from the fact most clothes today contain or are made of toxic synthetic fibers (such as nylon, polyester, acrylics, and spandex). The chemicals outgassing from these fibers affect you as you wear them and also contribute to toxic indoor air in your home. Often clothes are treated with dyes, formaldehyde finishes (permanent press), and mothproofing pesticides. Dry-cleaning clothing brings toxins close to your body and into your household. Clothes that have been dry-cleaned should always be aired out thoroughly before they are put into a closet or worn. Many people are sensitive to residues from laundry detergents and fabric softeners. Have you ever walked down the detergent aisle at the grocery store and had your eyes, nose, or throat feel irritated? Toxins in those boxes are outgassing. When washing your clothes, use environmentally friendly and unscented laundry products such as Seventh Generation. Do not use scented fabric softeners; these products might make your clothes smell "clean and fresh," but that smell is toxic. Buy clothes made of natural materials such as wool and cotton, and use natural cleaning products.

Keep your home or office well ventilated. Modern homes and office buildings are built a lot "tighter" than older construction, to save on energy costs. While reducing energy waste is good, reducing air circulation allows pollutants to accumulate to higher concentrations. This is why high-quality air filters (that will filter out both particulate matter and gaseous hydrocarbons) can be helpful. Use them in rooms where you spend a great deal of time such as your office or bedroom.

Obvious though it sounds, the most important thing you can do to keep your indoor air clean is to stop introducing pollutants in the first place. Before purchasing something new, consider if that product might contribute to your indoor pollution. After buying something, give it a chance to outgas before putting it in your living environment. Do not use products that have powerful chemical odors, such as mothballs or air fresheners. Use heat and/or sunshine to help expedite the outgassing process whenever possible.

Prescription Drugs

A major category of avoidable toxins is prescription drugs. When we finally get sick from our poor nutrition and toxic overload, we go to conventional physicians who, not knowing any better, proceed to increase our toxic load, making us even sicker. Prescription drugs are so toxic that *properly prescribed drugs are the third leading cause of death in America.* If we outlawed prescription drugs, we could eliminate the third leading cause of death, saving hundreds of thousands of lives each year while also increasing quality of life. In addition, we would reduce healthcare costs by hundreds of billions of dollars, while improving the health of our population.

Prescription drugs are one of the leading causes of disease and of death because they cause nutritional deficiencies and they are toxic. Drugs merely suppress the symptoms of disease, while the true causes are not addressed. Meanwhile, entirely new nutritional deficiencies and toxicities are being created, and the body's detoxification system is being overloaded. When you take a prescription drug, you are making yourself sick. Dr. Mehmet Oz, a professor of surgery at Columbia University and author of *YOU: The Owner's Manual* had this to say, "For every dollar we spend on prescription drugs, we spend a dollar to fix a complication."

Perhaps there might be justification for using drugs if they served a useful purpose, but many are little better than placebos in treating the diseases they are supposed to be addressing. At great cost, they do enormous amounts of harm, creating whole new health problems. The top-selling drug in the world is a cholesterol-lowering drug. Yet here is what a 1996 study in the *Journal of the American Medical Association* had to say about this class of drugs: *All members of the two most popular classes of lipid-lowering drugs (the fibrates and the statins) cause cancer in rodents, in some cases at lev-els of animal exposure close to those prescribed to humans.*

By the time you are on more than a couple of prescription drugs, every cell in your body is being poisoned and no one in the world knows what is going on—you are in biochemical chaos. Health is when the body is in balance—chaos is disease. Prescription drugs cause chaos and disease. When your body is in chaos, you are a sitting duck for *cancer*, or any other disease. The healthiest person alive will get sick if they take prescription drugs, but sick people are already compromised and have less ability to metabolize these chemicals and protect themselves from their toxic effects.

Since the year 2000, sales of prescription drugs have more than tripled. Americans represent 4 percent of the world's population, yet they take half of all the prescription drugs produced in the world. Since drugs cause disease, this helps to explain why the health of the American people is so poor when compared to other nations. Half of all Americans now take at least one prescription drug. One out of four children takes at least one prescription drug. Many of our elderly take a dozen or more drugs per day. It's no wonder they are losing their minds, unstable on their feet, feeling fatigued, and their health is in a downward spiral. These drugs represent a huge toxic load on us and on the environment. Alarming amounts of prescription drugs are now showing up in our water supply, poisoning fish and animals that depend on that water, not to mention poisoning young children who drink it.

Fortunately, drugs are unnecessary. It is difficult to think of a drug for which there is not a safer, less expensive and more effective alternative. Meanwhile most physicians still believe that drugs are the answer, but in reality, drugs are the problem. *Prescription drugs both cause and drive cancer.*

Personal Care Products

Almost all personal care products such as toothpaste, antibacterial soaps, shaving cream, aftershave, nail polish, deodorant products, skin lotions, hair sprays, hair dyes, fragrances, shampoos, and conditioners contain toxic chemicals that *add* to your toxic overload and put stress on your immune system. At least one-third of the chemicals used to make these products have already been identified as causing cancer or other serious health problems. In addition, these chemicals acting in combination are much more toxic than any one acting alone. Some of these chemicals are endocrine disrupters that affect hormone balance, leading to numerous problems, including mood swings and cancer. Suntan lotions contain at least half a dozen chemicals that have been found to be carcinogens or endocrine disrupters. Most people don't even conceive that products as common as toothpaste or shampoo are significant sources of dangerous toxins that are making them sick and contributing to their cancer. It is important to seek out and use only safe personal care products.

Especially important are products you put in your mouth or on your skin. Toxins you swallow are subjected to enzymes in your stomach, and then pass through the liver, so they are broken down before they reach the rest of your body. When toxins are absorbed through the mucous membranes in the mouth or through the skin, they can enter the bloodstream and your tissues without the above protective effects. The same toxin can be 100 times more toxic when absorbed through the skin or mucous membranes than when swallowed, so be especially cautious when using products like mouthwash, toothpaste, shampoo, and skin lotions. Most such products are highly toxic, and with daily use, cause serious damage as they bioaccumulate in your cells and tissues.

Most skin creams contain a mixture of toxic chemicals including mineral oil, paraffin, and petrolatum. These are petroleum products that are suspected carcinogens and hormone disrupters. Parabens are the usual preservatives in these products, and they too have hormone-disrupting qualities and are suspected carcinogens. Sodium lauryl or laureth sulfate are included in over 90 percent of personal care products. They break down the skin's moisture barrier, easily allowing other chemicals to penetrate the skin, and they combine with other chemicals, forming powerful carcinogens. These sulfate compounds are often disguised on the label by saying "comes from coconut" or "coconut-derived." Acrylamide is found in many hand and face creams, and it has been linked to tumors in laboratory research. Dioxane is a powerful carcinogen and it can be found as a contaminant in ingredients such as PEG (polyethylene glycol), polysorbates, laureth, and ethoxylated alcohols. Other common toxic ingredients include phenol carbolic acid and propylene glycol.

Toothpaste is something most people use daily without realizing it is a dangerous source of toxins. Read the warning label on the box to get an idea of how toxic this stuff is: if you swallow more than a little, you should seek medical assistance. Toothpaste contains a deadly mixture of numerous toxins, such as fluoride, artificial colors, flavors and sweeteners, synthetic detergents like sodium lauryl sulfate (SLS), and various carcinogens, all of which can pass through the mucous membranes and bioaccumulate in the body, leading to toxic overload and disease. The mucous membranes in your mouth are *very* permeable, so if you expose yourself to toxic toothpaste daily, you subject yourself to a *lot* of toxins.

Shampoo is another toxin-loaded product that many use daily. Shampoos contain synthetic detergents such as SLS, which disrupts the nervous system, hormone system, and normal cell chemistry. In addition, SLS is frequently contaminated with 1,4-dioxane, which is toxic to the liver, kidneys, and brain, and is also listed as a probable human carcinogen. Dioxane has even been found in baby shampoo. These toxins pass through the skin and bioaccumulate in tissues to levels that cause serious cellular malfunction and disease.

Shampoos also contain preservatives such as paraben compounds. The EPA has linked parabens to hormonal, neurological, metabolic, and developmental disorders, and to cancer. Researchers have found parabens in every sample of breast cancer tissue. Propylene glycol is another problem. This chemical is used in antifreeze and can be found in numerous shampoo and skincare products. It is a skin irritant and is known to cause liver and kidney damage. Shampoos also contain a variety of artificial colors and other toxic and carcinogenic chemicals. Artificial colors have been shown to be carcinogenic not only when ingested but also when applied to the skin. Here is what the Center for Science in the Public Interest had to say in a June 29, 2010 press release regarding artificial colors, "The three most widely used dyes, Red 40, Yellow 5, and Yellow 6, are contaminated with known carcinogens. . . . Another dye, Red 3, has been acknowledged for years by the Food and Drug Administration to be a carcinogen, yet is still in the food supply."

A study by the University of Southern California published in a 2007 *International Journal of Cancer* revealed that monthly use of permanent hair dye doubled the risk of bladder cancer when used for 12 months. The risk tripled after fifteen years of use. Temporary or semipermanent dyes did not have the same risks, according to the researchers.

The largest category of cosmetic and personal care products is perfumes, colognes, and fragrances. Even high-end perfumes are made with cocktails of dangerous and untested chemicals that may produce problems from allergies to hormone disruption and cancer. According to the Environmental Working Group, most perfumes contain an average of ten known allergens that can trigger reactions from asthma to headaches to contact dermatitis, and an average of four chemicals known to disrupt the hormonal (endocrine) system. These endocrine disrupters have been linked to reproductive defects in male infants, sperm damage in men, and more recently, hyperactivity in children.

Fragrances are also extensively used in a wide range of household cleaning products. The industry uses more than 5,000 different chemicals to make synthetic fragrances. Among them are endocrine-disrupting chemicals like phthalates and toxic solvents like xylene and toluene. Toluene is found in most synthetic fragrances, and chronic exposure can cause anemia, low blood cell count, liver or kidney damage, and damage to a fetus. These ingredients are not regulated, and they do not need to be listed on the label. Some of these chemicals are known to cause allergies, do reproductive and hormonal damage, and cause *cancer*. If you must use a fragrance, use a natural essential oil. These are derived from flowers and natural herbs and are available at health food and specialty stores.

Fortunately, there are safe personal care products available, such as safe toothpastes, shampoos, skin creams, and deodorants. All you have to do is choose them. This will lower your toxic load, put less of a burden on your overworked immune system, and help you to better prevent and fight cancer.

Nanotechnology

Nanomaterials are an emerging technology and a new threat to health. Engineered nanomaterials are structures and systems that are sometimes as small as atoms and molecules. These new materials are enabling significant breakthroughs in designing new materials for industry, medicine, and consumer products.

Nanomaterials are already used in hundreds of consumer products including sunscreens, cosmetics, stain-resistant clothing, and electronic products. However, there is growing concern about the toxicity of these small particles. Because of their small size, they can be inhaled, ingested, and absorbed through the skin, entering the bloodstream and penetrating cells throughout the body, causing cells to malfunction and even interfere with DNA processes. Evidence already indicates that titanium dioxide nanoparticles used in sunscreens may be toxic to algae and water fleas that are vital parts of marine ecosystems. Nanoparticles have not been adequately tested for safety, so avoid products made with them.

Support Detoxification

Our bodies are not only exposed to external toxins from our foods, the air, and water, but our cells generate a huge amount of toxins every day in the form of waste products from normal metabolism. Fortunately, we have exquisitely designed detoxification systems to safely dispose of these chemicals. Unfortunately, we are overloading these systems. Overloading is bad enough, but our poor diets also lack the adequate supply of nutrients these detox systems need to do their jobs.

The liver is our major detoxification organ. Anything we can do to ease its toxic burden will make the liver's job easier and be beneficial to our health. At any given time, about 25 percent of all the blood in your body is in your liver to be detoxified. This begins with a sophisticated filtering system that captures and digests foreign debris. Next, enzymes produced by the liver deactivate and eliminate toxins. However, these enzymes can be deactivated by environmental toxins such as lead and mercury, or never manufactured in the first place because of nutrient deficiency. Either of these will result in toxic overload. Liver-enzyme detoxification has two phases. In Phase I, the liver produces enzymes that take harmful toxins such as alcohol, pesticides, herbicides, and prescription drugs and oxidizes them in preparation for removal from the body. This process creates potentially harmful free radicals that must be neutralized with dietary antioxidant nutrients. In Phase II, more enzymes are used to combine the oxidized chemicals from Phase I with other molecules, which then can be excreted harmlessly in the bile or urine. In both phases, the food we eat supplies the raw materials needed to produce all of these enzymes, antioxidants, and other chemicals required. These elegant systems do a fabulous job, but they depend on a constant supply of nutrients, which we must get from our diet, but usually do not.

You can support your liver's Phase I detoxification process with antioxidant nutrients. Supplement with vitamins C, E, and A, along with CoQ10, carotenoids, bioflavonoids, selenium, manganese, copper, and zinc. Some of these nutrients neutralize free radicals directly—others activate enzymes that neutralize them. Red, yellow, and green vegetables are loaded with these antioxidant nutrients. You can assist Phase II detoxification with cruciferous vegetables such as cabbage, broccoli, cauliflower, green onions, kale, and Brussels sprouts. These vegetables enable the liver to eliminate powerful carcinogens, helping to protect against cancer. These dietary suggestions, combined with high-quality supplements, will keep your liver's toxic defenses at peak function. Juicing vegetables every day helps by making more of these precious chemicals biologically available.

Reducing Stored Toxins

Americans are some of the most toxic creatures on the planet, and the amount of stored toxins in our cells and tissues has reached crisis levels. Unless you are taking active measures to reduce your toxic load, then each day, you will be adding to them. As you grow older, your toxic load will reach catastrophic levels. We cannot afford to continue adding to our toxic load, we need to be subtracting and taking the load off our liver and detoxification systems. There are different approaches to reducing stored toxins; let's have a look at some that you can use to reduce your toxic burden.

Saunas

Avoiding toxins is essential, but it is not the whole answer. Getting rid of stored toxins is the other half of the equation. One solution is a sauna. Heat causes toxins to be released by cells, and hyperthermic (sweat) treatments have been used by cultures around the world for millennia. The ancient Egyptians, Greeks, and Romans used them, and even American Indians used sweat lodges. Hyperthermic practices are known to reduce levels of oil-soluble toxins, such as pesticides and PCBs. The skin is the body's largest organ and an important part of the body's detoxification system. Saunas melt the fat layer in the skin, allowing the oil to ooze out of the oil glands along with its cargo of accumulated fat-soluble toxins. In addition, water-soluble toxins are lost in the sweat, carrying out heavy metals like lead and mercury. Over time, it is possible to reduce one's toxic load substantially as well as keep it low.

With almost every American in toxic overload, using a sauna on a regular basis has become a necessity for achieving and maintaining good health. Sherry Rogers, M.D., an internationally known expert in environmental medicine and author of *Tired or Toxic?,* maintains that saunas have become *"a household necessity."* According to Dr. Rogers:

> *A sauna used to be thought of as a luxury. But studies now confirm that diet and environmental chemicals cause 95% of cancers. Furthermore, as the first generation of man exposed to an unprecedented plethora of daily chemicals, we have learned that stored chemicals can mimic any disease. "Incurable" chronic diseases that were thought to have no known cause often disappear when toxic chemicals are gone.*

Our genes were designed 100,000 years before the petroleum age, which began a century ago. Since then, our environment has become a sea of petroleum-based, oil-soluble toxins. Never before exposed to these chemicals, nature did not design a way for us to get rid of them. We didn't need to develop a solution to a problem that didn't exist. As a result, the average person is bioaccumulating between 300 and 500 man-made chemicals, most of which did not exist before World War II. Styrene (found in plastic drinking cups and food packaging) is now found in 100 percent of human tissue in America. PCBs, dioxins, paradichlorobenzene (found in mothballs and deodorizers), sodium lauryl sulfate (found in soap, shampoo, and toothpaste), triclosan (found in antibacterial soap and underarm deodorants), and many others are all bioaccumulating in our tissues. Many of these chemicals are known carcinogens. Many of them are hormone disrupters. Human fat cells make hormones, and now those fat cells are bioaccumulating known hormone disrupters. This helps to explain why so many of us have hormonal abnormalities, why children are entering puberty at younger and younger ages, and why we have so many hormone-driven cancers such as breast and prostate cancers.

A sauna will cause you to sweat less than a steam room, thus allowing you to spend longer in the sauna than you would in a steam room. Longer is necessary because oils take more time than sweat to ooze out onto the skin. After completing the sauna, it is essential to wash off with a good castile soap immediately. This washes the toxins off so they don't reabsorb into the skin. Conventional saunas are effective, but the regular use of a far-infrared sauna is even more efficient, and is the most effective way to remove stored toxins.

Saunas are available at gyms and health clubs. If you use one of these commercial saunas, lie prone on the lowest bench. This will expose your body to a manageable temperature, allowing you to spend more time. I recommend starting slowly and gradually working your way up to an hour or more. Saunas played a critical role in reducing my toxic overload and restoring my health when I was at death's door. Even today, I still sauna twice a week for sixty to ninety minutes to keep my toxic load down. You can use your sauna time to do other healthy things such as eye exercises or meditation. I even use that time to catch up on reading and return phone calls.

Many people cannot tolerate conventional saunas due to uncomfortable, excessively hot air. Even under these harsh conditions, the heat penetration from conventional saunas is superficial, penetrating only a few millimeters. Infrared saunas are a completely different experience. The infrared heats you rather than the air so the penetration is over one and a half inches deep, which is desirable for healing tissue and releasing toxins. Meanwhile, the air temperature is kept at a comfortable and controllable level—105 to 115 degrees versus 130 to 180 degrees in a conventional sauna.

If you have not used a sauna before, it may take some getting used to. Work your way up in time slowly, and if you ever feel faint, dizzy, or sick, get out. Over time, you will get used to it, and your body will love it. It is important to keep hydrated when using a sauna. Drinking pure water before, during, and after is recommended. Excessive water loss can disturb normal heart rhythms and also cause dizziness, nausea, and fatigue.

Some alternative physicians use far-infrared saunas to reduce biochemical cancer markers in their patients. Beneficial results, similar to those using expensive European hyperthermic cancer treatments, have been obtained. Studies show that a combination of daily exercise, nutritional supplements, and a regular sauna has a powerful beneficial effect on health—the therapeutic value of this practice can be absolutely enormous.

Fasting

Fasting is the complete abstinence from all substances except pure water in a restful environment. Juice fasting, a popular variation, is abstinence from all food and drink except water and fresh vegetable juices. Fasting is a powerful way of detoxifying. People have been fasting for thousands of years, both for spiritual and health purposes. It is an integral part of many religions including Islam, Judaism, and Christianity. Fasting is known to have a beneficial effect on health. As far back as 400 BC, Hippocrates prescribed total abstinence from food while a disease was on the increase and a spare diet on other occasions. Ancient priests provided sanctuaries where people could go to fast. Animals fast when they are sick or injured, and when we are sick, our hunger diminishes.

Fasting promotes detoxification. The body normally eliminates or neutralizes toxins through the colon, liver, kidneys, lungs, lymph nodes, and skin. Fasting helps this process because when you are no longer eating food, the body turns to its fat reserves for energy. When fat reserves are used for energy, as the fats are used, they release their stored toxins, which are then eliminated through the usual organs mentioned above.

Fasting also triggers the healing process. The body uses lots of energy to digest food. During a fast, energy is diverted away from the digestive system, since it has nothing to do, toward body metabolism and the immune system. When fasting, the body naturally searches for dead cells, damaged tissues, fatty deposits, tumors, and abscesses, tearing them down so they can be burned for fuel or expelled as waste. During fasting, the body also rebuilds damaged tissues. Fasting allows the digestive system to repair itself, restoring good digestion and elimination. The elimination of problem areas restores the immune system and metabolic functionality to an optimum state, rejuvenating the body and giving it a more youthful tone. The benefits of fasting can have lasting effects on your physical, mental, and emotional health.

A simple water fast is one where all you consume during the fasting time is water. It is important to consume plenty of pure water to help flush toxins through your system as your body uses its energy to release them. Avoid water straight from the faucet. Distilled water from a pure, natural source or reverse osmosis water is the best for cleansing. Drink at least two liters per day. Stirring buffered vitamin C powder into water throughout the day provides extra antioxidant power to protect against free radicals while helping the body to detoxify. Organic lemon juice in pure water can also be helpful in the cleansing process, as lemon is especially supporting to the liver. If you desire to make fasting a habit, an excellent book to teach you about fasting is *Toxic Relief* by Don Colbert, M.D.

Some people prefer a juice fast. If you choose to juice fast, you may consume a few 8-ounce glasses of fresh, home-juiced, vegetable juice (*not* store bought, processed juice) throughout the day. In addition to these, you must drink plenty of pure water, including lemon water. If you have responsibilities to maintain during your fast, you may find you have a little more energy with a juice fast. The vegetable juice also provides antioxidant protection from the toxins being released into your system as your body detoxifies.

Employ fasting only after you are well underway with the other lifestyle changes. Making too many changes at first will bring on a rapid detoxification that may sicken you and, even worse, discourage you from continuing. *There are some individuals who should not fast due to blood sugar issues.* Once your health has begun to improve and you have adjusted to other dietary changes, you may be able to begin occasional fasts.

Although fasting is not recommended in every situation, (cancer of the liver is one instance where fasting is contraindicated), in many situations fasting is the only known solution. Fasting dissolves tumors. As the body searches for energy sources, abnormal growths such as tumors are more likely to be self-digested by the body's natural enzymes. To overcome a severe disease like cancer, it is usually necessary to continue through a series of fasts to remove all the tumor tissue. Many have overcome cancer with fasting. Fasting has also been beneficial for arthritis, asthma, high blood pressure, high cholesterol, lupus, chronic fatigue, colitis, Crohn's disease, diverticulitis, spastic colon, irritable bowel, cases of paralysis, neuritis, neuralgia, neuroses, insomnia, addictions, mental illness, and other health problems.

Aside from the usual nightly fasts while we are sleeping, giving our body more extended times of fasting is a healthy new habit to cultivate. Whether you begin by just fasting one meal a day, two meals a day, or one day a week, your body will have extra time to cleanse and detoxify. In fact, fasting is the one practice that has been proven to extend life. Several incredible studies have been carried out proving the efficacy of fasting. Dr. Roy Walford, author of *The Anti-Aging Plan,* did a study in which he fasted mice. His study showed that the mice that fasted two days a week *doubled* their life span and were healthier.

Making a habit of fasting one day a week is not difficult, and by doing so, your body gets fifty-two days a year to rest and detoxify. That adds up to over seven weeks a year. The main reason for this habit is detoxification and health, but imagine how much less food is consumed in a year with a total of seven weeks without food. Some people prefer to fast three or four days in a row each month. Unless you have blood sugar problems, this amount of fasting is safe and beneficial. Once a year, I fast for seven to ten days in a row, and feel fabulous afterwards. In fact, it was a ten-day fast that helped to turn around my own serious health problems after I almost died from liver failure caused by a toxic prescription drug. Longer fasts are preferable to short ones because once the body is in the fasting state, systemic cleansing is able to reach into the harder-to-get-at body tissues. For this reason, most of the recoveries from serious illnesses have taken place with longer fasts. A medically supervised fast of thirty to forty days may be required. There are excellent clinics where you can go for such fasts. Long, unsupervised fasts can be dangerous, so consult your natural health practitioner or doctor before you start such a fast, and be sure you have supervision.

As your body eliminates more and more toxins, you will notice increased energy, better health, and sharper mental functioning. Regular fasting is one habit that will reward you with benefits including weight reduction and a longer life!

Enemas

Another effective approach to detoxification is coffee enemas—not recommended if you are allergic to coffee. Coffee enemas are known to work well in conjunction with vegetable juicing in healing the body of cancer. Such enemas were already an established part of medical practice when the famous cancer pioneer Dr. Max Gerson introduced them into cancer therapy in the 1930s.

Coffee enemas stimulate liver enzymes that are vital for detoxification. Increasing the activity of these enzymes has a powerful antioxidant effect, while it also helps break down carcinogenic substances. Coffee contains substances called choleretics, which help to dilate and open up the bile ducts to allow drainage of toxins from the liver. An additional benefit of detoxifying the liver is that pain relief quickly occurs following the coffee enemas as the liver toxins are released.

For cancer patients, some practitioners recommend coffee enemas every two hours during the first days of treatment. A typical formula is to add three teaspoons of *fresh ground, organic coffee* to approximately one quart or one liter of purified water. Boil for five minutes, and then cover and simmer for an additional fifteen minutes. Strain through a typical coffee filter and cool to body temperature. Use a typical enema bag, and try to retain the coffee for fifteen minutes. Much has been written on how to do coffee enemas, and this information is available on the Internet.

Vitamin C Flush

A vitamin C flush is like an internal enema that benefits the entire digestive system and the body as a whole. The procedure consists of taking vitamin C until you reach a watery stool or an enema-like evacuation of liquid from the rectum.

When possible, it is best to start first thing in the morning on an empty stomach. Allow yourself that day to finish the flush. Most people saturate their ascorbate need within a few hours. Occasionally, the need is much greater, and it may take most of the day to complete the flush.

Dissolve the fully reduced, buffered mineral L-ascorbate powder in a half glass of water. Plan to count and record each dosage. After allowing any effervescence to abate, drink the beverage. The amount of L-ascorbate needed depends on how quickly your body uses it up. Below are suggestions for how to best determine your needs based on how healthy you are:

- A healthy person begins with a level half teaspoon dissolved in 1–2 ounces of water or diluted juice every fifteen minutes.
- A moderately healthy person begins with 1 teaspoon every fifteen minutes.
- A person in ill health begins with 2 teaspoons every fifteen minutes.
- If after four doses there is no gurgling or rumbling in the gut, you should double the initial dosage and continue every fifteen minutes.

Caution: Do not stop at loose stool. Continue with these instructions until a quart or so of liquid is expelled from the rectum. You want to energize the body to "flush out" toxins and reduce the risk that they may recirculate and induce problems. After the flush, stop consuming the buffered ascorbate for the day. However, if your flush dosage is more than 50 grams of vitamin C, you should consume a dosage of vitamin C of at least 10 percent of that during the remainder of the day.

Caution: It is critical that the vitamin C used be very pure, and contain a proper balance of the major essential buffering minerals: 1) potassium, 2) magnesium, 3) calcium, and 4) zinc. The label should read: 100% L-ascorbate, fully reduced, corn free, buffered mineral ascorbate.

In Conclusion

Toxins are now a major force in causing our epidemic of chronic disease and cancer. Reducing your toxic overload is essential for preventing or reversing cancer. The buildup of toxins in your body reduces cell oxygenation, and many toxins damage DNA, causing cell mutation. Toxins interfere with critical metabolic processes by interrupting critical communications, giving inappropriate instructions to genes and shutting down essential metabolic machinery. The resulting biochemical chaos interferes with the body's ability to self-repair, self-regulate and keep you healthy—chaos is disease.

We all need to learn how to avoid toxins and stop putting them into our bodies. As much as possible, eat only organic foods and use only safe personal care products. We need to improve our diets and eat less garbage and more cruciferous vegetables that support our detoxification pathways. A high-quality supplement program, including plenty of antioxidants, is a must. We should also avoid drinking, taking showers with, or swimming in chlorinated water.

Getting rid of stored toxins is essential, or they will continue to build up until they cause major malfunction and disease. For women who wish to have children, this is especially important to protect the children from birth defects, neurological damage, and cancer.

Toxins are known to both switch cancer on and to drive cancer. To prevent and reverse cancer, minimizing toxins is essential. Safe and effective products, including supplements, saunas, soap, tooth-paste, shampoo, deodorants, skin cream, cleaning cloths, and air, pool, and water filters for your home are available at: www.beyond health.com.

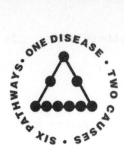

ONE DISEASE · TWO CAUSES · SIX PATHWAYS

6

THE MENTAL PATHWAY

The first place we must win the victory is in our own minds. . . .
If you don't think your body can be healed, it never will be.

—*Joel Osteen, author of* Your Best Life Now

The simple truth is, happy people generally don't get sick.
One's attitude toward oneself is the single
most important factor in healing or staying well.

—*Bernie Siegel, M.D., author of* Love, Medicine and Miracles

O ver 2000 years ago, Plato said in *Charmides,* "This is the great error of our day in the treatment of the human body, the physicians separate the soul from the body." Things haven't changed much since then; physicians still ignore the power of the mind and spirit for healing disease.

The power of the mind to heal or make you sick is almost limitless. Your nervous system controls all the other systems in your body. It is the master computer that checks and balances your entire health. Every thought and emotion triggers the release of chemical messengers throughout the body. In other words, there is no such thing as "just a thought." *Every thought has a physical consequence, for better or for worse.* That's powerful!

The Power of Mind Over Matter

One of the greatest mysteries in traditional medicine is the spontaneous remission of chronic diseases. But it is not so mysterious if one is aware of the tremendous power that thoughts and emotions have over physical processes in the body. Emotions are one of the most important factors contributing to all disease—especially cancer. A change in your thinking or belief can actually change how your genes express—same genes, different results. What you think can mean the difference between having cancer and not having cancer. Just as you are what you eat, *you are what you think.* Just as you can choose what you eat, you can choose what you think. *If you are sick, you must change what you eat* and *what you think.*

Even the CDC has stated that 85 percent of all diseases have an emotional component, and this estimate is most likely conservative. Feelings of anger, apathy, gloom, and resentment weaken the immune system and damage health. Positive thoughts of love, compassion, joy, humor, and the like support good physical health. Your mind is the biggest pharmacy on the planet, and it matters a great deal how you use it. Modern research has shown that your thoughts, emotions, and beliefs trigger the brain to produce a large variety of biologically active chemicals. The activities of the mind affect every body function and have a direct effect on how your cells operate.

In the mid-1970s, Hans Selye, M.D., was the first to demonstrate that animals subjected to stress experienced depressed immunity, elevated blood pressure, elevated triglycerides, and stomach ulcers. Since then, thousands of human studies have shown a direct link between mental state and disease, including cancer. Almost everyone lives with stress, but how you handle stress makes a big difference. People react to stress in different ways. Depending on how each chooses to respond, the same stressful event will make one person sick while having no effect on another. Depending on how *you* react, you can think your way into cancer and you can think your way out of it. The power of the mind to heal or make you sick is absolutely enormous.

As a result of decades of research, we now know that cell chemistry can be directly influenced by human intention. This knowledge helps to explain the placebo effect, spontaneous remission, and the value of faith and prayer in human health. Thousands of years of human history tell us that the mind has a major impact on the body. There are even hundreds of research studies indicating that when conventional medicine's drugs and surgery work, it is because of the belief that the patient has in their efficacy. Belief is so powerful that it can even overcome the toxic damage done by drugs and surgery and still make you well. How much better and less expensive it would be to harness that belief and skip the drugs and surgery!

Lack of purpose, low self-esteem, helplessness, hopelessness, anxiety, loneliness, depression, extreme mental or physical stress, or stressful life events, such as loss of a loved one, have all been proven to be immune-suppressing and cancer-promoting factors.

Depression has been found to double the risk of cancer. In 2003, the National Cancer Institute sponsored a roundtable at the PsychoNeuroImmunology Research Society's annual meeting. Data was presented finding that the survival of cancer patients could be accurately predicted based on their mental attitude and their will to live. People who beat the odds have a fighting spirit, live fully in the moment, and anticipate the future.

Our genes run the show, but the same genetic code produces different results based on the instructions we give to the genes. A strong and unambiguous intention to heal gives the genes the instructions they need to produce health-enhancing chemicals. Positive thoughts cause the creation of happy brain chemicals such as enkephalins and endorphins. Both these chemicals increase the production of immune T cells. But in addition to producing more T cells, positive thoughts cause something magical to happen—the vigor with which the T cells attack cancer cells is also increased. Positive thoughts increase immunity, protecting against infections and cancer. Negative thoughts have the opposite effect!

Everyday emotional stress can trigger the growth of tumors. Yet many people stress themselves needlessly about things over which they have absolutely no control. Why do this? All it does is do harm—to you! It's not worth the price. A woman once came to me for help for her cancer and numerous other health problems. I found out that twenty years prior she had gone through a nasty divorce. Then, every day for the past twenty years, she had relived the stress of that divorce—running the same movie over and over in her mind—the same high stress every day. Why? All it did was make her very sick and give her cancer. It is a scientific fact that your thoughts directly influence your physical health, so why not make that work *for* you instead of *against* you?

Turning Cancer Switches On

Stress can switch on and drive cancer. In response to stress, your body releases a flood of hormones into your blood. Hormones are part of your body's communications system. They deliver messages to genes and cells and act as genetic switches, turning genes on or off. They directly influence important cellular processes, including those that regulate cell growth and help to protect against tumors. Stress causes the release of growth-promoting hormones that help to switch cancer on. Stress hormones make blood platelets sticky, causing them to form clots, contributing to strokes and heart attacks as well as helping to switch cancer on and drive it. Stress hormones also activate an inflammatory response, which promotes the growth and spread of tumors. At the same time, vital functions such as digestion, tissue repair, and immune response are put on hold and slowed down. In 1908, Dr. Eli Jones in his book, *Cancer: Its Causes, Symptoms and Treatment,* identified *stress* as the number one cause of cancer. Modern studies support his thinking. Patrick Quillin, Ph.D., in his book, *Beating Cancer with Nutrition,* said, "In my years of experience, about 90% of the cancer patients I deal with have encountered a major traumatic event 1–2 years prior to the onset of cancer."

Recent studies indicate that the mind and the immune system are so intertwined that negative thinking depresses the activity of immune system cells, natural killer (NK) cells, and T- and B-lymphocytes. When a person gives up and feels that life is no longer worth living, the immune system gives up as well.

In addition to switching cancer on, stress drives cancer. Norepinephrine, a hormone produced during periods of stress, drives cancer. Norepinephrine increases the growth rate of cancer by stimulating tumor cells to produce two collagen-dissolving enzymes that break down the tissue around the tumor cells, allowing the cells to more easily move into your bloodstream. Once in the bloodstream, these cells travel to other organs and tissues and form additional tumors. Norepinephrine can also stimulate tumor cells to release a chemical called vascular endothelial growth factor, which promotes angiogenesis (the growth of the blood vessels that feed growing tumors). The stress hormone epinephrine has been found to cause changes in prostate and breast cancer cells in ways that may make them resistant to apoptosis (normal programmed cell death). Promoting angiogenesis and inhibiting apoptosis is a prescription for cancer growth.

Cortisol is another stress hormone. A study in a 2000 *Journal of the National Cancer Institute* measured survival in metastatic breast cancer patients and found that, up to seven years later, their daily cortisol levels were predictive of who would or would not survive. Both cortisol and norepinephrine block the action of cancer-protective NK cells. A study in a 2005 *Journal of Clinical Oncology* found that women with cancer who had positive attitudes had *much* more active NK cells than those who had sunk into depression and hopelessness.

Adrenaline is another hormone that we produce more of when we are stressed. Adrenaline depresses immunity by decreasing available antibodies and reducing both the number and activity of lymphocytes. The membranes surrounding the cells of our immune system contain receptors for various neurochemicals produced in the brain, so the brain is directly communicating with immune cells. When we are happy, the brain produces a type of neurochemical that causes the immune system to strengthen and build. When we are depressed, the brain produces another type of neurochemical that effectively shuts down the immune system, our first line of defense against cancer.

A 2010 study in *Cancer Research* found a 30-fold increase in the spread of cancer throughout the bodies of stressed mice compared to those that were not stressed. The stressed animals showed significantly more metastases throughout the body than did the control group. The cancer actually acted differently in the stressed mice. What happens is the growth of cancer cells damages tissue, sending a message to the immune system to repair the damage. The immune system responds by sending immune cells called macrophages. The macrophages turn on inflammation genes, which is part of the body's normal response to injury. Inflammation is necessary for cancer to cut through connective tissue and spread. In addition, blood vessels that are grown to aid healing instead feed the cancer by delivering the oxygen and nutrients it needs to grow and spread. When stress chemicals are present, many more macrophages are sent to the area of the tumor, making everything much worse with more inflammation and promoting the spread of the cancer. Erica Sloan, a research scientist at the UCLA Cousins Center for Psychoneuroimmunology and one of the study's authors, reported, "What we showed for the first time is that chronic stress causes cancer cells to escape from the primary tumor and colonize distant organs."

Recall from Chapter 3 that almost every American over age fifty has microscopic clusters of cancer cells (microtumors) throughout their bodies just waiting for the opportunity to grow and metastasize. Stress provides that opportunity!

As the evidence builds, conventional medicine is finally beginning to understand how profoundly stress and negative thinking can harm your physical health and make you vulnerable to all kinds of health problems. There are good, scientifically sound reasons why people with positive outlooks live longer and healthier lives, while enjoying life far more than those with negative outlooks. Stress-reduction techniques, such as meditation, are essential to cancer patients. Meditative practice works to balance the body, not only helping to prevent cancer, but also helping prevent the recurrence of cancer.

Turning Cancer Switches Off

One of the greatest gifts you can give yourself is to choose happiness. Too often we think that happiness is something that comes from outside us, but it really starts on the inside. There are people who have every advantage in life and they are still not happy. Wealth, status, and material goods do not create happiness. It is a positive attitude that matters. Older people with positive attitudes have a 55 percent lower risk of death from all causes. Your attitude is something you choose, and the more you stay genuinely positive, the better your health outcome is likely to be.

Many decades ago, I served a tour of duty in a U.S. Army combat infantry division. I knew from the nature of the job that I would be separated from friends, family, and loved ones, and that there were going to be some unpleasant experiences. I knew I was going to live through these unpleasant experiences because I didn't have a choice. The only real choice was to be unhappy and miserable or happy while experiencing them. I chose happy and happily lived through some very miserable experiences. Your life is no different. Unless you die young, you have to live it, and when life is filled with pain, sorrow, and disappointment, you can still choose to be happy regardless of the outward circumstances! Think about and be grateful for the blessings you have. It's the choice that supports your immune system and your health. It's also more fun. Remember, happy comes from the inside, not the outside. It's a big mistake to depend on things outside of us for our happiness.

Once you make up your mind to be happy, life is better and everything is easier. Admittedly, no one is going to be happy all the time, but if you choose to be happy most of the time you will be. It will not only make you healthier, but will help you get through even the worst of times. The more you smile, laugh, and look on the bright side, the better your life will be.

One way to be happy is to have purpose in your life—pursuing what motivates you and what makes you feel excited. Think about what gives you the most satisfaction, and do something with it. Without purpose, life can be really dull, and your immune system will respond accordingly.

Knowing you can choose to be happy is liberating. You don't have to feel bad because you're getting older, or because your life isn't going exactly as you planned. Once you make your mind up to be happy, you actually don't have to feel bad for any reason.

How to Use Your Mind to End Cancer

The will to live is your most important medicine. A radical change in thought can bring about a radical change in your body. Remember, genes are obedient servants. The same gene can express in thousands of different ways, depending on what you ask it to do. When you change your thoughts, you change the instructions given to your genes, and that changes how your genes express. The same genetic code you have always had will now be interpreted differently, which can mean the difference between having cancer and not having cancer.

In reality, when it comes to your potential for health, *you* are in the driver's seat. What it comes down to is two things—*attention* and *intention*. To affect the physical world, you have to pay attention to what it is you want to change and then form an intention of how you would like it to change. This is the basis of the power of prayer. Spiritual practice has been known for millennia to bring about measurable changes in health. Dr. Larry Dossey, in his book, *Healing Words,* describes the benefit of prayer as "one of the best kept secrets in medical science." Dr. Dossey defines prayerfulness as a feeling of love, compassion, and empathy toward another, and he explains that prayer is a powerful and legitimate (if often overlooked) method of healing.

Numerous scientific experiments have now proven what many people have preached for thousands of years—attention and intention can change your physical world. Change is best achieved when people enter into a calm, meditative state and then focus their attention and intention on what they want. The meditative state is one in which normal thinking is suspended and you enter into the realm of pure awareness. If you haven't meditated in the past, it will take some practice to get rid of the mental chatter, quiet your mind, and focus, giving attention to your intention. Learning how to meditate is an investment in your future health, and every cancer patient should do it.

In short, miracles can happen when people are in a calm mental and emotional state and apply attention and intention in order to change the physical world around them. In fact, tumors have been observed to shrink dramatically within hours of holistic treatment when the patient is highly motivated. *When you change your consciousness from one of disease to one of health, you can't lose.*

When my body was in progressive deterioration during the depths of my illness with liver failure, autoimmune syndromes, chemical sensitivity, chronic fatigue, and many other problems, I began to realize that for survival, I needed to employ my mind as well as my body. I began quieting my mind and saying to myself over and over: *Every day, in every way, I get stronger and stronger and better and better.* I kept repeating these words until I could feel strength coming into my body. I gave it a lot of attention and intention.

At first, when I said this to myself, my mind fought back, saying, *That's a lie! You feel worse today than you did yesterday.* I realized my own thinking was negating my positive affirmations, so I began to reply to my mind by saying, *I know I am worse today, but I am giving you an instruction.*

Once I became comfortable giving my body instructions, my own objections began to disappear, and my body began to respond. I would say my affirmation, sometimes out loud, with passion and expectancy many times daily. After a few weeks, my subconscious mind began to implement the instructions. One day, after saying these affirmations, I felt the best that I had felt since the onset of my illness more than a year before. The feeling lasted only five or ten minutes, but the fact that it happened proved I was on the right path. Soon the feelings of strength came more often and lasted longer. My badly damaged immune system was responding!

I began to understand that the subconscious mind's reactions to the thoughts of the conscious mind can have a major impact on health or disease. The subconscious takes orders from the conscious mind and implements them. Minds do what they are programmed to do, even though much of that programming is unintended. I began to realize my power to influence my health simply by choosing the daily thoughts I was putting into my mind. By focusing on my illness, I had been putting thoughts of disease into my mind, thereby creating more disease. The mind is always working, so why not make it work *for* rather than *against* you? Keep your images and suggestions as positive, simple, clear, and concise as possible. Then repeat them as often as possible. Allow the subconscious to accept them as a "command." When the mind speaks, on some level, the body listens.

Love, compassion, spiritual awareness, and all the life-affirming and positive emotions have extremely powerful implications for health. While these complex and non-tangible concepts are often difficult to define, explain, or measure, they are perhaps the most "real" considerations in our lives. The will to live, choosing to be happy, and maintaining a state of inner peace and calm are keys to better heath and a cancer-free life. In fact, there are recorded cures of cancer patients who did little more than change their diet and reduce their stress by meditating for a few hours every day. Ian Gawler, author of *You Can Conquer Cancer*, writes of his own personal experience and how his cancer was cured through meditation. Regular meditation is known to reduce stress, reduce inflammation, help regulate blood sugar levels, and enhance immune function. Each of these is vital to preventing and reversing cancer.

Disease happens when the body is out of balance. The body has many "natural rhythms," including something called *heart rate variability*. Regular meditation helps to normalize these biological rhythms, bringing the body back into balance and good health. When the body's rhythms are rebalanced, fewer inflammatory chemicals are produced, more anti-inflammatory chemicals are produced, and NK cell activity is enhanced. This is why it is not a surprise that the health literature contains many cases of people curing their cancer though nothing more than diet and meditation. In truth, everyone should take time out to meditate every day. There are many good books on how to do this. What type of meditation you choose doesn't matter. Choose one that speaks to you, since they all take you to the same place and give you the same benefits.

Cancer is a complex disease. Because of this, we have to use every tool at our disposal to fight it. Your mind is one of the most powerful tools of all, and it doesn't cost anything to use it. Put it to work and choose happy, loving thoughts and the belief that you will get well. Letting this seep into your subconscious through relaxed meditation can work miracles.

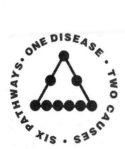

ONE DISEASE · TWO CAUSES · SIX PATHWAYS

7

THE PHYSICAL
PATHWAY

It is only in the past generation that most people have become sedentary.
. . . man has inherited an organism which is not adapted to such a life.

–Jean Mayer, Pan American Health Organization, 1971

One of the most powerful cures for cancer is streaming over
our heads each and every day, free of charge. It's sunlight. . . .
If it were a mainstream drug, it would probably make the cover
of *Time* magazine and be heralded as the greatest
medical breakthrough in the history of modern science.

—Mike Adams, Natural News.com 2006

The Physical Pathway addresses a world of physical factors that can have profound effects on your health. This includes how you breathe, the amount of physical activity you engage in, your electromagnetic exposure, the amount of sunlight and sleep you get, and even the amount of noise you are exposed to. You may be amazed to see the enormous impact these physical factors can have on the cancer process—best of all, you have control over them.

As I have said before, cancer is a complex disease. There are a lot of factors involved in switching on the cancer process, and that combination of factors can be different for every person. On the Physical Pathway, like on any of the Six Pathways, the more things you do right to support normal cell chemistry, the more you will move yourself toward health and away from disease.

Exercise

An active lifestyle not only lowers your risk of getting cancer, it also reduces the risk of cancer coming back. As you now know, your health depends on giving your cells the nutrition they need and protecting them from toxins that can interfere with their metabolic machinery. However, here is another factor: *the need to move and stretch your cells.*

Moving and stretching cells facilitates the delivery of nutrients and the removal of toxins, addressing both deficiency and toxicity. Ever notice that bedridden people get sicker? Movement is life. If you aren't moving, you are dying. In addition to helping deliver nutrients and promoting detoxification, exercise balances hormones, reduces inflammation, and improves immune function. You can't do without it. Cancer patients should get as much exercise as they possibly can.

While almost half of all Americans will develop cancer in their lifetime, only 14 percent of those who are physically active will develop cancer, and *thirty minutes of exercise every other day has been shown to cut the risk of breast cancer by 75 percent.* The Harvard Nurses' Health Study, started in 1976 and expanded in 1989, is one the largest and longest running investigations of factors that influence women's health; it has shown that regular exercise after a breast cancer diagnosis can reduce the risk of death from this disease. Exercise is a wonder drug!

Here is how this wonder drug works: It helps to block the prime cause of cancer, oxygen deficiency, by providing more oxygen to tissues. Exercise helps to balance hormones by reducing the excess of estrogens and testosterone that are known to promote breast, prostate, uterine, ovarian, and testicular cancers. High blood sugar and insulin drive cancer. Exercise reduces insulin and blood sugar levels, starving cancer cells of the food they desperately need to stay alive and grow. IGF (insulin-like growth factor), which contributes to inflammation and to tumor growth, is also reduced. Exercise also lowers the amount of inflammatory cytokines in the blood, which cause and drive cancer. Exercise pumps the lymph system, improves lymph flow and promotes the removal of toxic wastes from the body. In addition, exercise supports the immune system, stimulating natural killer (NK) cell activity. NK cell activity is critical to preventing and curing cancer. People with the lowest NK cell activity not only have the most cancer, they have the most aggressive cancers, and these are the same people cancer is most likely to kill. There isn't a drug or a medical treatment in the world that can do all this! Best of all, this miracle treatment doesn't cost you a dime. The American Cancer Society recommends at least thirty minutes of moderate to vigorous physical activity five or more days a week.

Historically, getting the physical activity that we need for good health was not a problem because our work required that we moved. Now, however, we are the most sedentary people in history, and our health is failing. All exercise is good, whether it is walking, swimming, or tennis, but with our busy lifestyles, many people say they can't find the time to exercise. Fortunately, there is a way to cheat—a form of exercise that virtually anyone can do at home, and it is extremely effective. *Rebounding* is a unique form of exercise that involves bouncing up and down on a mini-trampoline—and its effects are almost magical. It is simple, surprisingly easy to do, safe, a lot of fun, and it can be done by almost anyone regardless of age or physical condition. You can rebound while you watch the evening news or while talking on the telephone. Rebounding tones, conditions, strengthens, and heals the entire body in as little as fifteen minutes per day, although more is better.

Jumping up and down on a rebounder moves and stretches every cell in your body simultaneously, so it is a concentrated form of exercise. When you bounce on a rebounder, your entire body (internal organs, bones, connective tissue, and skin) becomes stronger, more flexible, and healthier. Blood circulation, oxygen delivery, lymphatic drainage, and toxin removal are vastly improved.

Visualize for a moment a balloon filled with water. Hold the balloon by its stem and observe how gravity pulls on the water, slightly stretching the balloon. Now move your hand rapidly up and down and observe how the extra gravitational force causes the balloon to significantly stretch and distort. When you bounce up and down on a rebounder, this is what happens to every cell in your body—cells are like little, microscopic water balloons. Rebounding alternately puts pressure on and takes pressure off of body cells, like squeezing a sponge. This moving and stretching of the cells facilitates nutrient delivery and toxin removal, which is exactly what you need to be healthy. All of this without having to take the time to go to the gym, work up a sweat, or end up with sore muscles and possible injuries. One caveat is that poor quality rebounders may shock the joints and tissues and cause injury. Look for barrel springs that are fatter in the middle and tapered at the ends.

Breathing

Oxygen metabolism in the body is complex, depending on numerous factors regarding how you deliver oxygen to your cells, including how you breathe. Deep breathing supplies more oxygen, and shallow breathing less. Most of us do shallow breathing.

Since cancer is an oxygen deficiency disease, a first line of defense against cancer is proper breathing, taking oxygen into our lungs so it can be supplied to our cells and tissues. Failure to breathe correctly deprives our cells of needed oxygen and changes our body chemistry.

Just as we can control what foods we eat, the toxins we are exposed to, the thoughts we put into our mind, and how much exercise we get, we can also control how we breathe and how much oxygen we supply to our body. The way you breathe can substantially affect how you look and feel, your resistance to disease, and even how long you live. Proper breathing technique will help to optimize your health as well as keep you relaxed and more mentally alert.

We were all born knowing how to breathe. However, the stress of modern living has caused many people to develop poor breathing habits. The most common problem is shallow or rapid breathing, also called *overbreathing*. Despite the name, overbreathing actually results in less oxygen being available to cells. Overbreathing is usually caused by *stress,* and it manifests as shallow chest breathing, irregular breathing, rapid breathing, or holding of the breath. On occasion, overbreathing is not a problem, and we all do it. Yet the stress of modern life causes many of us to breathe too rapidly, more times per minute than we should, and take breaths that are too shallow.

Overbreathing causes constriction of the blood vessels. This can result in up to a 50 percent reduction of oxygen and glucose to the brain—immediately affecting one's ability to learn, think, remember, and perform physically. Many people feel dizzy or lightheaded when stressed, due to oxygen shortage. By causing an oxygen shortage at the cellular level, numerous side effects can be experienced, including heart palpitations, irregular heartbeat, dizziness, muscle spasms, muscle fatigue, high blood pressure, poor memory, asthma attacks, poor concentration, anxiety, and other symptoms. Most importantly, an oxygen shortage at the cellular level causes cancer.

Overbreathing not only causes an oxygen deficiency, it also causes a carbon dioxide deficiency. Rapid breathing causes the body to lose too much carbon dioxide; the body needs to maintain normal levels of both oxygen and carbon dioxide. Oxygen is transported to tissues by bonding with hemoglobin in red blood cells. Normal oxygen respiration creates carbon dioxide as a metabolic waste product. Local concentrations of carbon dioxide signal the red blood cells to release their oxygen so your cells can obtain a new supply of oxygen. When you expel too much carbon dioxide through rapid breathing, there is insufficient carbon dioxide present to cause the hemoglobin to release its oxygen. Your cells and tissues then become oxygen-deficient. *This is another way by which stress causes cancer.*

When you are breathing carbon dioxide out too fast, your blood ends up with too little acid-forming carbon dioxide, which causes the pH of your blood to become too alkaline. To rebalance blood pH, the body takes alkaline minerals out of the blood and dumps them in the urine. The chronic loss of alkaline minerals, such as calcium and magnesium, creates a deficiency in the cells. While losing alkaline minerals helps to balance blood pH, the mineral loss from the cells makes the fluid inside your cells too acidic, and also contributes to osteoporosis. Acidic cells compromise your ability to obtain and use oxygen, creating a deficiency of oxygen respiration and causing cancer.

To breathe correctly, it is important to bring air *down* into the lungs, by using the *diaphragm,* a deep abdominal muscle that nature intended for breathing. Breathing downward with the diaphragm (belly breathing instead of chest breathing) is an effortless and efficient way to breathe. Unfortunately, people often use their chest and upper back to breathe; chest breathing takes more effort and is less efficient. Breathing downwards (as opposed to outwards with the chest) moves the viscera (guts) down and away, making more room for the lungs. This creates the capacity for more air in your lungs and more oxygen for your tissues, whether you are exercising *or* at rest. Each breath should begin downwards in the belly, only moving up into the chest when necessary.

Correct breathing should be effortless, through the nose rather than mouth, and relatively slow—at a resting rate of less than 15 breaths per minute, preferably 8 to 10. Here is a simple test to check how you are doing: Relax and count the number breaths you take per minute. Lie on your back on the floor, put a book on your abdomen, breathe through your nose, and watch to see if the book goes up and down with each breath. Concentrate on "belly breathing" until the book moves up and down. Count the number of breaths and try to keep breaths per minute less than 15 and preferably less than 10. The key word is *effortless*. Let your body do the breathing for you, as it was designed to do. During aerobic exercise, keep the breath down in the belly and out of the chest as much as possible. Breathing has such profound effects, both physically and psychologically, it is little surprise that many ancient traditions—such as meditation, yoga, and martial arts—rely first and foremost on breathing technique. Daily deep-breathing exercises are very calming and will help to keep you oxygenated and healthy.

Sunlight

Sunlight not only prevents cancer, it helps to reverse cancer. Sunlight is like a magic elixir for the body. It's one of nature's most powerful healing agents. Our ancestors were out in the sun all the time, and they didn't get cancer. Yet we are repeatedly advised to avoid the sun. This bad advice has cost countless thousands of lives by perpetrating an epidemic of vitamin D deficiency and all the many diseases resulting from that deficiency including: heart disease, multiple sclerosis, osteoporosis, type 1 diabetes, infections, autoimmune diseases, depression, asthma, and cancer. Science doesn't even begin to understand all the marvelous benefits of sunlight, yet the disease industry continues to perpetuate the myth that the sun causes cancer. Exactly the opposite is true. Cells have light-activated receptors that, when triggered, initiate a number of beneficial and cancer protective biological reactions. Scientists are beginning to examine whether the acupuncture meridians function as a photon transfer system, resembling fiber optics, delivering light throughout the body.

Vitamin D plays a critical role in preventing cancer. It is one of our most important nutrients, and we were designed to get up to 90 percent of our vitamin D through the interaction of sunlight with cholesterol-like compounds in our skin. If sunlight were bad for us, why would Mother Nature make us dependent on it? We are designed to need sunlight, and the more sunlight you get, the healthier you will be, with less risk of getting cancer. In fact, cancer is more prevalent in northern latitudes where less sunlight is available. Northerners get more of all kinds of vitamin D deficiency diseases. More than 40 percent of the American population is deficient in vitamin D, and that goes up to about 60 percent by the end of the winter. One reason flu spreads so quickly in the winter is because people are vitamin D deficient, and vitamin D is crucial to immune function.

Vitamin D acts like a hormone and interacts with genes, giving them crucial instructions that prevent cancer. Without sufficient vitamin D, the risk of cancer skyrockets. Research indicates that people with the lowest blood levels of vitamin D are four times more likely to die of colon cancer. Likewise, a 2008 study in *Carcinogenesis* found that women with breast cancer were three times more likely to have low vitamin D levels.

Caution! This is not an invitation to rush out and get sunburned. Sunburn damages DNA and can cause cancer. Too much of a good thing can be bad for you. People with light skins need less sunlight than those with dark skins. In fact, people with dark skins need a lot more sunlight to get the same benefits. Use the sun sensibly. Don't abuse it and it will be your partner in health. When your skin starts getting pink, get out of the sun. It is best to get sun as often as possible in small, graduated doses. When outdoors for long periods of time, wear protective clothing and a wide brimmed hat.

Modern research shows that sunlight nourishes and energizes the human body, and helps in the prevention of infections from bacteria, molds, and viruses. Sunlight enhances the immune system by increasing white blood cell count as well as gamma globulin, a protein that helps the body fight infection. Significantly, sunlight stimulates the production of more red blood cells, increasing the oxygen content of the blood, which helps to prevent and reverse cancer.

Sunlight is also good for the heart. It enables the body to lower the resting pulse rate, lower blood pressure, and lower cholesterol as well as triglycerides in the blood. In fact, sunlight may decrease cholesterol by more than 30 percent. It also enhances the power of the skin to resist diseases such as psoriasis, eczema, and acne. Sunlight also lowers blood sugar and enhances liver function. It stimulates the liver to produce an enzyme that increases your ability to detoxify environmental pollutants. Further, sunlight stimulates the pineal gland to produce vital brain chemicals such as tryptamines, which cheer you up and prevent anxiety and depression.

Do not use sunscreens—sunscreens block out essential wavelengths, and most sunscreen products are toxic, even carcinogenic. Dating from antiquity, approaches to protecting against sun damage are using high-quality olive oil or coconut oil on your skin.

Even manmade light can be helpful. A 2002 study in the *International Journal of Molecular Medicine* found that exposure to dichromatic blue light for two 20-minute sessions per day inhibited the growth of melanoma cells.

Electromagnetic Fields

There is a growing body of evidence indicating that brain cancer is only one of the many health problems produced by our new wireless society. Invisible to the human eye, electromagnetic fields

(EMFs) are present everywhere in our environment. The human body is electromagnetic in nature, and its electrical system, which relays signals in nerves and stimulates heartbeats, is affected by external EMFs, increasingly coming from Wi-Fi networks, cordless phones, cell phones, and cell phone towers. Over the last century, exposure to manmade EMFs has been increasing steadily as growing demand for electricity, ever-advancing technologies, and changes in social behavior have created more and more artificial sources. At home and at work, from the generation and transmission of electricity to domestic appliances and industrial equipment, to telecommunications and broadcasting, all of us are now exposed to a complex mix of electric and magnetic fields.

Increasingly, people are becoming electromagnetically sensitive. It is estimated that 3 to 8 percent of the population in developed countries now experience serious electrohypersensitivity symptoms, while 35 percent experience mild symptoms. Some people can be totally debilitated just by walking into a Wi-Fi equipped area. One symptom of electrohypersensitivity is altered sugar metabolism similar to diabetes. In fact, some researchers believe we even have a new kind of diabetes caused by electromagnetic sensitivity. A groundbreaking study in a 2010 issue of the *European Journal of Oncology* found that cordless phones can interfere with your heart, causing abnormal rhythms. Dr. Thomas Rau, medical director of the world-renowned Paracelsus Clinic in Switzerland says in an interview at www.ElectromagneticHealth.org that he is convinced that electromagnetic loads lead to concentration problems, ADD, tinnitus, migraines, insomnia, arrhythmia, Parkinson's, and *cancer.*

The human body is an electromagnetic device, and it produces its own weak electromagnetic field. Cell membranes act as capacitors to store voltage and as semiconductors, diodes, and microprocessors, which control cell function by interacting with the environment. Anyone who understands how profound these facts are won't even question the fact that we are affected by external electromagnetic fields. The real questions are what effects EMFs have, how long the effects last, and how harmful they might be. The effects of EMFs are difficult to study; there are so many variables involved. However, you need to be aware of at least some of what we do know.

A 2007 study in the *Internal Medicine Journal* looked at a database of 850 patients diagnosed with lymphatic and bone marrow cancers between 1972 and 1980. The study found that living next to high-voltage power lines increased the risk of cancer. People who lived within 328 yards of a power line up to age five were five times more likely to develop cancer. In addition, people who lived that close to a power line at any point during their first fifteen years were three times more likely to develop cancer as adults. The study concluded that living for a prolonged period near high-voltage power lines is likely to increase the risk of leukemia, lymphoma, and related conditions later in life. The power industry had dismissed safety concerns after previous, short-term studies failed to show increased cases of leukemia in children living near power lines. This 2007 study is significant because it establishes that the cancer shows up in adults who were exposed as children. Obviously, these are long-lasting effects. Based on this study and others, it would be prudent not to live, work, or go to school within 300 yards of a high-voltage power line.

EMFs present challenges for those wishing to prevent cancer. We are all exposed to EMFs in our daily living. We can't escape them. Electromagnetic pollution may be the single largest change we have made to our environment. Cell phones, computer screens, TV sets, hair dryers, refrigerators, dishwashers, and even the clock radio by the side of your bed are putting out unhealthy levels of EMFs. Driving your car exposes you to a lot of EMFs. While we have little personal control over many of the EMFs in our environment, such as radio and TV broadcasts, there are some we have a great deal of control over. Cell phone use is one example. A Swedish study in a 2006 *International Archives of Occupational and Environmental Health* has found that heavy users of cell phones had a 240 percent increase in brain tumors on the side of their head on which the phone was used. The study defined heavy use as more than 2,000 total hours, or approximately one hour of use per workday for ten years. This is a good reason to limit cell phone use and to use the speakerphone option to avoid holding the phone next to your head. In 2007, the European Environment Agency, the official environmental watchdog of the European Union, warned that cell phone technology "could lead to a health crisis similar to those caused by asbestos, smoking, and lead in petrol."

Tragically, more and more children and teens are using cell phones. In the United States, nine out of ten sixteen-year-olds have their own cell phones, as do many primary schoolchildren. It is noteworthy that brain cancer has now surpassed leukemia as the number one cancer killer in children. The incidence of pediatric brain cancers in Australia has increased 21 percent in just one decade.

Because the negative effects of cell phone usage are not immediate, people think cell phones are safe. While cell phones have been used heavily for less than twenty years, it can take up to thirty years for brain tumors to develop as a result of their use. Children, however, are more susceptible to cell phone damage because their cells are still reproducing more rapidly. Their brains and nervous systems are still developing, and their skulls are thinner. A 2007 study in *Occupational and Environmental Medicine* by Dr. Lennart Hardell, a professor in oncology and cancer epidemiology in Sweden, found that teenagers with heavy use of cell phones have 500 percent more brain cancer as young adults, and that young people who used the cordless phones found in many homes had rates almost as great—more than 400 percent higher than those who avoided their use. In Europe and the U.K. the incidence of brain tumors has increased by 40 percent over the last twenty years. Some researchers are predicting an epidemic of brain cancer as cell phone use continues to grow.

Here is what Dr. Hardell had to say about cell phone use in general:

What we did find was an increased risk for tumors in the temporal area of the brain . . . on the same side as the person had used the mobile phone. We found overall an increased risk of 30 percent for brain tumors, increasing for those who had used the mobile phone for over 10 years to 80 percent increased risk. This is a significant finding.

Adding to our concerns, Israeli scientist Dr. Siegal Sadetzki concluded in a study published in a 2008 *American Journal of Epidemiology* that there is a link between cell phone usage and the development of cancer of the salivary glands. Heavy cell phone users were found to have an increased risk of about 50 percent for developing a tumor of the main salivary, compared to those who did not use cell phones. Other studies have indicated risks beyond brain and salivary tumors, finding cognitive problems, disorientation, eye damage, bone damage, Alzheimer's, and others.

Research sponsored by the telecommunications industry, found an almost 300 percent increase in the incidence of genetic damage when human blood cells were exposed to cell phone radiation. Dr.

Ronald B. Herberman, the head of the University of Pittsburgh Cancer Institute, has testified before the U.S. House Subcommittee on Domestic Policy that regular cell phone use doubles the risk of brain cancer. After reviewing the existing data, Dr. Herberman now advises against using cell phones in public places because it exposes other people to the hazardous EMFs that you are generating. Cell phones not only affect the user but, like secondhand smoke, also affect those around the user. Children especially should be protected from this EMF pollution; cell phones should not be used in close proximity to children. In 2009, Dr. Herberman issued an unprecedented warning to his faculty and staff: *Limit cell phone use because of the health risks.*

Lloyd Morgan, a director of the Central Brain Tumor Registry of the United States and one of the authors of the International EMF Collaborative's report, "Cell Phones and Brain Tumors: 15 Reasons for Concern," said: "Exposure to cell phone radiation is the largest human health experiment ever undertaken, without informed consent, and has some 4 billion participants enrolled. . . . I fear we will see a tsunami of brain tumors, although it is too early to see that now since the tumors have a thirty-year latency. I pray I'm wrong, but brace yourself."

In an April 16, 2010, interview in Lanka Journal newspaper, Dr. Vini Khurana, an associate professor of neurosurgery at the Australian National University, who had conducted a fifteen-month study of the link between mobile phones and malignant brain tumors, said that mobile phone radiation could heat the side of the head and thermoelectrically interact with the brain. He also said that Bluetooth devices and unshielded headsets could "convert the user's head into an effective, potentially self-harming antenna."

Studies in other nations confirm that living close to cell phone towers damages health. German researchers reporting in a 2004 *Umwelt Medizin Gesellschaft* found that people living within 1,200 feet of a cell tower experienced high cancer rates and developed their tumors on average eight years earlier than the national average. Breast cancer topped the list. Spanish researchers reporting in a 2003 *Biology and Medicine* found that people living within 1,000 feet of cellular antennas developed illnesses at average power densities of only 0.11 to 0.19 microwatts per centimeter, which is thousands of times lower than those allowed by international exposure standards. Researchers in Israel reported in a 2004 *International Journal of Cancer Prevention* that people who lived near a cell tower for three to seven years had a cancer rate four times higher than the control population. People living close to cell phone towers suffer extreme sleep disruption, chronic fatigue, nausea, skin problems, irritability, brain disturbances, and cardiovascular problems.

Rooftop transmitters, which readily pass microwave radiation into structures, can be especially dangerous. Across the world there are reports of cancer clusters and extreme illness in office buildings and multitenant dwellings where antennas are placed. In 2006, the top floors of a University of Melbourne office building were closed after a brain tumor cluster drew media attention to the risks of microwave communications transmitters on top of the building. Radiation in living spaces near cell phone transmitters has been measured at up to 65 microwatts per square centimeter; the FCC's maximum safety limit is 580 microwatts, so people are told the cell towers are safe. However, this can't be true! The Spanish researchers above found problems at 0.11 to 0.19 microwatts, and then remember that during the cold war the Soviets bombarded the U.S. embassy in Moscow with a constant 0.01 microwatts of microwave radiation, and this made international news because of all the health problems it caused at the embassy.

Countless Wi-Fi systems, both indoors and out, accommodate wireless laptop computers, personal digital assistants, Wi-Fi-enabled phones, gaming devices, video cameras, even parking and utility meters. Hundreds of cities already have or are planning to fund Wi-Fi networks, each consisting of thousands of small microwave transmitters bolted to buildings, street lamps, park benches, bus stops, and even buried under sidewalks. All this has been planned with virtually no studies or warning signs about radiation exposure. Not a single environmental or public health study has been required as the industry unleashes this new wireless technology from which no living thing will escape.

Dr. Robert Becker, author of *The Body Electric: Electromagnetism And The Foundation Of Life,* is noted for his decades of research on the effects of electromagnetic pollution. He warns: "Even if we survive the chemical and atomic threats to our existence, there is the strong possibility that increasing electropollution could set in motion irreversible changes leading to our extinction before we are even aware of them."

To prevent cancer, limit your cell phone use to only the most essential calls, and then limit the call to less than two minutes. Cell phones are a fact of life. They aren't going to go away. The challenge is to use them sensibly. Make no nonessential phone calls. When cell phones are on they are emitting radiation, even when you are not using them. Do not carry a cell phone close to your body while it is on. Keep your phone turned off when it is not being used; turn it on as needed to check for messages. Do not hold a phone next to your brain. Use the speakerphone feature to make your calls, keeping the phone as far away as possible. Keep children away from the immediate vicinity when you make a call. Do not allow children under the age of eighteen to use a cell phone except in emergencies. Use of cell phones inside buildings or in cars increases cancer risk, because it increases the radiation a phone must emit in order to function. Don't live within 1,200 feet of a cell phone antenna. Use of text messages and nonwireless headsets can reduce, but not eliminate, cancer risk. The evidence is becoming overwhelming that cell phone use is hazardous to your health, but do not count on the government to protect you. Federal exposure limits have been deliberately set so high that no matter how much additional wireless radiation is added to the national burden, it will always be "within standards."

When buying a home or choosing an apartment, choose one that is not immediately adjacent to high voltage transmission lines, cell phone towers, or transformers. Be prudent in the use of appliances. When possible, use rechargeable battery-powered appliances rather than plug-in models. Do not stand immediately next to an electrical appliance when it is turned on, especially for an extended period of time. Turn on the dishwasher when finished in the kitchen and you are ready to leave the room. Avoid electric blankets or use them only to warm up the bed before you get in it. Keep telephone answering machines and electric clocks away from your head while you are sleeping. Increase distance from televisions (at least six feet away) and avoid appliances that come into close contact with your body such as hairdryers and nonbattery electric razors.

Sleep

Getting a good night's sleep is essential to good health and another piece of the puzzle to prevent and cure cancer. The body is designed for certain sleep patterns, and disturbing those patterns can seriously alter the balance of hormones in your body. The reality is our bodies have been programmed over millennia to sleep when it's dark and be awake during daylight. This is how our ancestors lived, and if you do otherwise, you are sending conflicting signals to the body, upsetting its normal biochemistry and balance.

Unfortunately, a good night's sleep is increasingly losing out to late-night TV, the Internet, e-mails and the other distractions of modern life. According to a poll by the National Sleep Foundation, the majority of Americans are not getting enough sleep. Only 40 percent of the respondents reported getting a good night's sleep every night, or almost every night. Lawrence Epstein, past president of the American Academy of Sleep Medicine and author of *The Harvard Medical School Guide to a Good Night's Sleep* said, "We have in our society this idea that you can just get by without sleep or manipulate when you sleep without any consequences. What we're finding is that's just not true."

The necessary amount of sleep varies from person to person. Some people function quite well on just a few hours of sleep, while others barely function without getting a full ten hours. Most people need between seven and nine hours. Recent research indicates that, for the majority of us, sleeping less than eight hours a night has significant cumulative consequences.

People who get less than six hours are at greatly increased risk for disease. Adequate sleep is necessary for good health, and lack of sleep can cause and drive cancer. There is even a strong risk to overall mortality. A study by Harvard Medical School of over 82,000 nurses participating in The Nurses' Health Study found that getting less than six hours sleep per night increases the risk of premature death. Links have also been discovered between too little sleep and diabetes, obesity, hypertension, and high cholesterol.

The picture that is emerging is that not sleeping enough, being awake in the early-morning hours or waking up frequently at night throws the body's internal clock out of whack. "Lack of sleep

disrupts every physiologic function in the body," said Dr. Eve Van
Cauter of the University of Chicago in an October 9, 2005 article in
the *Washington Post*. She went on to say, "We have nothing in our
biology that allows us to adapt to this behavior."

Sleep regulates hormone balance, and hormone balance is essential to health. Studies indicate that lack of sleep increases the production of stress hormones, and stress hormones both cause and
drive cancer. Cortisol is one of the hormones affected. Cortisol
helps to regulate the release of natural killer cells that help the body
battle cancer. Cortisol needs to be properly balanced, but night
shift workers have a shifted cortisol balance. People who wake up
frequently during the night are also more likely to have abnormal
cortisol rhythms that throw the body out of balance.

Melatonin is another hormone affected by sleep. Melatonin protects us from cancer and is known to interfere with tumor growth.
Melatonin also has antioxidant properties that help protect DNA
from cancer-causing mutations. The brain produces this hormone
during sleep. However, melatonin production is sensitive to the
amount of sleep we get and the amount of light we are exposed
to; this can be a problem, especially with the exploding number of
artificial light-producing electrical gadgets that are now part of our
daily lives. Many people keep these devices in close proximity during night hours and are continually exposed to light emissions during sleep that influence melatonin production. A wealth of research
is indicating this is increasing our risk of cancer.

Research shows that even the smallest amount of light from
devices such as iPods, laptops, electronic readers, and TV sets is
sufficient to cut melatonin production in half. This emphasizes the
importance of sleeping in a totally dark room to lower cancer risk.
Shift workers who are up all night produce less melatonin. Insuf-

ficient melatonin affects levels of other hormones and increases estrogen. High estrogen increases the risk of breast and prostate cancer. The truth is even minimal exposure to an artificial light source is sufficient to alter the expression of genes that are connected to the formation of cancer as well as of genes that assist in the fight against cancer. When melatonin production is delayed or halted by artificial light sources, our nighttime rhythms are disturbed and normal metabolic activity required for cellular repair is disrupted. The body requires seven to nine hours of uninterrupted sleep each night, with no light distraction, to complete the repair functions that are essential to maintaining optimal health.

Interfering with the body's natural rhythms is never a good idea—health is when the body is balanced and functioning normally. Female night-shift workers have higher rates of breast cancer than women who sleep normal hours, and they are more likely to have more rapid tumor growth and to die earlier from breast cancer. Tumors grow two to three times faster in laboratory animals with severe sleep dysfunctions. Because sleep helps to restore one's internal environment, people who sleep poorly or do not get enough sleep have higher levels of inflammation. People who get six or fewer hours of sleep typically measure higher levels of three inflammatory markers: fibrinogen, IL-6 (interleukin-6), and C-reactive protein. Chronic sleep problems result in chronic low-grade inflammation, and inflammation both causes and drives cancer.

Cell phones are another problem affecting sleep. A Swedish study published in the 2008 Progress in Electromagnetics Research Symposium Proceedings said there was now "more than sufficient evidence" to show that cell phone radiation delays and reduces sleep. Using cell phones before bed causes people to take longer to reach the deeper stages of sleep and to spend less time in them. Less time in the deeper stages of sleep interferes with the body's ability to do its daily repairs. Repair deficits impair your immune system, leaving you less able to fight off diseases of all kinds, as well as contributing to the aging process.

Despite what has been said above, there is no magic number of hours of sleep that covers everyone at every age and circumstance. Children and teens need more sleep than adults. Your sleep needs are individual to you, and you may require more or less sleep than someone of the same age, gender, and activity level. Listen to your body. To determine how much you need, make note of how you feel immediately upon awakening. If you still feel tired, you probably need more sleep. The first step in getting a good night's sleep is allowing yourself to do it. Stress is well known to interfere with sleep, and if you lose sleep, you won't be able to handle stress as well. This can lead to more stress and more loss of sleep in a vicious cycle.

If you are a cancer patient, you must make the time to go to bed by 10:00 PM in a dark and quiet environment and try to get a good eight hours of sleep. The body recharges the adrenal glands during the hours of 11:00 PM and 1:00 AM, which helps to balance your hormones, so you should be asleep during those hours. Adequate sleep is one of the most important factors in your health and quality of life, and it definitely influences cancer outcome.

Noise

Chronic noise has been linked to cancer through disrupted sleep patterns and the resulting hormonal imbalances. Research has proven that noise can cause health problems. Everything from aircraft traffic to barking dogs and loud music can interrupt sleep patterns and result in abnormal hormone secretions. One analysis at

Stanford University concluded that noise-caused sleep disruptions upset hormonal balance and created abnormal immune responses, resulting in cancer-supporting conditions. However, the damage caused by noise goes beyond sleep loss. For example, workers chronically exposed to loud noise suffered calcium and magnesium losses, which can be significant for the effect they have on a variety of health problems from osteoporosis to cancer.

The body reacts to noise by secreting inflammatory chemicals (cytokines). Some researchers believe that one reason cytokine production rises as we grow older is exposure to a lifetime of noise. Bottom line: noise disrupts normal hormone balance, normal immune response, and creates inflammation in the body. All of these support the cancer process.

We have created a society where noise is normal. This is just one of the fundamental changes we have made in our modern world, and it is one of the reasons why cancer is now normal. As much as possible, reduce the amount of noise in your life.

Things to Remember

Many factors switch on and drive the cancer process, and the factors in the Physical Pathway are among them. By controlling these factors in your favor, as well as those in the other five Pathways, you can move yourself toward a disease-free, cancer-free life.

- Be sure to get at least thirty minutes of exercise every other day as a minimum.
- Rebounding even twenty minutes a day as you watch TV or listen to music will do wonders for your health, and at no inconvenience.

- Watch your breathing throughout the day. Proper breathing will help you relax, lower your stress levels, and supply more oxygen to your cells.
- Get frequent sunlight on most of your body. When this is not possible, take a high-quality vitamin D supplement.
- Minimize your exposure to radiation of all kinds, from medical x-rays to cell phones to airport scanners (decline to go through the scanner; request a manual search).
- Go to bed before 11:00 PM, and try to get eight hours of sleep every night.
- Avoid noise, especially chronic, loud noise.

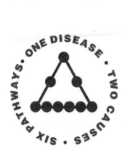

8

THE GENETIC
PATHWAY

Every year over 97% of your body is completely replaced,
even the structure of the DNA in your genes, reconstructed entirely from
the nutrients we eat. The quality of those nutrients determines
the quality of your renewed cellular structure, the level
at which it can function and its resistance to disease.

—*Dr. Michael Colgan, author of* The New Nutrition

Nutrition can alter the course of high risk genes, not only by turning these
genes off but also by inhibiting the resulting bad effects produced by them.

—*Russell L. Blaylock, M.D., author of* Health and Nutrition Secrets That Can Save Your Life

G enes are essential to life itself and play important roles in the cancer process. Research has proven that there are genes that turn cancer on, promoting its growth, and genes that turn cancer off, inhibiting its growth. However, there is still a lot of misunderstanding about genes and what they do or do not do.

Genes are like blueprints. They are a set of instructions that tell our bodies how to develop from one single cell into an entire human being. Only about one-quarter of our genes express (turn on) automatically, determining, for example, whether our eyes are blue or our hair is curly. Most genes merely offer a set of thousands of possibilities—what *can* happen, not what *will* happen. For something specific to happen, these genetic blueprints require an instruction, some sort of *trigger* (environmental or psychological), in order for them to choose which option to express. You are in control of these triggers through your diet, lifestyle, and thoughts. Therefore, you control your genes—including those that govern the cancer process.

Just because a certain trait, good or bad, runs in the family does *not* mean that every person in the family will possess that trait in their genes, or that they will express it even if they do possess it. We often worry far more than we need to about genetic inheritance. Are there genes that make you more susceptible to cancer? Yes. Will these genes cause cancer? No. They make the cancer process possible, but they don't cause it. To cause cancer, you have to do something to activate those cancer-promoting genes. They wait for you to tell them what to do. Unactivated, they sit there and do nothing. Consider that a century ago cancer affected only 3 percent of the American population. Now almost 50 percent of Americans will develop cancer in their lifetime. Our genes haven't changed in the last century, but our diet, environment, and lifestyle have changed radically. It is not possible to blame our increases in cancer on inherited genes. The real problem is we are giving different instructions to the genes.

Most important to whether or not you get cancer is the environment you create for your cells based on what you eat and how you live your life. You cannot control your heredity, but you *can* control the environment you create for your cells. The environment is a trigger that causes genes to express in different ways, and you are creating that environment every moment of every day. You are changing how your genes express with the foods you eat, the air you breathe, the water you drink, the toxins you expose yourself to, and the thoughts you think. *You* are in control of your health destiny.

Rather than thinking of genes as an absolute and unchanging set of instructions, one might think of them as a variety of possibilities—a set of "what if" instructions. *If* certain circumstances are present, *then* your genes will express in a particular way; if other circumstances are present, those same genes will express in a different way. Biochemist Roger Williams, author of *Nutrition Against Disease,* maintained that genes alone are entirely useless threads of chemicals. They alone do not determine our sickness or health. They act more like computer programs that sit dormant, essentially doing *nothing,* until you tell them what you want them to do.

Unfortunately, in today's world, we are telling our genes to give us cancer. We are damaging our genes, giving them improper instructions, and in every way possible causing them to malfunction in ways that cause the symptoms we call cancer. Not only are we instructing our genes to give us cancer, but through our wrong diet, exposure to toxins, stress, lack of sleep, and other factors, we are also shutting down the tumor suppressor genes that are there to protect us against cancer. We are doing everything just right to switch on and drive the cancer process.

To prevent or cure cancer, you have to:

• Stop damaging your genes
• Support DNA repair
• Give your genes the correct instructions

Genes are the blueprints of life, directing the initiation and termination of biological processes, including cell growth, apoptosis, angiogenesis, and the respiration process. Modern diets and lifestyles damage our genes, causing mutations. Genetic damage involves *changes* in the coding itself, different from changing the *expression* of existing genetic coding. When the DNA in a normal cell is damaged, this change in the metabolic software may favor the growth of cancer cells. A mutation is like a damaged computer program. The program will no longer work as originally intended. The operating instructions for oxygen respiration in the cell may be damaged, resulting in a deficiency of oxygen respiration, which leads to cancer.

Mutations caused by chemicals and radiation can cause dramatic and unpredictable changes in the coding. Genes are crucial plans for creating, repairing, and reproducing an organism. Randomly changing these plans is a bad idea. What would happen if you started making random changes to the blueprints for a house? Doors, windows, walls, and even whole rooms could end up in strange places. The house would no longer function normally; so it is with genetic damage.

Damaging genes with mutations is one way to alter genetic function; another is changing the instructions we give to normal, undamaged genes. Genes are obedient servants, doing what you ask. If you change what you ask for, you get different results. Genes will give you cancer if you ask for it, and if you want cancer to go away, you have to stop asking. There are mechanisms other than mutations that can inhibit oxygen respiration and cause cancer. One of these is *epigenetic* change, a change that alters the instructions given to the genes without altering the genes themselves. Such changes in gene expression are the result of diet, lifestyle, and exposure to environmental chemicals.

Epigenetic changes are turning out to be a big problem. We now know that environmental chemicals can cause cancer, even without causing actual mutations or structural damage to DNA. Certain chemicals react with DNA in ways that do not damage or mutate the gene, but alter the way the gene expresses, which can have a huge effect on gene behavior. For example, gene products that suppress cancer growth may not be produced, allowing cancer cells to grow out of control. Worse, there is evidence that these epigenetic changes may also be passed on to future generations. This is one more reason to make the effort to avoid exposing yourself to environmental toxins and to do what is necessary to reduce your existing toxic load.

Another cause of epigenetic changes is poor nutrition. A mother's malnutrition, without changing the genes themselves, can permanently alter the expression of genes in her offspring, including genes that influence susceptibility to cancer. Part of our cancer epidemic can be explained by our consumption of nutritionally deficient processed foods over several generations—even the nutrition of your grandparents can affect how your genes express and your susceptibility to disease. The toxins we are exposed to and what we eat have far-reaching consequences beyond the damage they do to ourselves and our own children. The future of the species is also being affected.

Inflammation damages DNA, causing mutations, and when there is a lot of inflammation, this damage exceeds the capacity of our DNA repair capabilities. Inflammation is a foundation stone of all chronic diseases, and cancer is totally dependent on it. Inflammation produces what we call "oxidative damage," which plays a huge role in the cancer process, activating cancer genes and facilitating the spread of cancer. Inflammation can be controlled with a good diet, minimizing toxins, managing stress, and antioxidant supplementation.

Stop Damaging Genes

There are genes that slow cell division (tumor suppressor genes) and those that speed it (proto-oncogenes). Such genetic on/off switches help to keep the body balanced. Damage to these genes can result in the uncontrolled growth of cells, which is cancer. To protect yourself from DNA mutations, limit your exposure to things that are known to damage DNA such as:

- *Ionizing radiation*: About half the average person's exposure to ionizing radiation comes from *diagnostic x-rays* and *medical radiation treatments*. Avoid this kind of radiation unless absolutely necessary. It is paradoxical that physicians, who put so much stock in the genetic origins of disease, inflict massive amounts of genetic damage with toxic pharmaceutical drugs and radiation.
- *Nonionizing radiation*: Such radiation, while not causing mutations, may also have genetic repercussions. As a general rule, avoid close proximity or prolonged exposure to all types of

electrical devices, electrical boxes, transformers, cell phones, cell phone towers, and high-voltage power lines.

- *Toxins*: These include man-made industrial chemicals, prescription drugs, tobacco, and chemical residues in meat and dairy products such as hormones, PCBs and dioxins. Foods heated to high temperatures or blackened (such as in barbecuing) contain chemicals capable of causing gene mutations and cancer.

Ionizing radiation damages DNA and is directly carcinogenic; we know with certainty that the x-rays used for mammograms cause breast cancer. Our physicians and dentists have irresponsibly exposed us to radiation, and that has been a major contributor to our cancer epidemic. Up to 90 percent of x-rays are not medically justified. Decline all routine x-rays, and allow only those x-rays that are absolutely necessary.

Exposure to environmental toxins can damage DNA, causing mutations that can permanently alter the way cells work, and such damage can also damage a cell's ability to recognize and repair faulty DNA. In other words, toxins can even damage the instructions that operate your DNA repair machinery. Numerous natural and man-made chemicals have been identified as causing genetic mutations and cancer. In a matter of minutes, exposure to these chemicals can potentially cause permanent damage to DNA. Such chemicals include many common household products, pharmaceuticals, pesticides, herbicides, food additives, fluoride, and metals such as mercury and lead. We live in a sea of carcinogens and must learn how to avoid them.

To avoid carcinogens, avoid foods heated to high temperatures, and especially food that has been blackened. They contain powerful carcinogens, including *benzopyrene* and *heterocyclic amines*.

Benzopyrene binds to DNA and causes severe genetic mutation. Heterocyclic amines are the most abundant carcinogen in fried meats. Women with high intakes of grilled, smoked, or barbecued meats are 75 percent more likely to develop breast cancer, and there is a 60 percent increased risk of pancreatic cancer in those who like their meat well-done. Peanuts and corn products are often moldy and high in aflatoxins, which are potent carcinogens. Avoid fluoride contaminated tap water, toothpaste, and processed foods because fluoride inhibits DNA repair enzymes.

If DNA is damaged and not repaired before the cell divides to form a new cell, the damage will become permanent and show up in all the new cells. The effects of this can range from minor to devastating, as the damage is cumulative. If genetic mutations take place in a sex cell, there is a 50/50 chance of passing these on to future generations. Damaged cells and genes can lead to premature aging and a variety of conditions including fatigue, poor resistance to infections, psychological stress, social maladjustment, and cancer.

Inherited genes are not causing our epidemic of premature aging, disease, and cancer; it is damage to our genes that is causing these problems. Life in the twenty-first century is now damaging our genes and creating mutations in unprecedented ways and at an alarming rate. Due to our poor diets, exposure to carcinogenic chemicals, and x-rays, most of our older population and many of our younger people now have clusters of cancer cells throughout their bodies. Given the right conditions, these cells will grow and then metastasize. The full development of cancer usually takes between five and forty years.

Fortunately, genetic damage can be repaired. Not only must we avoid damaging our genes in the first place, we also must provide our genes with the raw materials (nutrients) they need to repair themselves.

Support DNA Repair

Genes are damaged all the time. This is normal, and it is why we have DNA repair systems. However, due to our poor diets and our massive exposure to toxins and radiation, our DNA repair systems are having a difficult time keeping up with all the damage. Critical DNA repairs are not getting done, and sometimes the genetic damage even disables the repair machinery itself.

Certain nutrients are known to support the DNA repair process. These include vitamins B3, B6, B12, and folate, as well as zinc and L-carnitine. Most Americans are deficient in these nutrients. According to the USDA, 73 percent of Americans are deficient in zinc, 40 percent are deficient in B12, and 80 percent are deficient in B6. Supplementing your diet with high-quality supplements is essential. You have to supply the nutrients the body needs to do its job or the job will go undone, and you will accelerate the aging process, enable the cancer process, and get sick.

Giving Your Genes the Correct Instructions

When turned on, a single gene is capable of producing as many as 30,000 different proteins, each of which has a different role in the body and creates a different outcome. What determines which protein the gene will produce? The instructions it receives from its environment—and *you* create that environment. In one way or another, *you tell your genes when to turn on or off, which proteins to produce, and when to produce them.* You are in control!

A lot of people think that genes cause cancer, that cancer runs in their family, and therefore they are going to get cancer. This is an old way of thinking, and it is wrong. A study of twins, reported in a 2000 *New England Journal of Medicine,* concluded, "The over-whelming contributor to the causation of cancer in the populations of twins that we studied was the environment." The *environment* you create for your genes is far more important than the genes themselves in determining whether or not you get cancer.

The environment gives the genes instructions telling them how to express. If we think about genes as computer programs, computer programs are designed to do specific tasks such as word processing, e-mails, spreadsheets, or computer games. Within its intended area of function, each program is capable of doing a variety of different tasks, depending on what you ask it to do. The chemical environment you create inside each cell determines what you ask your genes to do.

You create those environments with your diet and lifestyle. Your level of physical activity, and the amount of sunlight, fresh air, and sleep you get all influence the chemical environment produced in each cell. The pH inside your cells, the amount of sodium in your cells, the amount and kind of toxins in your cells, the hormones and hormone-like chemicals you have consumed, the electromagnetic environment you're exposed to, and your thoughts, beliefs, and emotions all create an environment that interacts with your unique set of genes to tell them what to do, resulting in how they express. One way or another, all this is under your control.

Hormones are genetic switches, activating certain genes and inac-tivating certain others. If you want to control cancer, it is extremely important that you normalize hormone balance. The correct hor-mone balance is cancer protective, and the wrong balance will speed the growth of cancer. Hormone balance is why getting the right amount of sleep is so important and why stress hormones can kill you. One reason why sugar is such a dangerous toxin is because it unbalances your hormones. It is also why consuming meat and dairy products, and the hormones they contain, contributes to cancer.

Scientists have discovered that vitamin D directly influences over 200 genes. Included are genes connected to cancer and autoimmune maladies like multiple sclerosis. This illustrates how grave vitamin D deficiency can be, and by the end of winter, more than half of all Americans are vitamin D deficient.

Studies have shown that lifestyle changes among cancer patients involving diet, exercise, and human interaction can and will alter the expression of hundreds of cancer-related genes in a healthy direction. Meanwhile, stress hormones have been found to change gene expression for the worse. Further, stress hormones affect virtually every cell in the body, and the negative programming can remain even after the hormones have returned to their normal levels. In other words, whether you are mentally stressed or able to maintain a more positive outlook can influence the expression of your genes, and thus directly impact your capacity to develop, avoid, or cure cancer.

Ultimately what matters is not what genes you have, but how they are expressed. You don't have control over which genes you inherited, but you do have control over how they express. Through your lifestyle choices, you tell your genes to turn on or off and which proteins to produce and when to produce them. It can be said that genes run your life, but you run your genes—*so you run your life.*

Things to Remember

To prevent and reverse cancer, stop damaging your genes, support your DNA repair, and give your genes health-enhancing instructions. These recommendations are important to keep in mind because genes play an essential role in cancer. As we know, cancer is uncontrolled cell growth. There are genes that regulate cellular proliferation, but they have to be given the correct instructions. To make sure these genes operate normally, maintain healthy thoughts and emotions and keep your internal cell chemistry in balance through proper nutrition and the avoidance of toxins. The accumulation of mutations in genes damages their ability to control cell growth and is one reason why cancer rates rise with age. Protecting yourself from epigenetic changes and DNA mutations is critical for preventing disease and prolonging life.

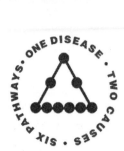

ONE DISEASE · TWO CAUSES · SIX PATHWAYS

9

THE MEDICAL PATHWAY

The central tragedy of the prevailing dogma of medicine is that it has convinced the public that diseases can only be treated with drugs and surgery, and that disease prevention and reversal with nondrug natural measures is not scientific.

—*Majid Ali, M.D., former professor of pathology, Columbia University*

Conventional cancer treatment is a search-and-destroy mission: find a tumor, cut it out, poison it with chemotherapy, or obliterate it with radiation. If there is an approach to cancer that obviously does not work, this is it. . . . the death rate for cancer has not budged over the last fifty years; in fact, it has increased. Despite the fact that this approach doesn't work, it is . . . almost universally accepted.

—*Julian Whitaker, M.D., Whitaker Wellness Institute*

Think about this: *If conventional cancer treatments worked, there would be no reason to fear cancer.* People fear cancer because conventional treatments are failures. They fail to cure cancer because they do nothing to address its true cause. They even fail to extend life or improve quality of life.

Why Medicine Isn't Working

Conventional cancer treatment consists of managing symptoms with radiation, drugs, and surgery. These therapies will indeed remove or shrink tumors, but they do nothing to address the underlying cause, and nothing to shut down the cancer process. In fact, they promote the cancer process and cause more cancer than they cure. This is the reason why most cancer patients who choose to do nothing live longer than those who undergo conventional treatments. In her book, *Knockout*, actress, author, and breast cancer survivor Suzanne Somers interviews internationally renowned New York cancer expert Nicholas Gonzalez, M.D., who says, "As soon as patients have chemo and radiation their chances of success, although not completely eliminated, are lessened."

Conventional cancer treatment is little different from our outdated medical system as a whole; it is ineffective and dangerous. Most physicians are well intentioned and enter medicine with the desire to help people. But the education they receive is, for the most part, hopelessly obsolete, unscientific, and invalid—the results are disastrous. Looking at medical education in America, Sir George Pickering, M.D., a professor of medicine at Oxford University and one of the twentieth century's most respected experts in medical education, said in a 1971 *British Medical Journal:*

Medical education in the U.S. is, to a large extent, worship at the improbable shrine of worthless knowledge. We produce "scientific illiterates" . . . who are not scientific in their approach to clinical questions or new technologies.

Our physicians get no training in scientifically advanced *molecular medicine,* which emphasizes cellular and molecular interventions with nontoxic nutrients. Instead, they learn "drug and cut" medicine: how to prescribe toxic, health-damaging drugs and do invasive, health-damaging surgery—neither of which cure disease. This Medical Pathway chapter will help you to avoid the pitfalls of this deeply flawed system.

Here is an illustration of the pitfalls. In early 2009, my friend Frank Wiewel, the president of People Against Cancer (an organization dedicated to finding effective alternative treatments for cancer), told me of a phone conversation he had just had with one of the top oncologists in America. When the call came in, Frank immediately recognized the name of this prominent cancer specialist. When Frank asked to what he owed the honor of the call, the physician answered, "I have cancer." More than a bit taken aback, Frank asked, "Why are you calling me?" The physician replied that she wanted his help in finding an alternative treatment for her cancer saying, "We are woefully aware of our own inadequacies in the treatment of advanced cancer." Why would oncologists be seeking out alternative treatments for their own cancer? *Because they know what they do doesn't work!*

Despite trillions of dollars spent on disease care annually, the incidence of cancer and other chronic diseases continues to increase. This is happening because we really don't have a health industry; we have a disease industry, an industry that is totally dependent on millions of people getting sick and staying sick. In this system, there is no economic incentive to keep people well or to restore health. There is no incentive to cure cancer. What if cancer were cured? What would happen to all those cancer doctors, drug companies, hospitals, diagnostic centers, treatment centers, researchers, cancer nonprofits, and all the other businesses that serve the cancer industry? Perhaps this is why conventional medicine has made it illegal in many states for physicians to offer alternative care for cancer. Despite clinically proven benefits, alternative therapies are not allowed. This forces cancer patients to use conventional treatments that make big profits for the cancer industry, even though over a half century of use has proven them to be dangerous and ineffective.

Most people have the misconception that their doctor is using the best technology that modern science has to offer. Nothing could be further from the truth. Several studies, including one by the U.S. Office of Technology Assessment, have concluded that only 10 to 15 percent of conventional medical treatment has any basis in science, and it is in this small area, primarily crisis intervention and trauma care, that medicine excels. This means that 85 to 90 percent of medical practice has never been proven by scientific method to be safe and effective. The most recent study to document the unscientific basis of current medical practice was published in 2011 in the *Archives of Internal Medicine*. It found that even when doctors follow existing medical guidelines to the letter, 86 percent of the time they are using treatments that have little or no scientific support.

When doctors follow the existing guidelines, they mistakenly believe they are practicing "evidence-based medicine," but there is no science behind the guidelines. In reality, the guidelines are based on the assumptions or opinions of the members of a guideline-drafting panel. Patients trust their doctors and the doctors trust the medical authorities, assuming that the professors who taught them and sit on the panels know what they are doing. But they don't. As a result, doctors and patients underestimate the amount of harm that most drugs and surgeries do and overestimate the benefits. In fact, there is little or no evidence that many widely used treatments and procedures actually work better than various cheaper and safer alternatives.

Conventional medicine has been unable or unwilling to translate the enormous scientific advances of the last century into clinical practice. There is a good reason for this. Because of their inadequate training, most physicians have no idea how to read, interpret, and understand a scientific paper. In addition, most studies in the medical literature are poorly directed, deeply flawed, funded by organizations with vested interests, and often announce conclusions that are not supported by the data in the study. This is bad science, and it is why the eminent scientist Linus Pauling called most cancer research "a fraud."

Conventional medicine is now so far behind the science, and the situation is so serious, that the prestigious Institute of Medicine of the National Academy of Sciences studied the matter and issued a report in 2001. This report, *Crossing the Quality Chasm,* concluded that "between the health care we now have and the health care we could have lies not just a gap but a chasm." The report also said:

> *The nation's health care delivery system has fallen short in its ability to translate knowledge into practice and to apply new technology safely and appropriately. . . . If the system cannot consistently deliver today's science and technology, it is even less prepared to respond to the extraordinary advances that surely will emerge during the coming decades.*

Conventional medical practice in America is so far off course at this point, there is no way it can be salvaged—it needs to be discarded and replaced with what the Academy called "a fundamental, sweeping redesign."

Where did we ever get the idea that we could help sick people by feeding them toxic chemicals or chopping them into pieces? People are sick because they have nutritional deficiencies, not because they have drug and surgery deficiencies. Deficiency and toxicity are the two causes of disease, and prescription drugs are toxins, which create deficiencies. Sick people need nutrients, not drugs, and they also need a body with all of its organs in place and functioning.

Conventional medicine waits for disease to happen. Then it attempts to suppress the symptoms with toxic drugs and invasive surgery, doing enormous, often irreparable—and even fatal—damage to the body. This irrational approach not only runs up the costs, it keeps you sick, makes your disease chronic, leaves you sicker than when you started, and may even kill you. This hopelessly outdated system needs to be replaced with science-based medicine. We must move away from the obsolete paradigm of *diagnosing and treating disease* to a new paradigm of *preventing and curing disease.* We need to focus on creating health instead of managing disease. This advanced approach not only increases longevity and quality of life, it drastically cuts costs, which is what we sorely need.

More than three out of four healthcare dollars are spent treating entirely preventable chronic diseases. It costs a lot more to fix something after it is broken than to prevent it from breaking in the first place. Yet conventional medicine makes almost no attempt to prevent disease. It also does an extremely poor job in treating chronic disease, and it does an even worse job treating cancer, with oncologists seemingly oblivious to the fact that their treatments do more harm than good.

Americans spend more than twice as much per capita as most other countries on health care. Given the money we spend, by any measurement of results, we have the worst performing healthcare system in the world. The World Health Organization ranks us only thirty-seventh in the world in overall health. As our healthcare spending has increased at twice the rate of other developed countries, our life expectancy has not improved and is projected to sharply decline in the coming decades. The United States is now ranked number forty-nine in life expectancy, down from number twenty-four in 1999 and number five in 1950.

Our healthcare system is not only inefficient; it is dangerous and deadly, with alarming rates of medical errors. Yet most people trust their doctors. A 2006 Harris Poll conducted by telephone between July 7 and 10 by Harris Interactive compared how likely people are to trust another person, based on the other's profession. Doctors topped this list. Eighty-five percent of the people polled believed they could trust their doctors. The problem is that our doctors are operating in an outmoded, unscientific paradigm. Considering that fact, it is actually quite predictable that their success rate would be so poor.

From medical errors to adverse drug reactions to unnecessary procedures, conventional medicine is literally killing us, and the numbers are right there in the medical statistics. A number of analyses, including those in Dr. Carolyn Dean's 2005 book, *Death by Modern Medicine;* Dr. Gary Null's 2010 book, *Death by Medicine;* the 1991 Harvard Medical Practice Study; the 1994 *Journal of the American Medical Association* article, "Error in Medicine," and others have shown that American medicine has caused more harm than good. The authors of these analyses took statistics right from the most respected medical and scientific journals and investigative reports by the Institute of Medicine. They have clearly demonstrated that medical intervention is the leading cause of death in America, killing more than 1 million people per year. According to the 2011 Health-Grades Hospital Quality and Clinical Excellence Study, the incidence rate of medical harm is now over 40,000 each and every day.

When diseases are not cured, they remain chronic and the symptoms require constant management. This may be good for the disease industry's business, but it isn't good for you. Let us have a look at some of conventional medicine's standard procedures and see how they affect the cancer patient.

Surgery

Surgical removal of the primary tumor is the standard treatment for the majority of tumors. Surgery can be effective in a limited number of cases. Virtually all of conventional medicine's few cancer cures can be attributed to surgery alone in cases where the cancer had not yet metastasized. However, the majority of cancer patients already have metastasized cancer by the time they are diagnosed, and once a cancer has metastasized, surgery is ineffective and merely palliative. Worse, there is a growing body of evidence proving that cancer surgery can increase metastasis. (Metastasis is the process by which cancer cells travel and become established in other parts of the body, growing new tumors.)

The usual thinking is that if you remove the tumor, you remove the cancer. Unfortunately, this thinking is wrong because the tumor is merely a symptom—a side effect of the cancer process. The only way to truly win in the battle against cancer is to shut down the cancer process. If the cancer has metastasized and all you do is remove the tumor, more cancer will be produced because the process is still operating. As you will see below, adding radiation and chemotherapy to the surgery doesn't help either. Even in early-stage cancer, surgery promotes cancer metastasis. Metastasis is far more serious than the original tumor; it is these metastatic lesions that represent a true lethal threat. Anything that promotes metastasis should be avoided, or at least not undertaken lightly.

Although we hear much about it, metastasis is a complicated process that requires a lot to be successful; it should be very rare, as the body has numerous defense mechanisms to prevent it from happening. Unfortunately, surgery creates a situation where these natural defense mechanisms are bypassed and metastasis is encouraged. Oncologists do not inform their patients of this reality, so patients opting for surgery are not making fully informed decisions. Doctors often wildly exaggerate the benefits of surgery while minimizing the probability of harm. Patients are led to believe that they are getting rid of their cancer, when in fact they may be helping it to spread.

For metastasis to happen, cancer cells must first break away from a primary tumor. They must then break through the connective tissue surrounding the tumor. Then the cancer cells must use special enzymes to help them get access to a blood or lymphatic vessel. Once in the blood or lymph system, the cancer cells can travel throughout the body. However, as they travel, the cancer cells become extremely vulnerable to circulating immune cells whose job it is to kill such abnormal cells. Assuming they survive, the cells must then successfully adhere to and penetrate through a blood vessel, successfully penetrate surrounding connective tissue, and then arrive at and establish their new home. Fortunately for us, the survival rate of cancer cells going through this process is exceedingly low. Unfortunately for us, there are things our physicians do to change this poor success rate and vastly improve the ability of cancer cells to metastasize—one of them is surgery.

Surgery can effectively bypass many of the body's protective mechanisms and increase the metastasis success rate. A 2009 study in the *Annals of Surgery* concluded that cancer surgery can greatly lessen the obstacles that cancer cells face when trying to metastasize. During surgery, both the tumor and the blood vessels are disrupted, making large numbers of cancer cells immediately available to the bloodstream. The next problem is that surgery has been shown to increase cancer cell adhesion. To survive and grow, cancer cells have to be able to adhere to blood vessel walls in order to penetrate them, and then adhere to each other in order to form tumors. Otherwise, they will just float freely in the fluids. A study in a 2004 *International Journal of Cancer* determined that cancer cells released by surgery had 250 percent higher adhesive capacity than cancer cells not exposed to surgical conditions.

Surgery, anesthesia, and blood transfusions all powerfully suppress the immune system, and this can last for several weeks after the surgery. This gives the cancer a chance to spread without opposition; it also increases the risk of all kinds of post-operative infections. The immune system plays a critical role in preventing metastasis by attacking roaming cancer cells before they have the opportunity to form a new tumor.

The principal anti-metastasis tool, mentioned in previous chapters, is a white blood cell called a natural killer (NK) cell. It is well established in the medical literature that low levels of NK cells are associated with increased risk of metastasis and death from cancer, and that the level of biological activity of NK cells is a good predictor of cancer survival in general. Surgery results in a substantial reduction in NK cell activity. This is tragic, because when cancer cells have been dumped into your bloodstream by the surgery, you have the highest need for NK cell protection. A study in a 1993 *British Journal of Surgery* found that NK cell activity in women who had breast surgery was reduced by 50 percent within a day after surgery.

Angiogenesis is another problem with surgery. Angiogenesis is the process whereby new blood vessels are formed. This is a critical process as we grow from an infant into an adult; it is also a critical process for metastasis to happen. A growing tumor needs a fresh blood supply or it cannot grow. Tumors cannot grow beyond the size of a pinhead without an expanded blood supply. To protect you from harm, your body responds to the presence of a primary tumor by producing anti-angiogenic chemicals that inhibit the formation of new blood vessels. This inhibits the growth of new tumors. In this way, the presence of the primary tumor acts to inhibit metastasis, restricting the growth of cancer elsewhere in the body. But when the primary tumor is surgically removed, these chemicals are no longer produced. Metastasis is no longer inhibited, and clusters of cancer cells around the body are free to grow. Making matters even worse, in order to heal the surgical wound, it is necessary to grow new blood vessels, so the body will produce chemicals that support angiogenesis. This also supports the growth of new tumors.

Yet another effect of surgery is to increase inflammation in the body. Surgery places enormous stress on the body, causing a substantial increase in the production of inflammatory chemicals, including interleukin-1 and interleukin-6. Both of these increase the production of a highly inflammatory enzyme called cyclooxygenase-2 (COX-2). High levels of COX-2 have been shown to decrease survival rates in cancer patients. COX-2 stimulates the production of new blood vessels that feed tumors and also increases cancer cell adhesion.

Even a needle biopsy is dangerous. Needle biopsies are widely used and accepted as a safe procedure for diagnosing cancer. But they are not safe, and as early as 1940, medical experts warned that needle biopsies could cause cancer cells to break away from a tumor and spread to other parts of the body. A 2007 study in the *British Medical Journal* indicates that biopsies do exactly that—spread the cancer. If you have a needle biopsy, you are 50 percent more likely to have your cancer spread. The body tries to wall off tumors to protect you. When you poke a hole in this protective capsule, cancer cells can spill out directly into the bloodstream or lymphatic system and spread throughout the body.

Chemotherapy

With very few exceptions, chemotherapy is a dismal failure. It doesn't cure cancer, extend life, or improve quality of life. It does much more harm than good. Yet chemotherapy is given to about 80 percent of all cancer patients. The idea of chemotherapy is to use extremely toxic chemicals to kill cancer cells. Unfortunately, these chemicals kill more good cells than bad ones, damaging the entire body and drastically weakening the immune system. The medical literature acknowledges that chemotherapy is effective only about 2 percent of the time, and only for very specific cancers including Hodgkin's disease, testicular cancer, and acute lymphocytic leukemia. Chemotherapy does not work the other 98 percent of the time (even when it does work, it greatly increases the risk of developing new cancers years later). Of all the cancer drugs approved by the FDA over the last quarter century, only five have been demonstrated to extend life, but only for weeks or months, not years. This life extension comes at an average cost of $250,000, plus enormous pain and suffering.

When a doctor tells you that chemotherapy is effective, it doesn't mean it cures cancer. It means temporary shrinkage of the tumor.

Cancer cells will be poisoned, they will die, and the tumor will shrink. However, not all the cancer cells die, and the survivors will start growing again once the treatment is stopped. Further, the remaining cancer cells will now grow much faster and more aggressively. All that is achieved is a temporary shrinkage that comes at enormous economic and personal cost. The personal cost includes "side effects" such as vomiting, hair loss, mouth sores, catastrophic destruction of intestinal tissue, mental impairment, and immune suppression to the point of developing life-threatening and even fatal infections. Another tragic side effect is the enormous damage done by chemotherapy to the body's genes and metabolic machinery. This diminishes the patient's ability to respond to more effective nutritional-based approaches, thus limiting the options for getting well.

The economic cost of drug treatments for cancer is high. The anticancer drug Folotyn can cost $30,000 per month. Folotyn has not been shown to prolong life, but only to temporarily shrink tumors. For a bargain price of only $8,800 per month you can take Avastin, the bestselling cancer drug in the world. Avastin has never been proven to help anybody live longer or improve quality of life. For $10,000 a month you can choose the highly controversial Erbitux.

The *New York Times* reported in 1975 that Nobel Laureate James Watson, best known as the co-discoverer of the structure of DNA, declared at a cancer symposium at M.I.T. that the American public had been "sold a nasty bill of goods about cancer." Here is how nasty: A 2009 study in *Cancer Cell* indicates that anticancer drugs like Avastin and Erbitux actually *promote* metastasis. The side effects of these drugs are horrendous: they often kill you and now we know they promote metastasis. The chemotherapy drug Taxol causes cancer cell "microtentacles" to grow longer and tumor cells to attach to new sites more rapidly, playing an important role in spreading the cancer. If you are treated with Taxol before surgery to shrink the primary tumor, the number of circulating tumor cells in your body increases by up to 10,000 times.

Chemotherapy destroys healthy cells throughout your body right along with cancer cells. Cells lining the gastrointestinal tract are damaged. This causes malabsorption of nutrients and leaky gut that triggers food allergies and immune responses that further weaken the already overloaded immune system. Chemo also damages the liver, kidneys, and nervous system, leading to cognitive impairment called "chemo brain." These drugs are so toxic and carcinogenic that they will cause cancer in healthy people, even in minute quantities. This is why the healthcare workers who make their living producing, mixing, and administering these toxic chemicals have high rates of cancer. Even their extremely small exposures, over a period of years, are enough to give them cancer.

For all the expense and damage, if chemo drugs did some good, perhaps their use could be justified. Unfortunately, except in very rare situations, they do nothing to benefit the patient—life is not prolonged beyond a few weeks or months of low-quality existence.

Even painkillers, often given to cancer patients, cause cancer to spread. A growing body of research, including an article in the June 25, 2010, issue of *Scientific American,* is showing that opiate-based painkillers stimulate the growth and spread of cancer cells. Opiates, such as morphine, promote cancer by making cancer cells replicate faster and speeding the development of new blood vessels needed by tumors to grow. Cancer patients who do not receive these drugs have longer survival times.

Radiation

Radiation causes cancer. Numerous studies, including a 2007 study in *Prostate Cancer and Prostatic Diseases,* show that patients who receive post-surgical radiation treatments actually die sooner than those who undergo surgery alone. It is a fact that ionizing radiation increases the cellular mutations that lead to cancer, and there is no scientific evidence that radiation treatment will cure cancer or prolong life. Radiation is one of the best-known causes of cancer, and it is well known that radiation treatment causes secondary cancers, as well as doing major damage to other tissues, such as causing substantial bone loss. Yet, despite the fact that radiation does only harm, it remains the most common treatment for breast cancer following surgical removal of the tumor. Like chemotherapy, radiation may provide a short-term benefit, such as shrinking a tumor, but it does long-term harm. In fact, radiation treatment increases the risk of developing new tumors by over 100 times.

One major problem is that radiation treatment suppresses the immune system, and the immune system is your first line of defense for keeping cancer under control. Radiation damages bone marrow, which is the very heart of the immune system. Radiation and chemo alike do major damage to healthy cells and organs, weakening the body and in many instances causing damage so severe that it ends up killing the patient.

Diagnostic x-rays are a special problem. Americans are exposed to seven times more radiation from diagnostic x-rays than they were in 1980. Most of the average person's lifetime radiation exposure comes from diagnostic x-rays, yet there is no medical justification for as much as 90 percent of them, including routine x-rays like mammograms. Mammograms expose your body to radiation that can be 1,000 times greater than a chest x-ray. Mammograms not only increase the risk of developing breast cancer, they also increase the risk of its spreading. Regarding mammograms, a 1995 study in the *Lancet* concluded, "The benefit is marginal, the harm caused is substantial, and the costs incurred are enormous." Each additional radiation exposure, no matter how small, increases the risk of cancer. This is why you should refuse all but the most necessary medical x-rays.

There is a reason why radiologists and technicians who are around x-ray equipment every day have more cancer than the general population. X-rays cause cancer. John Gofman, M.D., Ph.D., was both a medical doctor and a nuclear physicist. He was one of the world's leading experts on radiation damage, and his groundbreaking book, *Radiation from Medical Procedures in the Pathogenesis of Cancer and Ischemic Heart Disease,* was published in 1999. Gofman's three decades of research into the effects of low-dose radiation on humans indicated that medical x-rays play an essential role in about 75 percent of all breast cancers. Cancer statistics show that breast cancer has increased since the introduction of mammographic screening in 1983. In fact, one form of breast cancer, ductal carcinoma in situ, has increased more than 300 percent. A 2008 study in the *Archives of Internal Medicine* found the start of mammography screening programs throughout Europe was associated with an increased incidence of breast cancer.

In addition to radiation damage, there are other reasons not to do routine mammograms. Mammography compresses the breasts (often painfully), which could cause the spread of any existing malignant cells. Mammograms have a high rate of false positives. About 5 percent of mammograms suggest further testing; over 90 percent of those are false positives. This results in unnecessary expense, emotional trauma, needless biopsies, and other unnecessary surgical procedures. Mammograms also produce a high rate of false negatives; a false negative could cost you your life. According to the National Cancer Institute, for women in the forty to forty-nine age group, the rate of missed tumors is 40 percent! The truth is, mammograms don't save lives. Research shows that adding an annual mammogram to a careful physical examination of the breasts does not improve breast cancer survival rates.

Fortunately, there is a better way. Physicians practicing more advanced forms of medicine use a safe, accurate, and inexpensive diagnostic test called a thermogram. Thermography measures the temperature of the breast. It uses no mechanical pressure or ionizing radiation, and it can detect breast cancer as much as ten years earlier than a mammogram. A growing tumor requires its own blood supply. The increased blood flow makes that area warmer than the surrounding tissue. This temperature differential can be accurately measured, with no false negatives and few false positives, without any danger or discomfort to the patient.

Another serious problem is the widespread use of CT (computed tomography) scans, originally known as computed axial tomography (CAT) scans. The use of these x-ray scanners has increased dramatically over the last two decades, and an estimated more than 75 million scans are now being performed in the United States annually. CT scans can image the entire human body within seconds, producing high-definition images that provide physicians with an incredibly detailed view of the organs and tissues deep within us.

While CT scans can be beneficial for certain situations, like serious injury from multiple traumas, alarm is being raised in medical journals about the overuse of these devices and an enormous amount of unnecessary radiation exposure. Healthy people are being exposed to excessive, cancer-causing radiation for clinically dubious screening purposes. In particular, two studies regarding CT scans were published in the *Archives of Internal Medicine* in 2009, and they have significantly increased levels of concern.

Recall that, regarding cancer, there is no known "safe" dose of radiation. In light of this reality, consider that a single CT coronary artery angiogram can deliver the same amount of radiation as 310 chest x-rays. Making matters worse, the above researchers found enormous variations in the amount of radiation being delivered by different CT imaging facilities. Thirteen-fold variations have been found between the highest and lowest doses for the same type of scan. Some people have received grossly excessive radiation doses during their scans, to the point where their hair began falling out. The risk of developing cancer is proportional to the dose of radiation received, and CT scans deliver a lot. These researchers have estimated that the CT scans done in 2007 alone will result in approximately 29,000 future cases of cancer caused directly by the scans, and this estimate is most likely conservative. Anyone with a nutritional deficiency or a poorly functioning DNA repair system will be especially vulnerable to the ill effects of radiation. To prevent cancer, radiation should be avoided whenever possible, including x-ray scanners at airports.

Prescription Drugs

Prescription drugs are one of our leading causes of disease as well as the third-leading cause of death in the United States. One of the more tragic aspects of conventional medicine is the use of toxic chemicals called prescription drugs. Everyone wants a magic pill to cure disease, but there is no such thing. The risk of taking these drugs far exceeds their potential benefits, and they are major contributors to our cancer epidemic.

By making the body both deficient and toxic, prescription drugs damage the body's overall resistance to disease. This is why properly prescribed prescription drugs hospitalize over 2 million and kill an estimated 300,000 to 400,000 people every year. In addition, prescription drugs decrease the quality of life for tens of millions.

It is a tragedy that over 60 percent of American adults are on at least one drug to treat a chronic health problem, and many, especially our elderly, take multiple medications daily. Many of these drugs are prescribed to cope with side effects caused by the initial drug treatment. When you are on multiple drugs, the body is plunged into biochemical chaos, making it impossible to rebalance the body's chemistry and get well. This is an open invitation to cancer. People who are taking multiple drugs often improve their health dramatically when they stop taking the drugs. Just saying "no" to drugs is usually desirable and beneficial, but in most cases needs be done while working with a knowledgeable natural health practitioner.

Not only are prescription drugs toxic, they cause nutritional deficiencies, creating both deficiency and toxicity—the two causes of all disease. For example, cholesterol-lowering drugs cause CoQ10 deficiency, which can result in fatigue and congestive heart failure, as well as promote cancer. Chemotherapy drugs cause magnesium deficiency. Birth control pills lower vitamin C, folate, B2, B6, B12, magnesium, and selenium. Low levels of vitamin C and folate increase the risk of cancer. Hypertension drugs deplete vitamins C, B1, B6, and K, along with CoQ10, calcium, magnesium, and zinc. By taking drugs for a long period of time, the resulting nutritional deficiencies vastly increase your risk of every disease, including cancer.

Some people are alarmed at the thought of not taking their drugs. They think that they need their drugs to lower their blood pressure, treat their depression, or whatever. In truth, virtually no one *needs* a drug. It is difficult to think of a prescription drug for which there is not an alternative treatment that is safer, less expensive, and more effective. Drugs are toxic to the body; they make you sick, not well. Every time independent researchers take a serious look at a prescription drug, they find they are dangerous—so why take them? Find an alternative doctor who will treat you naturally. Your body will thank you with the gift of better health.

There is a dangerous misconception in America that when you are sick, you need a drug. *The only real solution to any health problem is to get well.* Getting well is about giving your cells the nutrients they need, reducing their toxic load, and restoring them to normal function. When you do this, whatever is wrong will disappear, including cancer. Despite decades of negative results and the unnecessary tragic deaths of millions of people, our physicians continue the obsolete practice of prescribing toxic drugs that poison the body. They should be prescribing nutrients and detoxification to nurture the body and restore health. Let's have a look at some common drugs that can increase your risk of getting cancer.

Birth Control Pills

One class of drugs that has been found to cause cancer is birth control pills. A 1991 study in the *Journal of the National Cancer Institute* found that women who take birth control pills for five years or more increase their risk of getting liver cancer by 550 percent over those who have never taken the drugs.

Hormone Replacement Therapy

Hormone replacement therapy (HRT) is another cancer-causing medical treatment that ranks among conventional medicine's greatest blunders. Numerous studies have proven that HRT causes heart attack, stroke, and blood clots. Women on HRT are up to three times more likely to develop blood clots as well as cancer. After decades of well-founded suspicion, it has now been established that HRT causes cancer. A study of 46,000 women in a January 2000 issue of the *Journal of the American Medical Association* found that women who used the most common form of HRT for five years had a 40 percent increased risk of breast cancer, and that the risk increased by 8 percent with each year of use. A more recent 2010 study in the *Journal of the American Medical Association* found that not only does HRT increase the risk of breast cancer, but it makes it more likely the cancer will be aggressive and deadly. In addition to breast cancer, a 2006 study in the *Journal of the National Cancer Institute* found a link between HRT and ovarian cancer; other studies have found links to lung cancer. Since 2000, many physicians have stopped prescribing HRT, and studies show that the recent decline in breast cancer deaths is the direct result of fewer HRT prescriptions. The breast cancer death rate is dropping because fewer doctors are *giving* their patients cancer!

TNF Blockers

Another class of cancer-causing drugs is tumor necrosis factor (TNF) blockers. TNF blockers are used to treat inflammatory and autoimmune diseases such as Crohn's disease and rheumatoid arthritis. The FDA has ordered makers of these drugs to include a "black box warning" about an increased risk of cancer in children and adolescents. This is the most severe warning that the FDA can place on a product without withdrawing it from the market. The FDA was forced into this action after numerous reports of children developing cancer while taking these drugs started to pour in. The FDA analyzed these reports and concluded, in its August 4, 2009, Ongoing Safety Review of Tumor Necrosis Factor (TNF) Blockers, that "there is an increased risk of lymphoma and other cancers associated with the use of these drugs in children and adolescents." It would be foolhardy not to assume they are also risky for adults.

Antibiotics

Most people think of antibiotics as one of the greatest triumphs of conventional medicine. In truth, antibiotics are one of medicine's greatest fiascos. A properly functioning intestinal tract is one of your first lines of defense against disease, and declining levels of friendly intestinal bacteria precipitate the onset of chronic disease. Antibiotics destroy the natural balance of flora (bacteria, yeasts, and other microorganisms) in the gut, doing damage so fundamental that these toxic drugs have devastated the health of our population. Antibiotics contribute to virtually every imaginable disease from the common cold to asthma, allergies, autoimmune syndromes, damage to the brain and nervous system, and cancer.

Antibiotics are deadly poisons; their purpose is to treat infections by killing bacteria. But they also destroy beneficial bacteria, and this is catastrophic. Helpful bacteria in the gut play vital roles in both immunity and digestion. They also degrade toxins, produce vitamins, and help with nutrient absorption. Astonishingly, there are more bacteria living in our intestines than we have cells in our body (bacteria are much smaller than human cells). In a way, they are comparable to an organ in the body, like the heart or lungs. *Antibiotics cripple this organ.*

Seventy percent of the immune system is located in the intestines, and beneficial bacteria play key roles in its optimal function. Stripping your gut of its natural balance of healthy bacteria promotes an overgrowth of harmful microorganisms such as parasites, mycoplasma, fungi, yeasts like Candida, and hostile bacteria such as Pseudomonas, Clostridium, and Klebsiella. Once this happens, immunity is severely impaired.

The harmful microorganisms produce many toxins, including neurotoxins. These toxins cause dysfunction of the endocrine glands, resulting in hypothyroidism and adrenal insufficiency, as well as producing numerous cognitive and neurological problems similar to multiple sclerosis and amyotrophic lateral sclerosis. These same toxins also compromise the body's ability to kill cancer cells by damaging the gut lining; this lowers immunity by decreasing the production of intestinal immune cells.

Good health begins in the intestinal tract. With the exception of oxygen, all nutrition enters the body through the intestines. To be healthy, your food must first be properly digested, and good bacteria play important roles in digestion. If food is not properly broken down, it will ferment and putrefy in the gut, producing powerful toxins that poison you. Once food is properly digested, nutrients from the food must be absorbed through the intestinal walls into the bloodstream. Good bacteria facilitate this absorption, while damage done to gut tissue by harmful flora impedes it. Thus, destruction of helpful bacteria results in deficiency and toxicity—the two causes of all disease.

Food allergies, immunodeficiency syndromes, and a variety of intestinal disorders can result from altered flora. Damage done by antibiotics has led to an epidemic of digestive difficulties, with an enormous quantity of over-the-counter digestive aids sold every year. Sadly, most doctors are unaware that the antibiotics they themselves have prescribed have caused their patients' digestive problems.

The ill effects of taking antibiotics might not be too bad if they were temporary, but once the normal balance of gut flora undergoes this kind of major damage, it is extremely difficult, and perhaps impossible, to completely restore it back to normal. This can leave you permanently damaged, with your health compromised and lasting weakness where there was once strength. Even after one course of antibiotics, things may never be as they once were. Taking high-quality probiotic supplements or including raw, live culture sauerkraut or kimchi in your diet are your best choices for helping to cope with this damage.

Antibiotics do so much fundamental damage to your health that it should not be a surprise they cause cancer. A study in a 2004 *Journal of the American Medical Association* determined that women who have taken antibiotics are at increased risk for developing breast cancer, and as the number of prescriptions for antibiotics increased, the risk of breast cancer steadily climbed. The researchers suggested that antibiotics kill off bacteria needed to metabolize and remove estrogen in the gut. This causes an estrogen excess that stimulates the growth of cancer. Women who had taken fewer than twenty-five antibiotic prescriptions had a 50 percent greater risk of breast cancer, while women who had taken more than twenty-five prescriptions had a 200 percent greater risk compared to women who took no antibiotics. More and more studies are showing a relationship between antibiotic use and cancer. Some researchers believe that the long-term use of antibiotics may be the primary reason patients with Lyme disease are now frequently diagnosed with lymphomas.

Another harmful effect of antibiotics is the increase in numbers of antibiotic-resistant bacteria strains created by their use. These antibiotic-resistant bacteria are now ravaging our hospitals and moving out into the general population. They cause illnesses that are difficult, if not impossible, to treat with antibiotics.

Taking an antibiotic even once in your lifetime can start a chain of events that will devastate your health. Taking antibiotics often, or for long periods of time, is virtually certain to cause lifelong health problems, including cancer. Fortunately, there is no need for antibiotics. There are effective, natural, and much safer ways to prevent and cure infections, such as with immune enhancing vitamins like vitamins A, C, D, and E and with natural antibiotics like wild oregano and olive leaf extract.

Vaccinations

Another of conventional medicine's colossal blunders is vaccinations. The purpose of vaccinations is to prevent infectious disease. The problem is there is no scientific evidence that immunizations prevent disease and plenty of evidence they are dangerous. Vaccines are not tested to see if they are carcinogenic, yet we inject these dangerous, toxic concoctions into our children, without knowing whether or not they cause cancer. Recalling that cancer has become the leading cause of death by disease for our young people, perhaps we should be paying more attention. A growing number of researchers are now attributing the epidemics of leukemia, asthma, autoimmune disease, cerebral palsy, infantile convulsions, sudden infant death syndrome, and childhood cancer to vaccinations. Vaccinations cause cancer in adults as well. Two 2002 studies in the *Lancet* estimated that up to half of the 55,000 annual cases of non-Hodgkin's lymphoma can be attributed to polio vaccinations received decades ago.

The dramatic decline of infectious diseases, such as smallpox, diphtheria, and polio, is often cited as proof of vaccinations' effectiveness. The truth is the incidence of infectious disease decreased dramatically *before* the introduction of vaccines—in other words, vaccines get credit for something they did not do. For example, in 1950, the polio epidemic was at its height in Great Britain. By the time the polio vaccine was introduced in 1956, polio had *already* declined by 82 percent.

Here is what Australian researcher Viera Scheibner, Ph.D., had to say in her book *Vaccination* after investigating some 60,000 pages of medical literature on vaccination:

> *Immunizations, including those practiced on babies, not only did not prevent any infectious diseases; they caused more suffering and more deaths than has any other human activity in the entire history of medical intervention.*

Canadian physician, Dr. Guylaine Lanctot, author of the bestseller *The Medical Mafia* puts it this way:

> *The medical authorities keep lying. Vaccination has been an assault on the immune system. It actually causes a lot of illnesses. We are actually changing our genetic code through vaccination . . . 100 years from now we will know that the biggest crime against humanity was vaccines.*

Renowned pediatrician and author Dr. Robert Mendelsohn was equally direct in his book *Confessions of a Medical Heretic:*

> *Much of what you have been led to believe about immunization simply isn't true. If I were to follow my deeper convictions, I would urge you to reject all inoculations for your child. . . . There is no convincing scientific evidence that mass inoculations can be credited with eliminating any childhood disease.*

Medical researcher Juan Manuel Martínez Méndez, M.D., writing in the Aug/Sept 2004 *Townsend Letter* (a respected examiner of medical alternatives), said:

> *These chronic diseases, including hay fever, asthma, cancer, and AIDS, are the result of wrong interventions upon the organism by conventional medicine . . . the immune systems of the Western population, through strong chemical drugs and repeated vaccinations, have broken down . . . medicine, instead of curing diseases, is actually the cause of the degeneration of the human race.*

Vaccines contain mercury compounds, formaldehyde, and aluminum, all substances that are known to cause cancer. Aluminum causes cancer by displacing iron from its protective proteins, raising the level of free iron in the body and triggering intense inflammation, free radical generation, and lipid peroxidation. Vaccines also contain viruses, and certain viruses have been associated with cancer. For example, we know that a monkey virus SV40, found in polio vaccine, has been proven to cause cancer and to be responsible for an outbreak of lung, brain, bone, and lymphatic cancers in those who received polio vaccine decades ago. In addition, vaccines drive cancer by depressing immunity; strong immunity is critical to defending ourselves against cancer.

In addition to being dangerous, no vaccine has ever been proven in double-blind, placebo-controlled studies to be effective; the existing evidence indicates they are not effective. Given they are dangerous and of unproven effectiveness, it is unconscionable that by the time a child starts kindergarten he or she will have received forty-eight doses of fourteen vaccines. Of these, thirty-six doses will be given during the first eighteen months of life when a child's body and brain are undergoing massive development. This helps to explain the explosion of neurological and immune system disorders in American children, and almost certainly contributes to the explosion of childhood cancer.

Your Dentist

Still another colossal blunder is conventional dentistry's use of x-rays, toxic metals such as nickel and mercury, and carcinogenic local anesthetics. X-rays are known to cause cancer. It is widely acknowledged that there is no safe level of radiation, yet dentists use x-rays routinely. While there may be justification for this risk in certain situations, the use of routine x-rays has to be questioned by the patient.

A so-called "silver" filling actually consists of about 50 percent mercury. Despite the fact that mercury is one of the most dangerous toxins in our environment, damaging the brain, central nervous system, and kidneys as well as causing cancer, an estimated 100 million mercury fillings are still done each year in the United States.

No one has ever been able to prove that there is a safe level of mercury. Mercury damages the immune system. Beyond small amounts, most fish is now considered unsafe due to mercury contamination of the oceans. The EPA recommends ingesting a maximum of 0.1 micrograms per kilogram of body weight per day. This translates to no more than 6.8 micrograms of mercury per day for a 150-pound person. Average daily absorption from fish and seafood is estimated at 2.3 micrograms. Alarmingly, a single mercury filling, through evaporation and mechanical wear, can release 15 micrograms per day, every day. A person with eight fillings will be absorbing 120 micrograms per day! Fortunately, plastic composites are now used extensively in place of the mercury fillings. Anyone with mercury fillings should have them removed by a dentist who is skilled in the proper procedures for safe removal—you should have your own air supply during the removal so as not to breathe the mercury vapors.

About 75 percent of porcelain crowns are made with a stainless steel liner to give them strength. The stainless steel contains nickel; nickel is an allergen and is an even more powerful carcinogen than mercury. If you have porcelain crowns made with nickel, it would be best to remove them. Crowns made with gold are a better choice. Today porcelain technology has advanced to where crowns are available that have no metal at all; these would be the best choice.

Root canals are another problem. Virtually every root canal has been found to be infected. These low-grade infections produce toxins that poison the entire body, damaging immunity. In his book *Cancer: A Second Opinion*, Dr. Josef Issels calls root canals "toxin factories" that produce compounds called thioethers that can cause cancer in humans. If you have cancer, your root canals should be removed, but you need to find a skilled dentist who knows how to remove them safely.

Local anesthetics (including lidocaine) are commonly used by dentists and may be substantial contributors to our cancer epidemic.

These anesthetics break down in the body into cancer-causing compounds called anilines. In 1993, the FDA found that lidocaine, when exposed to human tissue, breaks down into 2,6-dimethylaniline, a compound that is known to cause virtually every kind of cancer in animals, and it does so more than 99 percent of the time. In September 1996, as a result of these findings, the FDA removed from the market all over-the-counter painkillers containing these local anesthetics and required that a warning be placed on all new prescription pharmaceuticals containing them. Unfortunately, pre-existing prescription anesthetics were not required to carry the FDA's warning, and most health professionals are still unaware of this problem. For those interested in learning more, Integrated Laboratory Systems published a report on this subject, *Final Toxicological Summary for Amide Local Anesthetics,* in October of 2000. Fortunately, there is a new anesthetic that is not cancer causing—Septocaine. You can request that your dentist use this product.

In Conclusion

There is good reason why Henry Bieler, M.D., the author of *Food Is Your Best Medicine* said, "This is the dark age of medicine." The healthcare system in America needs serious rethinking. Conventional allopathic medicine is less than 100 years old, but this fatally flawed system is a major cause of disease and has become our leading cause of death. It is a system that not only has failed to keep up with and put into practice the enormous advances in science over the last century, but it has become corrupted by multinational drug and food industry interests, which put their profits far ahead of improving your health and the human condition in general. It is a system that relies on treating only the symptoms of disease and never the causes. The reason healthcare costs so much is because conventional medicine doesn't cure anybody, patients stay sick, and money is spent to keep treating them, managing their symptoms.

Conventional medicine's treatment of cancer is a fraud. It doesn't work, and in fact, conventional medicine causes cancer. The science is there and the facts are indisputable. With a correct understanding of what is going on at the cellular and molecular levels, we already know how to prevent and cure almost any disease—including cancer. The way to cure any disease is to address the problems of deficiency and toxicity and restore malfunctioning cells to normal. When making healthcare choices for yourself or your loved ones, keep these facts in mind.

Best of all is to keep yourself in good health. Keep your immunity strong by eating a good diet, taking high-quality supplements, and avoiding environmental toxins, toxic prescription drugs, vaccinations, and antibiotics.

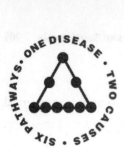

10

About Supplements

I take about sixty different supplements daily. . . .

I put back what my body needs to keep me at optimum health.

—Suzanne Somers, author of Knockout

Suzanne Somers used alternative treatments to cure her cancer, and in the quote above, she told Oprah Winfrey that she takes sixty different supplements daily. Oprah was stunned. In fact, most people are shocked at such a statement. But look at the results! She is cured and doing just fine. I take twenty-six different supplements daily, but again, look at the results. I brought myself back from the brink of medically certain death at age forty-eight. At age seventy-four, I am in superior health. I never get sick and feel and function like I am in my twenties, with boundless energy and a sharp mind. I have had only one cold in the last twenty-four years—and I have a good excuse for that one cold. Most people my age have multiple health problems and are on numerous prescription drugs. Nutritional supplements will help to keep you in good health at a fraction of the cost, and with no side effects—other than feeling great.

Supplements are now a necessity. In April 1998, the National Academy of Sciences issued a press release saying that most people will not get all the vitamins they need, *even* if they eat a good diet with lots of fruits and vegetables. In 2002, a landmark study published in the *Journal of the American Medical Association*, analyzing thirty-six years of data, concluded that everyone needs at least a daily multivitamin regardless of age or health. Recent data from the U.S. Department of Agriculture shows that the nutrition in fresh produce has declined as much as 50 percent over the last twenty-five years. Our soils are so depleted of minerals that the entire food supply is compromised; our food is not up to the task of keeping us in good health. It is now almost impossible to obtain the nutrition you need without supplementing, and once you have a chronic disease, your nutritional deficiency is so great that supplementing is the only way to fully restore health. To normalize malfunctioning cells, they must be supplied with all the nutrients they need to do their jobs. Accomplishing this usually requires an exceptionally large amount of nutrients.

In 2000, a study in the *Journal of the American Nutraceutical Association* concluded, "There is sufficient pertinent scientific clinical data to indicate that certain antioxidant and other nutrient supplements can reduce cancer risk, clinical cancer occurrence, and/or interrupt the carcinogenic process." This conclusion is very clear. You can prevent and interfere with the cancer process using supplements.

Frequently, people equate taking several supplements with "pill popping," a phrase often used to characterize those who consume prescription drugs in large quantities. This is a huge misconception, as prescription drugs are foreign to our body chemistry. Drugs do harm by putting a toxic load on the body, disrupting normal cell function, and forcing the body to spend precious energy and resources to detoxify these chemicals and repair the damage they do. Remember, because of their toxicity, prescription drugs are the third leading cause of death in America. On the other hand, high-quality, properly formulated supplements are foods, supplying the body with molecules that it needs and wants, supporting normal cell function, and helping to prevent and reverse disease. Think of it this way; when you take supplements, you are supplementing the nutrient-deficient foods you eat with the vitamins and minerals of which they have been stripped over time. By providing the body with what it needs to function properly, the need for medical treatment and drugs can be eliminated. The disease industry is mounting a worldwide effort to limit access to supplements, under the guise of promoting product safety. However, even poor-quality supplements are far safer than prescription drugs. According to the most recent information collected by the U.S. National Poison Data System (maintained by the American Association of Poison Control Centers), not even one death was caused by dietary supplements in 2008. While no man, woman, or child died from nutritional supplements, in that same year, millions were injured and hundreds of thousands were poisoned to death by prescription drugs, and that happens every year.

While supplements are necessary in today's world, it is challenging to know which supplements you need, which brands are best, and how much to take for optimal results. When I was sick and trying to restore my health, I found that most supplement brands were a waste of money and didn't work. Moreover, with my compromised immune system and chemical sensitivities, many of these

supplements had an adverse effect on me. These experiences motivated me to spend the next two decades studying vitamin chemistry.
Both enlightened and dismayed, I learned that making a vitamin
product that does what it is supposed to do requires much highly
specialized knowledge, as well as meticulous care and additional
expense—a rare combination in the supplement industry. I discovered that many top-selling brands are promoting biologically
ineffective products that are a waste of your hard-earned money.
However, because consumers lack the knowledge to make informed
choices, competition becomes a function of price and advertising
rather than quality. I also found that even higher price is not a guar-
antee of quality.

After learning how to cure myself of all of my life-threatening
conditions through improving my diet, taking supplements, and
eliminating toxins, I began to share the knowledge I had gained
with family and friends. In my extensive research on supplements,
I identified a manufacturer with high standards, and my family
and friends joined me in taking these supplements with measurable
results. Eventually, I developed my own line of superior-quality
supplements and got the manufacturers to produce them to my
exact specifications.

A 1999 article in the *Journal of the American Nutraceutical Association* stated that only 2.5 percent of the commonly available nutritional products they researched were effective. In other words, 97.5
percent of the supplements were ineffective! Without specialized
knowledge, it is next to impossible to wade through the shelves and
catalogs full of supplements and select from among the 2.5 percent
that are effective. You can download a free report, *The Roadmap
to Choosing Supplements*, that I wrote to help you make informed
choices. It is available at www.beyondhealth.com.

Many medical doctors still believe the average diet provides all the vitamins and minerals anyone needs, and they advise patients against wasting their money to make expensive urine. However, with the decrease in the nutritional value of many foods, and the increase in toxins in the environment, it is becoming increasingly difficult to argue against the necessity of nutritional supplementation. Any shortage will sabotage your body's biochemical balance and undermine your best efforts to stay healthy. *A chronic shortage of even one nutrient will cause disease, including cancer.*

Due to biochemical individuality, no two people have the same nutritional needs, and we all have different rates of absorption and utilization. One person may need many times the amount of a certain nutrient than another. Two people may live in the same house and eat the same diet, and one will be adequately provisioned and healthy while the other is malnourished and sick. When we take prescription drugs, such as antibiotics, we damage our gut tissue so that it selectively doesn't absorb certain nutrients. Given this, no one can afford to eat a marginal diet of processed foods and damaging foods such as sugar. We need to eat the most nutritious diet possible *and* take the highest quality supplements possible to be healthy, but few Americans are doing this.

People often ask what supplements they should take for a certain condition. Well-documented nutritional deficiency diseases such as scurvy, pellagra, and beriberi have simple cures because we know clearly what the deficiencies are. Other deficiencies however, are far more difficult to detect and correct. Remember that all nutrients act as a team. If one team member is chronically deficient, the entire team is compromised. The result is disease. Clearly, there is no magic pill that will solve all deficiency problems. A winning strategy is getting completely off the disease-causing Big Four, eating a diet high in fresh, organic vegetables, and getting on the best supplement program.

For the first time in 200 years, today's children have such compromised health that they are not expected to outlive their parents. The rise of chronic diseases among our children speaks to this fact. Children especially need supplements.

Remember that cancer is a biological process. Certain vitamins, minerals, and plant chemicals called phytonutrients are known to play special roles in preventing and shutting down the cancer process. For example, certain flavonoids and vitamins will interfere with enzymes that allow tumors to invade surrounding tissues. Other nutrients boost the immune system and support natural killer (NK) cell activity. Time and experience have proven a number of supplements to be especially effective in preventing and reversing the cellular malfunction we call cancer. When working to reverse cancer, high doses of vitamins and minerals are essential. The scientific evidence indicates that cancer cells will uptake vitamins in higher concentrations than normal cells; this supports apoptosis and interferes with the cancer process. Various combinations of vitamins and minerals working together are known to shut down the cancer process.

Ideally, it is always best to work with a knowledgeable physician who is experienced using nutrition to restore health. Unfortunately, especially outside of major population centers, such physicians are rare. Not every person needs to take all of the supplements mentioned below or in the doses I recommend. These are guidelines, and an enormous amount of additional information is readily available on the Internet. Always keep your doctor informed of what you are doing. However, the average physician has little or no training in nutrition, may not understand the need for supplements, and may not support your efforts. Don't let *anyone* discourage you from doing what is best for your body.

Let's have a look at some supplements you should consider.

Vitamin A

Vitamin A is essential for the normal functioning of the immune system and plays a well-known critical role in preventing and reversing cancer. In 2006 the National Institutes of Health (NIH) had this to say: "Dietary intake studies suggest an association between diets rich in beta-carotene and vitamin A and a lower risk of many types of cancer." A study of over 82,000 people by the NIH found that high intakes of vitamin A cut the risk of stomach cancer in half. A 2007 study in the *American Journal of Clinical Nutrition* said, "Vitamin A fights cancer by inhibiting the production of DNA in cancerous cells. It slows down tumor growth in established cancers and may keep leukemia cells from dividing." Yet people are warned that vitamin A is toxic. Nevertheless, each year the American Association of Poison Control Centers has repeatedly failed to show even one death from vitamin A.

There are different forms of vitamin A, called isomers, and these can act as hormones that affect the expression of genes that regulate the cancer process. Vitamin A also influences the development and differentiation of white blood cells, which play critical roles in the immune response. It also influences the activation of T lymphocytes, the major regulatory cells of the immune system. The skin and mucosal cells (cells that line the airways, digestive tract, and urinary tract) function as a barrier and form the body's first line of defense against infection; vitamin A is essential to maintaining the integrity and function of these barrier cells. In addition to supporting immunity, vitamin A supports apoptosis and helps to revert cancer cells back to their normal state.

Supplementation is advisable. I often recommend one tablespoon of high-quality cod liver oil, which supplies about 2,500 IU (international units) of vitamin A. The current recommended daily allowances (RDA) for vitamin A by the Food and Nutrition Board of the National Academy of Sciences are:

- Infants up to one year old—1,250 IU per day
- Children one through three years old—1,333 IU per day
- Children four through six years old—1,667 IU per day
- Children seven through ten years old—2,333 IU per day
- Males and females eleven years and older—3,333 IU per day
- Pregnant/lactating first six months—4,333 IU per day

Cancer patients may require megadoses as high as 300,000 IU per day, but this should be done under the supervision of a physician who uses vitamin therapy.

B Vitamins

B vitamins act as a team, and they are essential for growth, development, energy production, and a variety of other functions. The Bs play a major role in the activities of enzymes, such as in DNA repair enzymes. Keeping DNA in good repair helps to prevent cancer. B vitamins can be easily depleted when the body is under stress, and this leads to serious problems. When supplementing with B vitamins, take a high-quality formula containing the most biologically active forms.

Vitamin B1 plays a major role in energy production; supplement with 100 mg per day.

Vitamin B2 helps in the production of energy and also DNA repair; take 50 mg per day. The biologically active form of B2 is riboflavin-5'-phosphate; it should be included in a good formula.

Vitamin B3 (niacin) helps to prevent cancer because it is an essential component of the enzyme systems that repair damaged DNA. Several studies have shown B3 to be effective against existing cancer in doses of 100 mg three times daily to 1000 mg three times daily. A maintenance dose would be 100 mg per day.

Vitamin B5 helps the body to generate energy; supplement with 100 mg per day.

Epidemiologic studies have shown that vitamin B6 lowers the risk of cancer. B6 is critical to DNA repair. It also helps the body make several neurotransmitters, chemicals that carry signals from one nerve cell to another. B6 is essential for normal brain development and function, and helps the body make the hormones serotonin and norepinephrine (which influence mood) and melatonin (which helps regulate the body clock). High-quality supplements will include B6 in its biologically active pyridoxal-5'-phosphate form. Supplement with 200 mg per day.

Vitamin B9 (folic acid) is also critical to the DNA repair process. People with high levels of folic acid have a low risk of cancer. The recommended dose is 800 micrograms (mcg) per day.

Vitamin B12 plays a major role in DNA repair, and deficiency is a known risk factor for cancer. Adults older than 50 years should take at least 100 to 400 mcg/day of supplemental vitamin B12, and serum B12 levels should be measured periodically. Cancer patients may need 1,000 to 5,000 micrograms per day. Use care in selecting a B12 supplement, as most are in chemical forms that are not very biologically effective. A high-quality supplement will contain B12 in its hydroxocobalamin form.

Make sure the supplements you select have the biologically active forms of all these vitamins as listed above.

Vitamin C

Vitamin C can not only slow cancer down, it can eliminate it. Studies have shown that vitamin C supplementation is effective in preventing cancer, and that it can start a damaging chain reaction in existing cancer cells that destroys them. A 2008 study in the *Proceedings of the National Academy of Sciences* concluded that high-dose vitamin C treatment "significantly decreased growth rates" of ovarian, pancreatic, and malignant brain tumors, and that cancer-stopping levels of vitamin C can be "readily achieved in humans given ascorbate intravenously." For whatever reason, the cancer industry doesn't want you to know this, and organizations like the American Cancer Society actively discourage people from using vitamin C against cancer.

Vitamin C is one of the most important molecules you can put into your body, and most people don't get enough of it. It should be number one on your list of supplements. Vitamin C is a nontoxic anticancer agent, and high doses can go a long way toward preventing and reversing cancer. Vitamin C levels are lower in cancer patients, and this correlates with higher free-radical activity and oxidative damage to the body. The body uses vitamin C's special chemical properties (scientifically, it's called oxidation/reduction or "redox" properties) to instruct cells to divide, to differentiate into different types of cells, or to die. The body constantly produces stem cells that when first produced have no specific jobs. Vitamin C helps to instruct the cells as to the functions they should perform. As such, vitamin C plays an important role in influencing the cancer process; not the least of which is its role in apoptosis, telling cells when to die. In the absence of sufficient vitamin C, cells may divide out of control because they are not being instructed to die.

There are many excellent studies that prove the effectiveness of vitamin C against cancer. A 2005 study in the *Proceedings of the National Academy of Sciences* confirmed that vitamin C is selectively toxic to cancer cells and that tumor-toxic levels of vitamin C can be attained using intravenous administration. The researchers concluded, "These findings give plausibility to intravenous ascorbic acid in cancer treatment." A 2006 study in the *Canadian Medical Association Journal* found intravenous vitamin C to be effective in treating cancer, and a 2008 study in the *Journal of Cellular Physiology* found that intravenous vitamin C "plays a crucial role in the suppression of proliferation of several types of cancer." A 1990 study in the *Journal of Orthomolecular Medicine* reported the successful use of vitamin C to treat kidney cancer, and a 1995 study in *Medical Hypotheses* found that using 30,000 mg of intravenous vitamin C twice per week caused cancerous tumors in the lung and liver to disappear in a matter of weeks.

The recommended oral dose is bowel tolerance. To achieve bowel tolerance, slowly increase vitamin C intake until you get loose stools or diarrhea, then decrease the dose slowly until stools are normal. The body will absorb what it needs and any excess will act like a laxative, causing loose stools and gas. The amount will differ for each person. Orally, 20 grams (20,000 milligrams) per day in divided doses is not unusual, but doses of even 100 grams a day are not unheard of. High doses of intravenous vitamin C, in amounts needed to maintain normal blood levels, can be even more powerful and beneficial; this amount can be 50 grams per week or as high as 200 grams per day in some cases. Vitamin C is a less expensive, safer, and far more effective treatment than standard, toxic chemotherapy.

Both oral and, in particular, intravenous vitamin C are effective against cancer, and even topical vitamin C can be effective against basal cell skin cancers. When a vitamin C solution, made from vitamin C powder and water, is applied directly to basal cell skin cancers, they scab over and drop off. Selectively toxic to cancer cells, vitamin C does not harm healthy skin cells. This simple, home treatment was first publicly reported in 1971 by Frederick Klenner in the *Journal of Applied Nutrition*, yet the cancer industry hasn't made this information available to the public.

Basal cell carcinomas, which are slow growing and rarely metastasize, provide an excellent opportunity to try this topical treatment, provided one has proper medical diagnosis and follow-up. Preparation of a saturated solution of vitamin C is simple. Slowly add a small amount of water to about half a teaspoon of vitamin C powder. Use only enough water so that some of the vitamin C will not dissolve and undissolved powder is left on the bottom—this is called a saturated solution. Apply the solution with the fingertip or a cotton swab, several times daily. The water will evaporate in a few minutes and leave a coat of vitamin C crystals on the skin.

One problem with vitamin C is that most of the vitamin C on the market is not of the highest quality. Do not use commercial vitamin C. Vitamin C supplementation is essential, but taking good vitamin C is also essential. Good vitamin C should be described on the label as: *100% L-ascorbate, fully reduced, corn free*. If it doesn't say this, it is not the kind of vitamin C you should be taking to get maximum health benefits and maximum value for your money.

Vitamin D

Imagine if there were a magic potion that was: nontoxic, inexpensive, had no side effects, and worked to prevent aging, colds, depression, diabetes, flu, multiple sclerosis, obesity, and osteoporosis, *and was proven to prevent four out of five cases of cancer*. Most of us would take such a potion daily if it existed. Vitamin D is that amazing magical potion. Unfortunately, some researchers believe that up to 90 percent of all Americans are deficient in vitamin D, which helps explain our epidemic of chronic disease and cancer.

Research reported in a 2009 *American Journal of Clinical Nutrition* showed a startling 77 percent reduction in cancer risk in study participants who took calcium and vitamin D3 supplements. The vitamin D dose was 1,100 IU, almost three times the government's recommended daily allowance of 400 IU. Many vitamin D experts still consider this a low dose, and believe that 4,000 IU would be more appropriate. While a 77 percent reduction is almost miraculous, one can only wonder what might have been achieved had an even higher dose been used in the experiment.

Vitamin D improves health, prolongs life, and cuts cancer risk by influencing cell growth, promoting healthy cell differentiation, and supporting apoptosis (programmed cell death). It also inhibits angiogenesis—reducing the growth of new blood vessels that support tumor growth.

Low vitamin D and calcium levels disrupt cell-to-cell communications. Loss of cell-to-cell communications is one of the most important breakdowns that enable the cancer process to thrive. Efficient cell-to-cell communications are essential to healthy cell turnover, which prevents aggressive cancer cells from taking over. Not surprisingly, most cancer patients are vitamin D deficient.

Vitamin D deficiency plays a role in causing at least seventeen varieties of cancer, as well as heart disease, stroke, hypertension, autoimmune diseases, diabetes, depression, chronic pain, osteoarthritis, osteoporosis, muscle weakness, muscle wasting, birth defects, and periodontal disease. Over 200 critical genes are adversely affected by vitamin D deficiency. Some of these genes protect against cancer by inducing cell differentiation and controlling cell proliferation.

Breast cancer is particularly sensitive to vitamin D. We now know that the risk of breast cancer can be virtually eliminated if you get vitamin D levels up to about 60–80 ng/ml (nanograms per milliliter), which a blood test will indicate. Women with the lowest blood levels of vitamin D have the highest breast cancer risk, and those dying of metastasized disease are the most deficient of all. Even in those with active breast cancer, vitamin D can help to improve the prognosis. A study in a 2009 *Journal of Clinical Oncology* found that vitamin D can prevent breast cancer recurrence. The researchers found that women with vitamin D deficiency were 94 percent more likely to have recurrence and 73 percent more likely to die, compared with those with normal vitamin D levels in their blood. The current official recommendation is 200 IU per day for those under fifty, 400 IU for men and women between fifty-one and seventy, and 600 IU per day for those over the age of seventy. Vitamin D experts consider this to be too low. Everyone should have vitamin D levels measured periodically. The test is called a 25-hydroxy vitamin D [25(OH) D] test. Blood levels below 50 ng/ml are too low, and if you already have cancer, you will want to keep your levels in the 80–90 ng/ml range. Research in a 2010 *Journal of Nutrition* recommends an intake of 2,100 IU per day and 3,100 IU per day during the winter months. The anticancer properties of vitamin D appear to start kicking in at daily doses of about 1,100 IU.

Sunlight is the best source of vitamin D. People who live in northern parts of the country, where the winters are long, have a greater need for supplementation because there's less sun exposure. How much you need to supplement with vitamin D depends on how dark your skin is, where you live, how much sun you get, your individual genetic makeup, and your unique biochemistry. In 2010, the National Academy of Sciences' Institute of Medicine announced that 4,000 IU a day of vitamin D appeared safe for anyone over nine years old. A 2011 study in *Anticancer Research* concluded that adults needed to take between 4,000 and 8,000 IU a day to maintain the amount of vitamin D needed in their blood to help reduce the risk of disease.

People who have darker skin, who are older, who avoid sun exposure, or who live in the northern United States need higher amounts of vitamin D supplementation. Dark-skinned and older individuals require more supplementation because they are less efficient at producing vitamin D from sunlight. Most importantly, have your vitamin D level measured and keep it in the upper end of the normal range. Everyone should know his or her vitamin D level. It is now obvious that adequate vitamin D is the cheapest anticancer insurance you can buy. For cancer patients, it would be grossly negligent to disregard rather than optimize vitamin D blood levels.

Vitamin E

Vitamin E is a fat-soluble vitamin that acts as an antioxidant. It consists of a family of eight antioxidants—four tocopherols and four tocotrienols. Vitamin E's important jobs include protecting vitamin A and essential fatty acids from oxidation and helping to prevent damage to body tissues.

Cancer can be caused by oxidative, free-radical damage to DNA. Vitamin E helps to protect against the damaging effects of free radicals and, therefore, helps to protect against cancer. It also blocks the formation of nitrosamines, which are carcinogens formed in the stomach from nitrites in the diet. Further, vitamin E also protects against cancer by enhancing immune function.

Although some studies have claimed that vitamin E has no protective effect against cancer, these studies were poorly done and used synthetic vitamin E, which is known to be less effective than natural vitamin E. Contrary to these studies, the Nurses' Health Study, which I referred to earlier, found that women with a family history of breast cancer who consumed the highest quantity of vitamin E had a 43 percent reduction in breast cancer incidence compared to those with the lowest levels. A previously mentioned 2002 study in the *Journal of Cancer Research and Clinical Oncology* found that vitamin E supplementation reduced esophageal cancer risk by an astounding 87 percent. A 1996 study in the *Journal of the National Cancer Institute* found that men with a high vitamin E intake are 65 percent less likely to develop colorectal adenomas compared to men with low vitamin E intake. African-Americans who have the lowest serum alpha-tocopherol levels have the highest incidence of prostate cancer.

Tocotrienols, four of the eight members of the vitamin E family, have been shown to inhibit the growth of estrogen-sensitive cancer cells by as much as 50 percent in the laboratory. Tocotrienols have demonstrated a significant potential to both reduce breast cancer incidence and to inhibit the propagation of existing breast cancer cells. Several studies have indicated that tocotrienols are effective supporters of apoptosis.

Supplementing with vitamin E is important for overall health. I recommend taking both tocopherols (standard vitamin E) and tocotrienols. They should be taken at different times of the day so as not to compete for absorption. The daily dose for tocopherols is recommended at 400 mg per forty pounds of body weight, and for tocotrienols, 250 mg daily.

Beta-carotene

Beta-carotene is a member of a family of nutrients called carotenes. Carotenes are found in dark leafy green vegetables and in colored fruits and vegetables such as carrots, beets, and tomatoes. There is powerful evidence that the carotenes found in foods decrease the incidence of cancer. To maximize the bioavailability of the carotenes in the foods listed above, they should be eaten raw or steamed lightly. Beta-carotene is a powerful antioxidant that helps prevent free-radical damage to healthy cells. By preventing such damage and controlling inflammation, antioxidants play key roles in the prevention of cancer.

Beta-carotene is related to vitamin A, and it is a natural precursor to vitamin A. Unlike vitamin A, beta-carotene does not accumulate in the body and cause vitamin toxicity. In addition to protecting cells from oxidative damage, beta-carotene has been shown to enhance immune function. It has also been shown in animal studies to be selectively toxic to cancer cells. Beta-carotene injected into tumors has caused them to shrink. Supplementing with pure, high-quality beta-carotene is very safe and nontoxic. Cancer patients can take beta-carotene in doses of up to 100,000 to 300,000 IU per day. Carrot juice is a good source of beta-carotene, and natural-source supplements can also be taken. Synthetic beta-carotene should not be used as it can actually cause a carotene deficiency. Supplements should be made from natural forms, which can be listed on the label as being from natural beta-carotene, from D. salina, from an algal source, or from a palm source.

Flavonoids

Flavonoids are a family of natural chemicals called polyphenolic compounds. They are found in a variety of teas, vegetables, and fruits, as well as other foods, beverages, and supplements, and are responsible for the color in many fruits and vegetables. Rich sources of flavonoids include grains, nuts, and most legumes. Flavonoids act as antioxidants, which protect against free-radical damage to cells. In addition, they have antiviral, anti-allergic, antiplatelet, anti-inflammatory, and antitumor properties. Flavonoids also play a role in cell signaling, the complex system of communication that governs basic cellular activities and coordinates cell actions. About 5,000 flavonoids have been identified, and depending on their chemical structure, members of the flavonoid family of compounds are known as flavonols, flavones, flavanones, isoflavones, catechins, anthocyanidins, and chalcones. A single piece of fruit can contain hundreds of these beneficial nutrients, but only a few dozen of them have been extensively studied. Of these, quercetin and curcumin are two that stand out as especially useful; supplementing with these is recommended.

Flavonoids are powerful anticancer chemicals. They support apoptosis (normal cell death) and inhibit angiogenesis (growth of new blood vessels to feed growing tumors). Flavonoids are capable of shutting down the cancer process. In fact, plant flavonoids prevent cells from becoming cancerous, even when the cells are exposed to powerful carcinogens. Some of the chemicals found in plants can actually restore cancer cells to normal. Best of all, these powerful anticancer chemicals are found in common fruits and vegetables, especially in the cruciferous vegetables, such as broccoli, Brussels sprouts, cabbage, cauliflower, and kale. Generally, it's the fruits and vegetables with the deepest colors that have the most flavonoids.

Studies have shown that people with the highest flavonoid intake have the least amount of stomach, pancreatic, lung, and breast cancer. Not only do flavonoids neutralize free radicals, they boost immunity and strengthen blood vessels, thereby increasing blood flow and the availability of oxygen, among other beneficial effects.

Quercetin

Quercetin is a common plant flavonoid found in everything from tea to apples and onions. It is a powerful anticancer compound. A 2010 study in *Clinical Cancer Research* found that quercetin supports apoptosis, slowing the growth of cancer cells. Quercetin also inhibits angiogenesis.

Quercetin has anti-inflammatory and antioxidant properties, and it provides powerful antioxidant protection to DNA. It also acts as a building block for many other flavonoids. Natural sources of quercetin include apples, raspberries, other dark berries, black and green tea, buckwheat, onions, olive oil, red wine, red grapes, citrus fruit, cherries, broccoli, and leafy greens.

Quercetin acts like an antihistamine, preventing immune cells from releasing histamines, chemicals that cause allergic reactions. This helps to reduce symptoms of allergies, including runny nose, watery eyes, hives, and swelling. Quercetin also reduces blood pressure in people with hypertension, reduces the symptoms of prostatitis (inflammation of the prostate) and rheumatoid arthritis, and helps to prevent cardiovascular disease by reducing plaque buildup in arteries that can lead to heart attack or stroke. Quercetin also works with vitamin C to help the body maintain healthy collagen, which is necessary to help keep cancer from spreading. To prevent cancer, take 2,000 to 4,000 mg of high-quality quercetin in supplement form per day. People with cancer can take up to 25,000 mg per day in divided doses.

Curcumin

Curcumin is a nonflavonoid polyphenolic, which both prevents and reverses cancer. It is derived from turmeric, a spice that is a member of the ginger family. Tumeric's wide use in Indian cuisine is thought to be a reason why the rate of colon, breast, prostate, and lung cancer is ten times lower in India than in the United States.

Turmeric is a traditional Indian curry spice, and is also used as a yellow food coloring. For at least 6,000 years, turmeric has been used in traditional medicine from ancient Egypt to India. In 2010 alone, over 240 studies were published on the health benefits of curcumin.

Curcumin is a very effective anticancer substance because it interferes with the cancer process at multiple levels. It suppresses inflammation, thereby blocking a key biological pathway needed for cancer development. Curcumin shuts down nuclear factor-kappa B (NF-kB), a powerful master switch known to regulate the expression of more than 300 genes that promote inflammation. In fact, the anti-inflammatory activity of curcumin is comparable to steroidal drugs, without the dangerous side effects.

Curcumin promotes apoptosis by suppressing the production of the proteins in cancer cells that protect the cells from normal cell death. It also inhibits angiogenesis, starving tumors of the blood supply they need for their growth. Curcumin inhibits the growth of tumors by blocking enzymes necessary for dissolving the collagen that surrounds tumors. Further, curcumin blocks numerous molecules that are vital to cancer metastasis. Even topical application of curcumin as a paste on the skin inhibits the growth of skin cancer cells.

In human clinical trials, doses up to 10,000 milligrams per day have been found to be safe. Doses of 3,600 mg per day have been used to successfully interfere with the cancer process. As with any supplement, the quality varies tremendously. It is important to use a curcumin product that is well-absorbed after oral ingestion, biologically active, and free of toxic contaminants. See my article on curcumin at www.beyondhealth.com under "Health Resources."

Minerals

Nobel Prize winner Dr. Linus Pauling once said, "You can trace every sickness, every disease, and every ailment to a mineral deficiency." Unfortunately, mineral deficiency is epidemic today.

Selenium

Selenium is an essential trace mineral that, in very small amounts, supports the body's antioxidant activity. Selenium promotes a healthy immune system, has strong anticancer effects, and helps detoxify the body by removing heavy metals such as mercury, cadmium, and silver. Selenium is an essential building block for the special enzymes that knock out free radicals that can attack healthy cells and lead to cancer. It also helps to speed the elimination of cancer cells and to slow tumor growth. In addition, selenium plays a role in recycling antioxidants throughout the body, lowering the risk of cancer by preventing free radicals from damaging cells. Especially when combined with adequate amounts of vitamin E, selenium dramatically reduces the risk of pancreatic cancer.

A large body of evidence has found that increased intake of selenium is tied to a reduced risk of cancer. Low levels of selenium in the soil translate to low dietary intake and increased cancer risk. In populations with high risk for prostate cancer, selenium supplements decreased the risk and slowed the growth rate of tumors. Selenium supplements also halt the growth of polyps in the colon and reduce the risk of lung and liver cancers. Numerous studies have proven the benefits of selenium supplementation. In a region of China where selenium is low in the soil, esophageal cancer is epidemic. By supplementing with selenium, the risk was cut in half. Many cancer patients have low blood levels of selenium. People with the lowest blood levels had between 3.8 and 5.8 times the risk of dying from cancer compared with those who had the highest selenium levels. Taking 200 micrograms (mcg) of selenium daily for seven years cut the occurrence of all cancers in half and reduced the incidence of prostate cancer by 69 percent.

The amount of selenium we consume is dependent on the levels of selenium in the soil where our crops are grown. Countries with low soil levels of selenium include China, Denmark, Finland, and New Zealand. Rich food sources of selenium are grains and Brazil nuts. Fruits and vegetables also provide selenium.

The RDA for selenium is 55 mcg, but to protect against cancer, studies indicate that 100 to 300 mcg per day is necessary. Cancer patients have benefited by taking 200 to 1,000 mcg daily. Taking too much selenium can be toxic, and organic forms are far better than inorganic forms.

Other Minerals

Calcium has been shown to help prevent precancerous cells in the colon from developing further, and is often associated with a reduced risk for both rectal and colon cancer. No other mineral performs as many biological actions as calcium; it is involved in almost every biological function. Calcium provides the electrical energy for the heart to beat and for all muscle movement. It also plays an important role in pH control as well as in DNA replication, which is crucial for maintaining a youthful and healthy body. Due to our mineral-depleted soils, over 75 percent of all Americans are calcium deficient, which helps explain why our bodies are so acidic. One reason we are aging prematurely is because of deficiencies of calcium, and thus, inadequate DNA maintenance. Researchers suggest taking between 1,000 mg and 2,000 mg daily in supplemental form to help prevent cancer.

Alkalizing minerals such as calcium, magnesium, potassium, and zinc are all cancer protective. They help to keep the body alkaline, and cancer cannot thrive in an alkaline environment. Magnesium is especially important in helping to neutralize the acid being produced by the cancer process. Manganese is needed to form an antioxidant enzyme. Molybdenum is critical to a number of enzymes. All minerals work together as a team, so you need the whole team, and the entire team must be present in order to get anticancer benefits. The absence of even one mineral causes cellular malfunction and disease. This is why nutrition experts recommend that everyone take at least a high quality multivitamin daily.

Cesium

Unlike the nutrient minerals above, cesium is an alkalizing mineral that is used to treat existing cancer. While no therapy is appropriate for every cancer patient, studies have shown cesium to be effective in shrinking tumors with few side effects. Cesium is preferentially taken up by cancer cells, and it has the effect of raising the pH of cancer cells to above normal, which kills them. Cesium increases the pH of cancer cells to approximately 8.0, which is deadly for the cancer cell. At this pH, cancer cells will die within days and be absorbed and eliminated by the body. Cesium also limits the cellular uptake of glucose. Cancer cells need sugar to create energy, and cesium starves them. Practitioners who use this mineral therapy usually suggest a dosage of 1 to 6 grams/day of cesium chloride. Most cancer patients take 3 grams per day, always with food, as it can upset the stomach when taken alone. It is best to work with an experienced practitioner.

Iodine

Most people correctly associate iodine with healthy thyroid function, but may not be aware that every cell in the body uses and requires iodine. Iodine exhibits many cancer-fighting and cancer-preventing properties, such as supporting apoptosis. Unfortunately, in the United States, over the last three decades, body levels of iodine have dropped by nearly 50 percent. Not surprisingly, every cancer patient I have ever seen was iodine deficient.

Iodine deficiency is widespread for several reasons. Chemical farming techniques have depleted our agricultural soil of minerals, including iodine. Crops grown in such soils will be iodine deficient. In addition to soil depletion and low iodine intake, environmental toxins such as bromine, chlorine, and fluoride compete with iodine for use by the body, causing deficiency even if iodine intake is adequate. Decades ago, bakers used iodine as a dough conditioner. Since the 1980s, bakers have replaced iodine with bromine, which interferes with iodine and is a known carcinogen. This is yet another reason not to eat processed foods like bread or other commercial baked goods.

To keep the body in balance, there must be a balance between oxidants and antioxidants. Iodine functions as both a strong antioxidant as well as an oxidant in the body. This dual nature makes it a powerful anticancer agent. Dr. David Brownstein, author of *Iodine: Why You Need It, Why You Can't Live Without It,* maintains that iodine can cause tumors to shrink and die from the center out. He's found similar results with nodules and cysts in the thyroid, ovaries, and uterus after supplementation with iodine.

Iodine participates in the production of all of your body's hormones. It is also vital for proper immune function. Good food sources of iodine include fish and sea vegetables. You should know what your iodine level is, and if you are deficient, you should supplement. The test for deficiency is a simple urine test.

CoQ10

Coenzyme Q10 (CoQ10) slows tumor growth via several mechanisms. CoQ10 supports immune function, suppresses angiogenesis, and reduces inflammation, all of which are beneficial for the cancer patient.

Cells use coenzyme Q10 to help make the energy needed for the body to function. CoQ10 is also an antioxidant that protects cells from free radicals that can damage DNA. By protecting cells against free radicals, antioxidants help protect the body against cancer. CoQ10 also boosts the immune system by helping to supply the large amounts of energy the system needs to operate.

Low blood levels of CoQ10 have been found in cancer patients, and it has been known since the early 1960s that low blood levels of CoQ10 correlate with whether you have cancer and how the cancer will progress. It is even possible to predict survival in breast cancer patients by their CoQ10 levels. The higher the blood levels, the better the chances of survival.

By helping to create energy, boosting immunity, interfering with angiogenesis, and reducing inflammation, CoQ10 helps prevent and reverse cancer. Numerous alternative physicians have reported miraculous results in reversing cases of terminal cancer using large doses of CoQ10. The doses ranged from 300 to 1,200 milligrams daily, whereas normal doses might range from 60 to 100 mg.

Enzymes

Certain enzymes also help keep cancer under control. Cancer cells develop a thick protein coating that makes it difficult for the immune system to identify and attack them. Cutting through the protein coating makes cancer cells visible to the immune system so they can be destroyed. This can be accomplished through protein-dissolving enzymes called proteases (proteolytic enzymes). Two such enzymes the pancreas produces are trypsin and chymotrypsin. Poor diets, toxins, and genetic mutations can reduce the body's supply of these enzymes. Specifically, problems can begin with our high animal-protein diet. One reason consuming a high animal-protein diet is a risk factor for cancer is that meat requires proteolytic enzymes for digestion, making these enzymes less available for digesting cancer cells. Another is that meat acidifies the body, and pancreatic enzymes work best in an alkaline environment.

Supplementation can help to keep enzyme levels high. A number of alternative medical doctors are now using proteolytic enzymes as part of their cancer therapy, often in high doses as determined by the physician. These enzymes are natural and normal to the body. They do no harm, yet are effective in fighting cancer.

Lysine and Proline

In Chapter 3, I talked about the importance of maintaining strong, healthy collagen. Poorly constructed collagen fibers are more susceptible to damage, and this allows collagen-dissolving enzymes to cut through connective tissue, allowing cancer to spread. Vitamin C helps to support the production of collagen, while the amino acids lysine and proline are critical building blocks of collagen. You need all three in adequate supply, but most of us don't get enough lysine, even when supplementing with other nutrients. Supplementing with lysine and proline not only prevents cancer from happening, it also works to prevent the spread of existing cancer. A dose of 5,000 mg per day of each is recommended for cancer patients. For prevention, or for maintenance after the cancer has reversed, 500 mg of each per day is recommended.

Epigallocatechin Gallate

Epigallocatechin gallate (EGCG) is commonly called green tea extract. Green tea contains chemicals known as polyphenols, which have antioxidant and anticancer properties. The major polyphenols in green tea are called catechins, and the most important catechin appears to be EGCG, a powerful antioxidant. It also facilitates liver detoxification and protects DNA from damage by carcinogenic chemicals. Studies suggest that EGCG is effective both as a cancer preventive and a cancer treatment, both promoting apoptosis and inhibiting angiogenesis. For cancer patients, supplementing with 1,000 mg three times daily is recommended, as is consumption of organically grown, high-quality green tea. Drinking four to five cups of green tea daily may slow the growth of cancer, and even two cups per day may help to prevent cancer.

Grapeseed Extract

Traditionally, when people ate grapes, they ate the seeds as well. Today, we not only don't eat the seeds, we even have seedless grapes! As it turns out, grapeseeds are rich in cancer-inhibiting flavonoids, and grapeseed extract, available in pill form, has been demonstrated in the laboratory to support apoptosis, rapidly killing cancer cells. The recommended dose is 100 mg three times per day.

Modified Citrus Pectin

Pectin is a carbohydrate found in fruit, and is most concentrated in the peels of apples, citrus fruits, and plums. It is made of hundreds or thousands of sugar molecules, chemically linked together. To make modified citrus pectin, available in powder form, the pectin is chemically altered to break its big molecules into smaller ones that are more easily absorbed by the digestive tract.

Modified citrus pectin (MCP) will not cure cancer, but studies show that it helps to block metastasis and the spread of cancer around the body. MCP molecules appear to bind to receptors on cancerous cells, thereby preventing cancer cells from penetrating into nearby healthy tissue. MCP interferes with the binding properties of cancer cells and prevents them from adhering to each other and to the inner wall of blood vessels, which is necessary for metastasis. By inhibiting the spread of cancer, MCP keeps the body's immune system from becoming overwhelmed by an ever-increasing cancer load. The recommended dose is 15 grams per day in three divided doses.

IP-6

IP-6 (inositol hexaphosphate) is a natural compound found in cereal grains, beans, brown rice, corn, sesame seeds, wheat bran, and other high-fiber foods. IP-6 has many health benefits, including acting as an antioxidant, immune enhancer, and supporter of cardiovascular health. Additionally, it helps the liver transfer fat to other parts of the body and has been shown to have significant protective and growth-regulating effects on various cells and tissues.

IP-6 supports apoptosis, inhibits angiogenesis, inhibits platelet aggregation, and increases differentiation of malignant cells. Enhanced differentiation of malignant cells can result in restoring those cells to normal. This naturally occurring compound, available in pill form, offers a number of health benefits without any known toxicity. For people with cancer, a dose of 5 to 8 grams per day is usually recommended. To prevent cancer, a dose of 1 to 2 grams per day taken on an empty stomach should suffice.

To Sum Up

There is an enormous amount of research showing that antioxidant vitamins and other supplements reduce cancer risk. Supplements protect us by reducing free-radical oxidative damage to DNA, reducing the formation of carcinogens in the body, enhancing immunity, supporting cell-to-cell communications, signaling genes, and enhancing DNA repair in the body. They help to eliminate deficiency—one of the two causes of disease. Combinations of supplements work together to achieve an impact that goes far beyond what any one of them acting alone can achieve.

Most disease is caused by malnutrition, and the Standard American Diet is not capable of supplying sufficient amounts of nutrients to maintain optimal health. Even so-called "good diets" require supplementation. By supplying our cells with the nutrition they need, disease can be prevented and reversed. Researchers from the National Institute on Aging, reporting in a 1996 *Journal of Clinical Nutrition,* found that elderly people who supplement with vitamins C and E have a 50 percent lower risk of dying prematurely from any disease, compared to people who do not supplement. Everyone should be taking at least a high-quality multivitamin, plus extra vitamin C and E. Cancer patients require substantially more than this minimum.

Malnutrition is a fundamental cause of most disease, not only chronic diseases but also infectious diseases. Unfortunately, the average American diet does not supply a sufficient amount of minerals and vitamins to maintain optimal health. This is why we need to supplement. A survey by the American Medical Association, reported in a 2005 *Archives of Internal Medicine,* found that between the ages of eighteen and seventy-four less than one out of four of us consume five servings of fruits and vegetables per day, and this is only half of what we need for good health. Only 3 percent of American adults practice what is commonly considered a healthy lifestyle. Many Americans claim that consuming the required quantities of fruits and vegetables each day is impractical. However, getting cancer is far more impractical! Clearly, the right approach is to eat all the fresh fruits and vegetables you possibly can, *and* take high-quality supplements. A deficiency of just one nutrient can cause numerous different diseases, and supplementing with even one nutrient can cure them. The number one problem with supplements is the failure to take enough of them.

Be aware, however, that despite your good intentions, if you choose low-quality products (no matter how much they cost), they will be of little or no benefit.

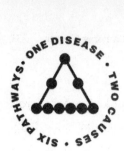

11

Preventing and Reversing Cancer

Cancer is one of the most curable diseases in this country today.

—Vincent DeVita, Jr., M.D.
Former director of the National Cancer Institute

It has been said that we have enough information
from worldwide studies to cure cancer, but no one
has sifted through all of the information
and put it into a clinically usable form.

—Russell L. Blaylock, M.D., author of
Natural Strategies for Cancer Patients

The person who says it cannot be done
should not interrupt the person doing it.

—Old Chinese Proverb

I f you have stayed with me through this book, I've taken you on a journey that has been at times shocking and disturbing, but also hopeful and promising. It is shocking to realize how many people have suffered and died because they put their faith in conventional medical treatments that are ineffective and dangerous. (The fact that poisoning, slashing, and burning are considered "conventional" treatments is itself shocking!) It is disturbing to learn how cancer survival statistics have been manipulated to the point of being meaningless, with the real cancer survival rates being no better than they were in the 1950s.

Yet there is hope and promise in the information I have presented. You can prevent and reverse cancer without resorting to draconian measures that are not even based in science. Albert Einstein advised that we can't solve problems by using the same kind of thinking we used to create them. To get well and stay well, we have to think differently. We have to stop thinking of food purely as entertainment and instead realize it is nourishment for our cells. We have to stop ignoring the toxins in our lives, despite the fact that they are relatively imperceptible and seem to have no immediate adverse effects.

We also have to stop thinking of cancer as a monster that attacks innocent victims for no reason. Instead, we must realize that cancer is a very predictable outcome of the poor choices we make—lifestyle choices that create an environment in the body that allows cancer to thrive. If we can create a cancer-thriving environment in our bodies by making bad choices, we can create an environment that does not support cancer by making good choices. *This is the new paradigm for preventing and reversing cancer.*

Finally (and this is the toughest one), we have to stop having blind faith in the institutions that are supposedly looking after our health. Despite the good intentions of the individuals involved, these institutions over time have succumbed to the sway of self-preservation at the expense of their mission. Do you truly believe that the Food and Drug Administration, the American Medical Association, the American Cancer Society, the National Cancer Institute, the pharmaceutical industry, and the health insurance industry have your health and well-being as their number one priority? Their very existence depends on the perpetuation of disease.

In today's reality, we cannot afford to delegate responsibility for our health to the institutions we have trusted in the past. We must take responsibility for our own life and put more faith in our body's natural ability to heal itself than we put in these institutions that are increasingly failing us. We do this by educating ourselves about the true nature of disease and what our body needs at the cellular level to function optimally.

If you are concerned about cancer, here is what you need to know. Cancer can be prevented; it can be cured. You can make yourself cancer proof by making *fundamental* changes in your diet and lifestyle, especially ones that increase cellular oxygen and help to maintain or restore normal oxygen metabolism in your cells. pH must be optimized and the correct oils must be consumed. Unless you have one of the rare truly genetic diseases, you can heal yourself of disease, but you have to be willing to do what it takes to make it happen.

Always remember that cancer is not a tumor to be removed by poisoning, slashing and burning your body. Cancer is the biological process that produces the tumor; it is a systemic problem in which the normal control mechanisms of the body are altered. This process is entirely dependent on you and what you put into your mind and body. To attack the tumor, which is conventional medicine's standard approach, is a losing strategy with a success rate that is so low it is a national disgrace.

Surgery, chemotherapy and radiation will all reduce your tumor burden, but they will not change the underlying conditions that allowed the cancer to happen. The tumor may disappear, but the cancer won't. Cancer is not the tumor, it is the process, and while that process is still operating—you still have cancer. To get cancer, you must change your internal environment to one that supports the cancer process. To cure cancer, you must restore normal body chemistry. When you do so, the cancer process shuts down and tumors simply disappear.

Since there are only two causes of disease—deficiency and toxicity—getting well is about eliminating deficiency and toxicity through nutrition and detoxification. The best strategy of all is to prevent cancer. Normal body chemistry will not support the cancer process; cancer cannot happen in a healthy body. To prevent cancer and make yourself cancer proof, keep your body chemistry normal.

At this point in time, the science is very clear and indisputable. Cancer *can* be prevented and it *can* be cured, but old mindsets are difficult to change. When correctly understood at the molecular level, all disease can be prevented and reversed. The greatest obstacle to success in curing cancer is the disbelief that it can be done. Yet as I talk to cancer survivors around the country, I get the same story over and over. The point at which patients start to improve is when they start alternative treatments—treatments that are aimed at helping the body to restore its normal balance and function in place of treatments aimed at removing or destroying the cancer. Indeed, there is only one disease—malfunctioning cells—and only one cure: restoring cells to normal and getting well.

As I said previously, cancer is happening because we have fundamentally changed our diets, our environment, and our lifestyle. Cancer is normal to the way we live because we are now eating a diet, existing in an environment, and living a lifestyle that promotes cancer. Disease happens when the body is no longer properly communicating, self-regulating, and self-repairing. In this unbalanced state, the body is out of control, and cancer is uncontrolled growth.

Your body is designed to be healthy. It has an awesome capacity to adapt, repair, and keep everything properly regulated, balanced, and running smoothly. It will do a fabulous job, until *you* screw it up. It is we who are creating this epidemic of chronic disease and cancer by choosing to eat a diet that will not even support healthy life in rats, by exposing ourselves to environmental toxins and electromagnetic radiation, and by throwing our complex metabolic machinery out of balance with chronic stress.

There are some factors affecting our health over which we have little or no control. For example, the diets and toxic loads of your parents can have a lifelong effect on your longevity, your overall health, and your susceptibility to cancer. However, all that is in the past and cannot be changed. Starting right now, the choices you make can reduce the negative impact of these parental influences on your health and longevity. No matter what hand of genetic cards you were dealt, right now it is how *you* play the game that matters. You have enormous control over your health, and you exercise that control all day, every day, with each choice that you make. Choose health every day in every way, and you can't lose. Use the information in the Six Pathways to help you make choices that support health.

To our conventionally trained physicians, cancer is something that just happens, and we have no control over it. The truth is by the time a tumor is diagnosed, the cancer process has been operating for a long time. It takes an average of seven years, and it can easily take twenty years, for a tumor to develop to an extent that a doctor can diagnose it. Your diet, your environment, and your lifestyle have been perpetuating unhealthy conditions in your body for years, even though you and your physicians may have believed you were in good health.

The good news about cancer's slow development rate is that there is ample opportunity to prevent it from ever becoming diagnosable. Too many Americans, especially those over 50, already have multiple clusters of cancer cells, microtumors, in their body. You may be one of them, but this doesn't mean you are doomed. These microtumors are waiting for the opportunity to grow, but they can't grow unless you provide the right conditions. By denying them the opportunity, you render those microtumors harmless. The process that generated these tumors can be shut down and the tumors that are already growing can be stopped.

The bad news about cancer's slow development is that it tends to contribute to the misperception that conventional cancer treatments are working, and that no lifestyle changes are needed after a tumor has been removed. If a post-operative cancer patient is "in remission" but has made no changes in diet or elimination of toxins to shut down the cancer process, there is a near certainty that the oxygen deficiency will continue and that new tumors will eventually be found, perhaps many years later.

Because cancer is such a complex condition, no single treatment will be 100 percent effective in every case. By the time cancer is diagnosed, your body is already enormously out of balance, in toxic overload, and weakened in many ways. This is why it is extremely important to take a comprehensive approach and follow all of the Six Pathways toward health to get the best results. To become cancer proof, you have to create health. You do this by restoring the body's internal environment to one that supports health rather than disease. You not only have to improve your diet and avoid toxins, you have to change your thoughts. The stress of negative thoughts and emotions creates deficiency and toxicity at the cellular level, and that creates disease.

We know that cancer is caused by a lack of oxygen respiration in the cell. However, there are many ways by which this can happen, and it is difficult to know exactly how this happened in a particular cancer patient. That is why, to reverse cancer, the cancer patient should do everything possible to switch the cancer process off. This includes: a good diet, high-quality supplements, detoxification, exercise, and positive thinking.

It is not easy to make a human being sick. We are hearty, resilient and adaptable organisms. This is why cancer was a rare disease historically. Medical historians have analyzed references to cancer in classical literature, and also searched for signs in the fossil record and in mummified bodies. Their conclusion is that tumors were extremely rare until very recent times. Their study of ancient bodies has determined that cancer is a man-made disease, one fueled by the modern excesses of pollution and poor diets. Unfortunately, after these modern excesses have succeeded in making us sick, the number of systems in the body that are compromised can become so great that the ability to repair is in jeopardy. This means that getting well requires a lot of dedicated effort—but it can be done. This chapter will help to summarize and streamline those efforts.

Good Nutrition

Everything your body does is dependent on nutrients that must be supplied by your diet. The single most important thing anyone can do to prevent and reverse disease is eat a good diet. Unless you focus on eating a healthy diet, poor nutrition will cripple any effort to get well or stay well. Cells have a grocery list of nutrients that they must obtain on a regular basis to function normally. A chronic shortage of even one can cause cancer. This is why we cannot afford to eat foods that are devoid of nutrients, and it is why our diet must consist primarily of raw/living plant foods.

Are you eating a lot of empty-calorie foods, or do you choose nutrient-dense foods that give you more bang for your caloric buck? Your honest answer to this question can mean the difference between health and disease for you. Each cell of your body is a complete living entity with its own metabolism. To function properly, each cell needs a constant supply of oxygen and other essential nutrients. When you don't supply these nutrients, when you poison the metabolic machinery with toxins, when you don't get enough movement or sleep, and when your digestion is impaired by taking antibiotics and other prescription drugs, your cells will start to degenerate. The normal process of cell replacement and rebuilding will slow down, your tissues will age, your resistance to disease will diminish, and you will become old and sick.

Eating a good diet is fundamental to good health, but to be realistic, there is no such thing as a diet that works for everyone. Some people will do extremely well on a strict vegetarian diet, but others will not. Some people need animal protein in their diet to feel well. Each of us is biologically unique with different requirements. The best advice is to listen to your body. See how you feel after eating a food. Do your eyes itch? Are you depressed, nauseous, tired, bloated or sluggish? Do you feel hot? Do you sweat? Do your muscles twitch? All of these are bad signs, telling you that particular food is not right for you. You are most likely allergic to these foods, and they suppress your immunity. If you listen carefully, your body will tell you what it wants or does not want. A lot of people today are following advice in books on nutritional typing, but I have yet to see one that really works for more than a small percentage of people.

The most important thing is to eat a diet high in nutrition. To reverse cancer, good nutrition alone is more effective than chemotherapy or radiation. A small number of cells in every person will turn cancerous. The body knows what to do and gets rid of those cancerous cells before they do harm. Problems begin when the number of cancer cells being created exceeds what the body can get rid of. Unfortunately, this has become the norm in our society. With our poor diets, increased toxic loads, chronic stress, electromagnetic pollution and health-damaging medical care, our immune systems have become significantly overworked and weakened, and cancer is now normal.

To prevent or reverse cancer you must be willing to make different dietary choices, and do what is necessary to transform your internal environment from one that promotes cancer into one that supports health. Give your cells the nutrients they need. Eat most of your diet raw, and if you must cook, lightly steam your food. Eat a diet rich in vitamins, minerals, flavonoids, and essential fatty acids. Get rid of immune-suppressing, cancer-causing foods such as the Big Four—*get the sugar out of your life*. Cancer cells need lots of sugar to survive and prosper, and every time you eat sugar, you are feeding the cancer. Anything that increases the insulin content of your blood is bad for you and should be avoided, such as any kind of sugar, white flour, white potatoes, white rice, and fruit juices.

Cancer cells cannot thrive where there is sufficient oxygen. Just as we couldn't survive on the moon with no oxygen, cancer can't survive where there *is* oxygen. What we need to do is increase the levels of oxygen in our cells, creating an internal environment that is hostile to cancer. Fortunately, there are relatively simple things any of us can do to increase the oxygen in our cells and make ourselves cancer proof. The following are the most important things you need to pay attention to:

Numerous studies have indisputably proven that the most important thing you can do to prevent and cure cancer is to eat lots of fresh fruit and vegetables, yet only about one in four do this. Health benefits appear to start at five servings per day, but 10 to 12 servings would be best. *There are chemicals contained in vegetables that shut down every known step in the cancer process.* The majority of cancer patients do not eat even two servings per day. People who eat the most fruits and vegetables suffer only half as much cancer of those who don't. This is why you should switch to a mostly vegetarian diet. People who eat almost no vegetables have four times as much pancreatic cancer as people who eat five or more servings per day. The correct combination of nutrients can actually change cancer cells back into normal cells.

By eliminating cancer promoters and maximizing cancer inhibitors, it is possible to turn cancer off. We know fresh fruits and especially vegetables are cancer inhibitors—eat lots of them. As much as possible, consume foods that are fresh, raw, and organic. Juicing vegetables breaks down plant cells to extract their nutrients, as much as tripling the amount of nutrition you get from the same vegetable than if you chewed it. Daily juicing of anticancer vegetables such as broccoli, cabbage, carrots, and kale will have a powerful anticancer effect on the body.

Eating more fresh fruits and vegetables results in eating less processed foods. Eating less processed food eliminates much of the sugar, salt and chemical additives from your diet. It also reduces the amount of processed oils in your diet, and processed oils may be the leading cause of cancer. Eliminating milk and dairy products lowers your fat intake; people with lower animal fat intake have less cancer. Milk is also rich in cancer-promoting hormones, which are known to drive breast and prostate cancer.

We know that sugar, excess omega-6 oils, and excess animal protein promote cancer—avoid them. Avoid all fruit juices, even if they are organic and fresh-squeezed; they contain too much easily absorbable sugar and this elevates insulin. Insulin must be controlled. This is why sugar must be eliminated from the diet. Excess omega-6 oils not only promote cancer, they also suppress the immune system, so avoid all those supermarket oils (corn, peanut, soybean, canola, sunflower, and safflower). Eat adequate amounts of omega-3 oils to offset this effect; supplement with flaxseed and fish oils. Turn cancer off by avoiding excess animal protein; this means very moderate consumption of meat, eggs, dairy, and fish. Cancer is highly iron dependent. Avoid more than small amounts of iron-rich foods such as red meat. As you can see, this is not rocket science. Anybody can do this.

Supplementing is an essential part of a good diet or any wellness program. Modern diets are deficient in essential nutrients. Things get worse when we deplete the body of its already inadequate stores of nutrients by eating an acidic diet, creating chronic inflammation, and provoking chronic immune responses from allergies and infections. The body's cellular machinery simply cannot operate in the absence of key vitamins, minerals, essential fatty acids and other nutrients. To rebuild health, these must all be supplied and restored to normal levels. One reason why so many people are unable to restore their health is that nutrient repletion and cellular repair require extraordinary amounts of essential nutrients. For example, an ongoing inflammatory process burns through a huge quantity of antioxidants daily—extraordinary amounts must be supplied to end this process. Cancer patients need to restore the integrity of cell membranes by avoiding the inflammatory processed oils and supplementing with lots of high-quality essential fatty acids in the correct ratios.

Certain supplements, such as a high-quality multivitamin, are a must. High doses of vitamin C are essential for most cancer patients. Optimizing levels of vitamin D and iodine has to be done. It may not be possible to beat cancer without adequate amounts of vitamin D. Virtually every cancer patient needs an oil change; supplementing with lots of omega-3 fatty acids is essential—lots of flaxseed oil.

Supplements are essential, but the supplements you take must be in forms that are capable of high biological activity. Be aware that most supplement products fail to do this. It is important that critical minerals such as boron, copper, iron, magnesium, manganese, molybdenum, selenium, vanadium, and zinc all have to be supplied in biologically active forms such as ascorbates, citrates, fumarates and malates.

Reduce Your Toxic Load

As much as possible, get the manmade synthetic chemicals out of your life. Use the Toxin Pathway chapter to identify sources of toxins and avoid them. Avoid processed foods that are loaded with toxins and consume fresh organic foods instead. Use only safe, non-toxic personal care products, avoiding conventional shampoos, skin lotions, perfumes, anti-bacterial soaps, and other such products. Drink pure water and avoid fluoride, as fluoride causes cancer and drives tumor growth. Do not use conventional laundry detergents.

After you have minimized the amount of new toxins you are putting into your body, then focus on removing the stored toxins you have already accumulated. Fat-soluble toxins bioaccumulate in the body's fatty tissues and the combined effect of numerous toxins acting together seriously disrupts your normal chemistry, making you sick and promoting cancer. The average person is accumulating hundreds of such chemicals, including pesticides, styrene, PCBs, dioxins, phthalates and fire retardants. Even people who have lived organically for years will still measure high in carcinogens, neurotoxins, and endocrine disrupters because they have not removed their previously stored toxins. The only reliable way to get rid of stored fat-soluble toxins is with regular saunas.

Managing Stress and Your Mind

The mind is probably our most underused and misused asset, but using our minds to heal is the wave of the future. Most of us, including our physicians, are still stuck in a mechanical universe based on Newtonian physics, where we regard the body as a mechanical machine that responds to physical things like drugs. Yet emotional health may be even more important than all the physical factors, and the sooner you address it, the better off you will be.

Old emotional wounds contribute to disease; to achieve optimal health, they must be resolved. Chronic stress substantially increases free-radical formation and severely depresses the immune system— both promote cancer. Regular use of stress-reducing techniques, such as breathing and meditation, is important.

Perhaps the strongest element of all is the will to live. There have actually been cancer cures based on this single factor. The problem is that not everyone who says they want to get well really does want to get well. For many, there are too many benefits for staying sick, such as getting a lot of attention or having the state take care of them financially. Some only want to live so they can be there for their family or others. That isn't good enough. You have to want to live for yourself. Your body's ability to heal will be at its greatest when you yourself have a strong desire to live. You have to have a reason beyond that of just being there for others; you need a sense of purpose. Many alternative cancer practitioners have observed that the patient's attitude, sense of hope, and degree of participation in their own healing are critical factors in their recovery process.

Many people with cancer have achieved remarkable cures through meditation, hypnotherapy, and guided imagery. You may want to seek out a professional who can help you with this, especially one who is experienced in working with cancer patients. Remember that your thoughts affect your physical body for better or for worse.

The truth is we are on the front edge of creating a whole new world based on quantum physics. Our physical world is made of energy. It is the immaterial energy that creates the physical realm. In this new world, it will be recognized that the energy of your thoughts has more importance than any perceived physical reality.

This new way of thinking opens up doors for healing that are more powerful than anything previously known. What is so exciting is that you can use this mental power right now to change your physical reality in order to stay healthy or restore health. Unfortunately, conventional medicine is so far behind the science and so hopelessly obsolete that this power is not being used in medical practice. You are on your own.

Instructing the body to get well and believing it will get well can work miracles, even in the sickest people. By changing the energy, you change the physical. Regardless of your intellectual abilities, you can learn to harness this energy to your great advantage. On the other hand, if you don't believe you can get well, you won't.

Controlling Inflammation

Chronic inflammation is a foundation stone in the development and progression of cancer. Inflammation is essential to the cancer process, as well as being a key factor in every chronic disease. Therefore, it is essential to know how much inflammation is in your body and to take positive steps to minimize it. One way of measuring inflammation is to test for C-reactive protein. Inflammation is so essential to the cancer process that measuring C-reactive protein has proven to be a reliable way of predicting survival in cancer patients.

Part of controlling inflammation is minimizing immune responses. Chronic immune responses such as allergic reactions are inflammatory, and they impair immunity. They also deplete the body of critical nutrient reserves and produce substantial amounts of acid byproducts, making the body too acidic. As much as possible, avoid allergic reactions. Don't eat allergenic foods like dairy, soy, wheat, and corn.

Once inflammation starts, unless it is shut down, it takes on a life of its own and continues in an endless cycle of increasing tissue damage and inflammatory responses. To end this cycle, you have to first stop doing the things that promote inflammation. Stop consuming inflammatory foods such as sugar, wheat, milk and dairy products, and the supermarket oils that contain excess omega-6 fatty acids. Avoid inflammatory toxins such as glutamates, food additives, prescription drugs, pesticides, fluoride, chlorine, and metals such as aluminum, arsenic, cadmium, lead, and mercury. Get rid of chronic infections, like gum infections. Allergens must be avoided. Existing levels of stored toxins must be reduced. Stress must be controlled. Vaccinations should be avoided.

Once you stop causing more inflammation, you have to work to shut down the existing inflammatory process. For someone who has been suffering from chronic inflammation, this can require massive amounts of antioxidants. Few people consider taking massive amounts, and most doctors recoil in horror at the thought. This is why most chronic inflammation is never shut down and remains chronic. Antioxidants shut inflammation down, and you must work to optimize the antioxidants in your body. Anti-inflammatory supplements include: omega-3 fatty acids, vitamins A, B complex (including folic acid, B6 and B12), C, D, and E, plus beta-carotene, CoQ10, curcumin, quercetin, selenium, N-acetylcysteine, zinc, and alpha-lipoic acid. Vitamin C should be taken orally to bowel tolerance, and intravenous administration may be required. These supplements shut inflammation down and are therefore anticancer supplements.

To stay well or get well, chronic inflammation must be prevented and reversed. To do this, remove as many pro-inflammatory factors as you are able and take massive quantities of antioxidants. By adding as many alkalizing foods and antioxidant supplements as possible, you will cause a biological shift in your body that will shut the inflammatory cycle down, enhance immune function, enhance cellular repair, and improve your overall defense capacity against disease.

Alkalizing the Body

Consuming an alkaline diet is a must. Cancer cells thrive in an acidic environment, but will wither away in an alkaline environment. We eat far too many acid-forming foods. For example, the typical American breakfast of sugary breakfast cereals, pancakes, waffles or toast, eggs, bacon, and coffee will add to your acid load, helping to make you too acidic. We eat way too much acidifying sugar, grains, dairy, meat, and cola drinks and not enough alkalizing fresh fruits and vegetables.

If you already have cancer, even juicing and blenderizing fresh vegetables daily may not be sufficient to restore normal pH. It can be difficult to alkalize with diet alone because of the acid produced by the cancer cells themselves. Supplementation is essential. Minerals such as potassium, magnesium, and calcium need to be taken in highly bioavailable forms.

Cellular acidosis (acidic cells) initiates a catastrophic chain of events that can destroy your body due to free radical damage, the buildup of toxins, impaired protein synthesis, repair deficits, and the slow loss of differentiated cells and the structural protein scaffolding that holds the body together. Swelling and water retention are often symptoms of this process.

The human body is about 60 percent water, and the normal pH of most bodily fluids, including the fluids inside our cells, is slightly alkaline. There is a good reason for this. Water that is slightly alkaline is capable of dissolving substantially more oxygen than water that is slightly acidic. Therefore, making body fluids more acidic will lower the oxygen-carrying capacity of the body and help to create oxygen deficiency.

The body is highly sensitive to changes in pH, and maintaining proper alkaline pH is critical to health. While most Americans are too acidic, a small percentage is too alkaline. Restoring your pH to normal is one of the most fundamental things you can do to prevent and reverse cancer, as well as other so-called diseases. Most people should be eating a diet that is 75 to 80 percent alkalizing—

primarily fresh fruits and vegetables. Some natural cancer therapies, such as the Gerson therapy, consist of consuming large quantities of vegetable juices that alkalize the body. Mineral supplements are also very helpful, but only if high quality.

Supplementing with the mineral cesium represents a unique opportunity to kill cancer cells, without doing harm to healthy cells, by changing the pH of the cells. There are areas in the world where cancer is almost unknown, such as the Hunza Valley in northeastern Pakistan, the volcanic regions of Brazil, and the Hopi Indian territory in Arizona. It is noteworthy that each of these areas contains high levels of the alkaline minerals cesium and/or rubidium in the soil and food.

Protecting Children

Some people like to think of children as "little adults," but this does them a disservice. Because their bodies are still developing, children are much more vulnerable than adults. Their chemistry is different, and they need special protection. Children are more easily damaged by environmental contaminants due to their smaller size and because their metabolic pathways are still immature. They are less able to detoxify environmental chemicals, so the same exposure will have a greater impact than on an adult. Children also have lower levels of chemical-binding proteins that help to flush toxins out of the body. In addition, children are less able to repair damage caused by toxins. All of the above make children far more vulnerable than adults to the same toxic load, and this can disrupt the development of a child's nervous, respiratory, immune, reproductive, and other organ systems, and cause cancer.

The rapidly developing cells of a child are much more susceptible to the effects of both deficiency and toxicity. In the first months of life, children are slower to metabolize, detoxify and excrete environmental chemicals. They have an increased risk of cancer from virtually all toxic exposures, whether to carcinogens or endocrine disrupting chemicals. The smaller body mass and rapid physical development magnify a child's risk from chemical carcinogens and radiation exposure. X-rays are dangerous to adults, but they are much more dangerous to children. Rapidly dividing cells are much more numerous in children than in adults, making children three to five times more affected by radiation than adults. Also, because they have longer to live, they have more time for a tumor to develop.

As much as possible, children need to eat a healthy diet, free of processed foods and low in the Big Four (sugar, wheat, processed oils, and dairy/excess animal protein). At the same time, exposure to carcinogens and endocrine disrupting chemicals must be minimized. Pound for pound, children take in more water, air, food, and environmental toxins than adults.

Very importantly, children must also be protected before birth. Prospective mothers have to be careful to consume a superior diet, be on a high-quality supplement program, avoid toxins, and actively detoxify. Mothers have a moral duty to detoxify before becoming pregnant. Today, children are being poisoned in the womb. They are being born "pre-polluted," damaged by the mother's environmental exposures. This is a major reason why our children are so sick and why they have so much cancer.

Children are exposed to toxins from the mother's blood before birth and from the mother's milk after birth. Tests of umbilical cord blood have found nearly 300 toxic chemicals, including flame retardants, food packaging chemicals, and pesticides. According to the EPA, more than 600,000 children are born every year with levels of methylmercury that puts them at risk for brain damage, learning disabilities and cancer. The mercury comes mostly from mercury dental fillings and fish consumption by the mother.

In Conclusion

Every 30 seconds someone receives a cancer diagnosis, and every 60 seconds someone dies from cancer. That someone *could* be you, but it doesn't have to be you! Cancer can be prevented and it can be reversed. All you have to do is understand what cancer is and why it happens, and that puts you in control. The state of your health is the result of the nutrition and the toxins you put into your body, how you live your life, and the thoughts you put into your mind. All of these are under your control. By exercising this control, you can prevent cancer from developing in your body, or you can reverse it if it has already taken hold.

Despite an enormous amount of false propaganda to the contrary, the death rate from cancer is essentially the same today as it was in 1950. Considering that over 100 billion dollars has been spent on cancer research, conventional medicine's treatment of cancer is a colossal failure. Conventional medicine fails to understand that curing cancer is not about removing tumors. It's about shutting down the biological process that created the tumor. If all you do is remove the tumor, the cancer process is still operating, so a new tumor will be produced. And that's what usually happens!

To prevent cancer, you have to maintain an environment in your body that does not support the cancer process. To reverse cancer, you have to reestablish an environment that does not support the cancer process. To accomplish this, the two causes of disease— deficiency and toxicity—must be addressed.

To prevent and reverse cancer there are certain things you must do:

- Get the Big Four (sugar, wheat, processed oils, and dairy/excess animal protein) out of your life.
- Switch to an organically grown, plant-based diet that is rich in raw, fresh fruits and vegetables, and get on a high-quality supplement program.
- Juice fresh vegetables daily.
- Be mindful that every cell must get all the nutrients it needs every day.
- Avoid putting cancer-causing toxins in your body, including glutamates, pesticides, and prescription drugs.
- Get the vaccinations, chlorine, fluoride, and excess salt out of your life.
- Normalize the pH in your cells by eating an alkalizing diet and taking alkaline mineral supplements.
- Change the oil in your body by avoiding supermarket oils and choosing high-quality flaxseed, olive, fish, and coconut oils instead.
- Get regular exercise. Rebounding or a brisk walk daily are good choices.
- Get regular sleep.
- Optimize your insulin levels by avoiding foods that increase insulin, such as refined grains, white potatoes, white rice, sweets, and sodas.
- Measure for and eliminate heavy metals such as lead and mercury.
- Optimize your vitamin D and iodine levels. People with low vitamin D have more cancer and their cancer is more aggressive.
- Eliminate the inflammation in your body—supplement with antioxidants.

- Do regular saunas.
- As much as possible, avoid electromagnetic fields and x-rays such as routine mammograms.
- Address and resolve your old emotional wounds that contribute to disease.
- Think positive thoughts and be grateful for all that you have.

If you do all of the above to the best of your ability, and do so as consistently as possible, you can rest assured that you are doing everything within your power to support your body's natural defenses against cancer. You have everything to gain and nothing to lose because this is a recipe for blocking tumor growth in your body. In fact, you may very well become cancer proof.

Once you choose to live a cancer-free life, since there is only one disease, you are really choosing to live a disease-free life. That's a choice worth making!

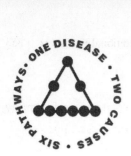

Additional Resources

Readers wishing to learn more from the author can read his previous books:

Never Be Sick Again: Health Is a Choice, Learn How to Choose It and *Never Be Fat Again: The 6-Week Cellular Solution to Permanently Break the Fat Cycle.*

The author publishes a free weekly e-mail newsletter called Newsclips. He also publishes a larger, more comprehensive subscription newsletter called Beyond Health News. Both can be obtained by going to: www.beyondhealth.com or by calling, in the U.S. or Canada, 800-250-3063. For calls from outside the U.S. and Canada, the regular phone number is 954-492-1324.

Also available on the website are two free reports. Click on the Free Reports button:

The Roadmap to Ultimate Health

The Roadmap to Choosing Supplements

In addition, under Educational Resources, there are archived articles by Raymond Francis on numerous subjects pertaining to health, all available for free.

Beyond Health International (BHI) is also a resource for many of the types of products mentioned in this book, including:

- Air Filters
- Water Filters
- Pool Filters
- Rebounders
- Saunas
- High Quality Supplements—BHI is world famous as a supplier of supplements with the highest obtainable purity and biological activity.
- High Quality Oils—Olive Oil, Flaxseed Oil, Fish Oil, and Coconut Oil.
- High Quality Personal Care Products—Toothpaste, Shampoo, Skin Cream, Cleaning Cloths.

Only products that have been carefully evaluated, tested, and approved by the author to follow the principles in this book are sold by Beyond Health. The Beyond Health brand of supplements has been researched by Raymond Francis and manufactured to his specifications to obtain exceptional quality, bioavailability, and beneficial biological activity in the body. BHI products can all be found by clicking the Products tab at www.beyondhealth.com.

Bibliography

Abbas, S. et al., "Serum 25-Hydroxyvitamin D and Risk of Postmenopausal Breast Cancer—Results of a Large Case-Control Study." *Carcinogenesis* 29, no. 1 (2008):93–99.

Agullo, G. et al., "Relationship Between the Structure and Inhibition of Phosphotidylinosito 3-Kinase: A Comparison With Tyrosine Kinase and Protein Kinase C Inhibition." *Biochemical Pharmacology* 53 (1997):1649–1657.

American Association for Cancer Research. Proceedings of the 4th Annual International Conference on Frontiers in Cancer Prevention Research, 2005.

American Chemical Society. Abstracts of the 239th ACS National Meeting, 2010.

Ames, Bruce. "Micronutrients Prevent Cancer and Delay Aging." a paper presented at the 1998 meeting at the Strang International Cancer Prevention Conference in New York City, 1998.

Anderson, R.C. "Toxic Emissions from Carpets." *Journal of Nutritional and Environmental Medicine* 5, no.4 (1995):375–386.

Atkins, R.C. *Dr. Atkins' Vita-Nutrient Solution.* New York: Simon & Schuster, 1998.

Bach, P.B. "Postmenopausal Hormone Therapy and Breast Cancer: An Uncertain Tradeoff." *Journal of the American Medical Association* 304, no. 15 (2010):1719–1720.

Bardocz, S. et al., "Decreased Levels of Heat Shock Proteins in Gut Epithelial Cells After Exposure to Plant Lectins." *Gut* 46, no. 5 (2000):679–87.

Barefoot, R. and C. Reich. *The Calcium Factor: the Scientific Secret of Health and Youth.* Wickenburg, AZ: Deonna Enterprises Publishing, 2001.

Barth, T. J. et al., "Redifferentiation of Oral Dysplastic Mucosa by the Application of the Antioxidants Beta Carotene, Alpha-Tocopherol and Vitamin C." *International Journal of Vitamin and Nutrition Research* 67 (1997):368–376.

Bartsch, H. et al., "Dietary Polyunsaturated Fatty Acids and Cancers of the Breast and Colorectum: Emerging Evidence for Their Role as Risk Modifiers." *Carcinogenesis* 20 (1999):2209–2218.

Bass, F.B. et al., "The Need for Dietary Counseling of Cancer Patients as Indicated by Nutrient and Supplement Intake." *Journal of the American Dietetic Association* (1995): 1319–1321.

Bernard, A. et al., "Outdoor Swimming Pools and the Risks Of Asthma and Allergies During Adolescence." *European Respiratory Journal* 19 (2008):827–832.

Bertram, J.S. "Carotenoids and Gene Regulation." *Nutrition Reviews* 57 (1999):182–191.

Bharti, A.C. et al., "Curcumin (Diferuloylmethane) Down Regulates the Constitutive Activation of Nuclear Factor-Kappa B and Ikappa Balpha Kinase in Human Multiple Myeloma Cells, Leading to Suppression of Proliferation and Induction of Apoptosis." *Blood* 10, no. 3 (2003):1053–1062.

Blatner, W.A. "Viruses Are Etiologically Linked to Approximately 20% of All Malignancies Worldwide." *Proceedings of the Association of American Physicians* 111, no. 6 (1999):563–572.

Blaylock, R. *Health and Nutrition Secrets That Can Save Your Life.* Albuquerque, NM: Health Press, 2002.

———. *Natural Strategies for Cancer Patients.* New York: Kensington Publishing Corp., 2003.

Block, G. "Epidemiological Evidence Regarding Vitamin C and Cancer." *American Journal of Clinical Nutrition* 32, no. 6 (1991):1310S–1314S.

Block, G. "Vitamin C Status and Cancer: Epidemiological Evidence of Reduced Risk." *Annals of the New York Academy of Sciences* 53(1992):280–290.

Block, G. et al., "Fruit, Vegetables and Cancer Prevention: A Review of Epidemiological Evidence." *Nutrition and Cancer* 18 (1992):1–29.

Block, J. B. and S. Evans. "Clinical Evidence Supporting Cancer Risk Reduction with Antioxidants and Implications for Diets and Supplementation." *Journal of the American Nutraceutical Association* 3, no.3 (2000):6–16.

Blot, W.J. et al., "Nutritional Intervention Trials in Linxian, China: Supplementation with Specific Vitamin/Mineral Combinations, Cancer Incidence, and Disease-Specific Mortality in the General Populations." *Journal of the National Cancer Institute* 85 (1993):1483–1492.

Blount, B.C. et al., "Folate Deficiency Causes Uracil Misincorporation into Human DNA and Chromosome Breakage." *Proceedings of the National Academy of Sciences USA* 94 (1997): 3290–3295.

Bobe, G. et al., "Dietary Flavonoids and Colorectal Adenoma Recurrence in the Polyp Prevention Trial." *Cancer Epidemiology Biomarkers and Prevention* 6 (2008): 1344–53.

Bollschweiller, E. et al., "Vitamin Intake and Risk of Subtypes of Esophageal Cancer in Germany." *Journal of Cancer Research and Clinical Oncology* 128 (2002):575–580.

Bonjour, J.P. et al., "Calcium Intake and Vitamin D Metabolism and Action in Healthy Conditions and in Prostate Cancer." *British Journal of Nutrition* 97, no. 4 (2007):596–597.

Boots, A.W. et al., "Health Effects of Quercetin: From Antioxidant to Nutraceutical." *European Journal of Pharmacology* 582, no. 2–3 (2008):325–337.

Bramsen, T. "Effects of Tranexamic Acid on Choroidal Melanoma." *Acta Ophthalmologica* 56 (1977):264–269.

Brenner, D.J. et al., "Computed Tomography—An Increasing Source of Radiation Exposure." *New England Journal of Medicine* 22, no.357 (2007): 2277–2284.

Brownstein, D. *Iodine: Why You Need It, Why You Can't Live Without It.* West Bloomfield, Michigan: Medical Alternatives Press, 2004.

Budwig, Johanna. *Flax Oil as a True Aid Against Arthritis, Heart Infraction, Cancer and Other Diseases.* Vancouver, Canada: Apple Tree Publishing Co. Ltd., 1994.

Bull, R. J. et al., "Water Chlorination: Essential Process or Cancer Hazard." *Toxicological Sciences* 28, no. 2 (1995):155–166.

Cade, J.E. et al., "Dietary Fiber and Risk of Breast Cancer in the UK Women's Cohort Study." *International Journal of Epidemiology* 36, no. 2 (2007):90–94.

Cameron, E. and L. Pauling. "Supplemental Ascorbate in the Supportive Treatment of Cancer: Prolongation of Survival Times in Terminal Human Cancer." *Proceedings of the National Academy of Sciences* 73 (1976):3685–3689.

———. "Supplemental Ascorbate in the Supportive Treatment of Cancer: Reevaluation of Prolongation of Survival Times in Terminal Human Cancer." *Proceedings of the National Academy of Sciences* 75 (1978):4538–4542.

———. "Survival Times of Terminal Lung Cancer Patients Treated With Ascorbate." *Journal of the International Academy of Preventive Medicine* 6 (1981): 21–27.

Campbell, T. Colin. The *China Study* Dallas, TX: BenBella Books, 2005.

Cannell, J.J. et al., "Epidemic Influenza and Vitamin D." *Epidemiology of Infections* 134, no. 6 (2006):1129–1140.

Cantor, K.P. et al., "Drinking Water Source and Chlorination Byproducts. I. Risk of Bladder Cancer." *Epidemiology* 9, no.1 (1998):21.

Carney, D.N. "Lung Cancer—Time to Move on from Chemotherapy." *New England Journal of Medicine* 346 (2002): 126.

Carone, B.J. et al., "Paternally Induced Transgenerational Environmental Reprogramming of Metabolic Gene Expression in Mammals." *Cell* 143, no.7 (2010): 1084–1096.

Carroll, K. et al., "Calcium and Carcinogenesis of the Mammary Gland." *American Journal of Clinical Nutrition* 54 (1991): 2065–2085.

Chan, June M. et al., "Dairy Products, Calcium, and Prostate Cancer Risk in the Physicians Health Study." *American Journal of Clinical Nutrition* 74 (2001): 549–554.

Chance, W.T. et al., "Immunostimulation Following Fish-Oil Based Parenteral Nutrition in Tumor-Bearing Rats." *Nutrition and Cancer* 26 (1996):303–312.

Chen, Q., et al., "Pharmacologic Ascorbic Acid Concentrations Selectively Kill Cancer Cells: Action as a Pro-Drug to Deliver Hydrogen Peroxide to Tissues." *Proceedings of the National Academy of Sciences;* 102, no. 38 (September 2005):13604–9.

Chen, Q., et al., "Pharmacologic Doses of Ascorbate Act as a Prooxidant and Decrease Growth of Aggressive Tumor Xenografts in Mice." *Proceedings of the National Academy of Science* 105 (2008):11105–11109.

Choi, M.A. et al., "Serum Antioxidant Levels and Lipid Peroxidation in Gastric Carcinoma Patients." *Cancer Letter*136 (1999):89–93.

Clark, L.C. et al., "Effect of Selenium Supplement for Cancer Prevention in Patients with Carcinoma of the Skin. A Randomized Controlled Trial." *Journal of the American Medical Association* 276 (1996):1957–1963.

Clark, L.C. et al., "Decreased Incidence of Prostate Cancer with Selenium (Se) Supplement: Results of A Randomized Control Trial." *FASEB Proceedings* Abstract 781, 1998.

Cocilovo, A. "Colored Light Therapy: Overview of Its History, Theory, Recent Developments and Clinical Applications Combined with Acupuncture." *American Journal of Acupuncture* 27, no. 1&2 (1999).

Cohn, P.D. "A Brief Report on the Association of Drinking Water Fluoridation and the Incidence of Osteosarcoma Among Young Males." New Jersey Department of Health, Environmental Health Service (1992): 1–17.

Colbert, L.H. et al., "Physical Activity, Exercise, and Inflammatory Markers in Older Adults: Findings from the Health, Aging and Body Composition Study." *Journal of the American Geriatrics Society* 52, no. 7 (2004):1098–1104.

Cole, W.C. and K.N. Prasad. "Contrasting Effects of Vitamins as Modulators of Apoptosis in Cancer Cells and Normal Cells: A Review." *Nutrition and Cancer* 29 (1997): 97–103.

"Common Pain Relief Medication May Encourage Cancer Growth." Science Daily, accessed November 19, 2009, http://www.sciencedaily.com/releases/2009/11/091118143209.htm

Connolly, J.M. and D.P. Rose. "Effect of Dietary Fatty Acids on Invasion Through Reconstituted Basement Membrane (Matrigel) by a Human Breast Cancer Line." *Cancer Letter* 75 (1993):137–142.

Connolly, J.M. et al., "Effect of Reduced Dietary Linolenic Acid Intake Alone or Combined with an Algal Source of Docosahexaenoic Acid on MDA-MD-231 Breast Cancer Cell Growth and Apoptosis in Nude Mice." *Nutrition and Cancer* 35 (1999):44–49.

Cook, N.R. et al., "Beta Carotene Supplements for Patients with Low Baseline Levels and Decreased Risk of Fatal Prostate Carcinoma." *Cancer* 86 (1999):1783–1792.

Cooper, C.L. *Stress and Breast Cancer.* New York: John Wiley, 1998.

Costello, A.J. "A Randomized, Controlled Chemoprevention Trial of Selenium in Familial Prostate Cancer: Rationale, Recruitment, and Design Issues." Supplement *Urology* 57 (2001):182–184.

Cummings, J.H. and S. A. Bingham. "Diet and the Prevention of Cancer." *British Medical Journal* 317 (1998):1636–1640.

Curl, C.L. et al., "Organophosphorus Pesticide Exposure of Urban and Suburban Preschool Children with Organic and Conventional Diets." *Environmental Health Perspectives* 111, no. 3 (2003):377–82.

Dalla Pellegrina, C. et al., "Effects of Wheat Germ Agglutinin on Human Gastrointestinal Epithelium: Insights from an Experimental Model of Immune/Epithelial Cell Interaction." *Toxicology and Applied Pharmacology* 237 no. 2 (June 2009):146–53.

Daviglus, M.L. et al., "Dietary Beta Carotene, Vitamin C, and Risk of Prostate Cancer: Results from the Western Electric Study." *Epidemiology* 32 no. 5 (1996):472–477.

Dawsey, S.M. et al., "Effects of Vitamin/Mineral Supplementation on the Prevalence of Histologic Dysplasia and Early Cancer of the Esophagus and Stomach from the Results of the Dysplasia Trial in Linxian, China." *Cancer Epidemiology Biomarkers and Prevention* 3 (1994):167–172.

Dean, Carolyn. *Death By Modern Medicine.* Belleville, Ontario, Canada: Matrix Verite-Media, 2005.

"Decline in Breast Cancer Cases Likely Linked to Reduced Use of Hormone Replacement," Science Daily, accessed December 15, 2006, http://www.sciencedaily.com/releases/2006/12/061214142620.htm

Diamond, Harvey. *You Can Prevent Breast Cancer.* San Diego, CA: ProMotion Publishing, 1995.

Diamond, Harvey *Fit For Life: A New Beginning.* New York: Kensington Books, 2000.

Dolecek, T.A. and G. Grandits. "Dietary Polyunsaturated Fatty Acids and Mortality in the Multiple Risk Factor Intervention Trial (MRFIT)." *World Review of Nutrition and Dietetics* 66 (1991):205–16.

Dorgan, J.F. et al., "Relationships of Serum Carotenoids, Retinol, Alpha-Tocopherol and Selenium with Breast Cancer Risk: Results from a Prospective Study in Columbia Missouri (United States)." *Cancer Causes and Control* 9 (1998):89–97.

Drake, I.M. et al., "Ascorbic Acid May Protect Against Human Gastric Cancer by Scavenging Mucosal Oxygen Radicals." *Carcinogenesis* 17 (1996):559–562.

Eckhart, E. "Several Kinds of Viruses Cause Cancer in Humans, Accounting For 10–20% of Cancer Worldwide." *Sci Prog* 81, Part 4 (1998):315–328.

Enstrom, J.E. et al., "Vitamin E and Vitamin C Supplement Use and Risk of All-Cause and Coronary Heart Disease Mortality in Older Persons." *American Journal of Clinical Nutrition* 64 (1996):190–196.

Environmental Protection Agency. "Human Exposure to Methyl Tert-Butyl Ether (MTBE) While Bathing with Contaminated Water." EPA/600/R–05/094 (2003).

Erasmus, Udo. *Fats and Oils.* Vancouver, Canada: Alive Books, 1986.

Ewen, S. and A. Pusztai. "Effects of Diets Containing Genetically Modified Potatoes Expressing Galanthus Nivalis Lectin on Rat Small Intestine." *Lancet* 354 (1999):1353–1354.

Faith-Magnusson, K. and K. E. Magnusson. "Elevated Levels of Serum Antibodies to the Lectin Wheat Germ Agglutinin in Celiac Children Lend Support to the Gluten-Lectin Theory of Celiac Disease." *Pediatric Allergy and Immunology* 6, no.2 (1995):98–102.

Farinati, F. et al., "Oxidative DNA Damage Accumulation in Gastric Carcinogenesis." *Gut* 42 (1998):351–356.

Fiala, E.S. et al., (1996) "Epigallocatechin Gallate, a Polyphenolic Tea Antioxidant, Inhibits Peroxynitrate-Mediated Formation Of 8-Oxydeoxyguanosine and 3-Nitrotyrosine." *Experimentia* 52:1210–1218.

Flagg, E.W. et al., "Epidemiological Studies of Antioxidants and Cancer in Humans." *Journal of the American College of Nutrition* 32, no. 5 (1995):419–427.

Fleischauer, A.T. et al., "Garlic Consumption and Cancer Prevention: Meta-Analysis of Colorectal and Stomach Cancers." *American Journal of Clinical Nutrition* 72 (2000):1047–1052.

Foster, H. "Lifestyle Changes and the Spontaneous Regression of Cancer: An Initial Computer Analysis." *International Journal of Biosocial Research* 10, no.1 (1988):17.

Freidenreich, C.M and M.R. Orenstein. "Physical Activity and Cancer Prevention: Etiologic Evidence and Biological Mechanisms." *Journal of Nutrition* 132, no. 11 (2002):3456S–64S.

Gann, P.H. et al., "Lower Prostate Cancer Risk in Men with Elevated Plasma Lycopene Levels: Results of a Prospective Analysis." *Cancer Research* 59 (1999):1225–1230.

Garewal, H.S. "Beta-Carotene and Vitamin E in Oral Cancer Prevention." *Journal of Cellular Biochemistry* 53 (1993):262–269.

Garland, C.F. et al., "Vitamin D and Prevention of Breast Cancer: Pooled Analysis." *Steroid Biochemistry and Molecular Biology* 103, no. 3–5 (2007):708–711.

———. "Vitamin D for Cancer Prevention: Global Perspective." *Annuls of Epidemiology* 19 (2009):468–483.

———. "Vitamin D Supplement Doses and Serum 25-Hydroxyvitamin D in the Range Associated with Cancer Prevention." *Anticancer Research* 31 (2011): 607–612.

Gerber, D.E. "Targeted Therapies: A New Generation of Cancer Treatments." *American Family Physician* 77, no.3 (2008):311–319.

Giovannucci, E. et al., "Intake of Carotenoids and Retinol in Relation to Risk of Prostate Cancer." *Journal of the National Cancer Institute* 87 (1995): 1767–1776.

Gofman, J. *Radiation from Medical Procedures in the Pathogenesis of Cancer and Ischemic Heart Disease: Dose Response Studies with Physicians per 100,000 Population.* San Francisco, CA: Committee for Nuclear Responsibility Books, 1999.

Guzyeyeva, G.V. "Lectin Glycosylation as a Marker of Thin Gut Inflammation." *FASEB Journal* 22 (2008):898.3

Haber, D. "Roads Leading to Breast Cancer." *New England Journal of Medicine* 343 (2000):1566.

Hall, L.M. et al., "Vitamin D Intake Needed to Maintain Target Serum 25-Hydroxyvitamin D Concentrations in Participants with Low Sun Exposure and Dark Skin Pigmentation is Substantially Higher than Current Recommendations." *Journal of Nutrition* 140, no. 3 (2010):542–550.

Hansson, L.E. et al., "Nutrients and the Risk of Gastric Cancer: A Population-Based Case Control Study in Sweden." *International Journal of Cancer* 57 (1994):638–644.

Hardell, L. et al., "Pooled Analysis of Two Case-Control Studies on Use of Cellular and Cordless Telephones and the Risk for Malignant Brain Tumours Diagnosed in 1997–2003." *International Archives of Occupational and Environmental Health* 79, no. 8 (2006): 630–639.

Hardell, L. et al., "Long-Term Use of Cellular Phones and Brain Tumours: Increased Risk Associated with Use for > or =10 Years." *Occupational and Environmental Medicine* 64, no. 9 (2007):626–632.

Havas, M. et al., "Provocation Study using Heart Rate Variability Shows Radiation from 2.4 GHz Cordless Phone Affects Autonomic Nervous System." *European Journal of Oncology* 5 (2010):273–300.

HealthGrades. *HealthGrades Hospital Quality and Clinical Excellence Study.* Denver, CO: Health Grades, Inc., 2011.

Heinonen, O.P. et al., "Prostate Cancer and Supplementation with Alpha-Tocopherol and B Carotene: Incidence and Mortality in a Controlled Trial." *Journal of the National Cancer Institute* 90 (1998):440–446.

Heisel, S.J. et al., "Natural Killer Cell Activity and MMPI Scores of a Cohort of College Students." *American Journal of Psychiatry* 143, no. 11 (1986):1382–1386.

Henderson, William. *Cancer Free.* Bangor, ME: Booklocker.com, Inc., 2008. PDF e-book.

Henson, D. et al., "Ascorbic Acid: Biological Functions and Relation to Cancer." *Journal of the National Cancer Institute* 83, no. 8 (1991):547–550.

Hickey, S. and H. Roberts. *Ascorbate: The Science of Vitamin C.* Morrisville, NC: Lulu Press, (2004).

———. *Cancer: Nutrition and Survival.* Morrisville, NC: Lulu Press, 2005.

———. "Selfish Cells: Cancer as Microevolution," *Journal of Orthomolecular Medicine* (2007).

Hickey, Steve and Andrew W. Saul. *Vitamin C: The Real Story* Laguna Beach, CA: Basic Health Publications, Inc., 2008.

Hidaka, H. et al., "Curcumin Inhibits Interleukin 8 Production and Enhances Interleukin 8 Receptor Expression on the Cell Surface: Impact on Human Pancreatic Carcinoma Cell Growth by Autocrine Regulation." *Cancer* 95, no.6 (2002):1206–1214.

Hogson, D.H. et al., "Chronic Restriction Influences Tumor Metastasis in the Rat: Parametric

Considerations." *Nutrition and Cancer* 28 (1997):189–198.

Hoffer, A. "Orthomolecular Treatment of Cancer" in *Nutrients in Cancer Prevention and Treatment* (Humana Press, Totowa, New Jersey, 1995): 373–391.

Hoffer, A. and L. Pauling. "Hardin Jones Biostatistical Analysis of Mortality Data for a Second Set of Cohorts of Cancer Patients with a Large Fraction Surviving at the Termination of the Study and a Comparison of Survival Times of Cancer Patients Receiving Large Regular Oral Doses of Vitamin C and Other Nutrients with Similar Patients Not Receiving These Doses." *Journal of Orthomolecular Medicine* 8 (1993):1547–1567.

Holick, M.F. "Vitamin D Deficiency." *New England Journal of Medicine* 357 (2007): 266–281.

Hong, R.L. et al., "Curcumin Inhibits Tyrosine Kinase Activity of p185neu and Also Depletes p185neu." *Clinical Cancer Research* 5 (1999):1884–1891.

Hoover, R.N. et al., "Cancer—Nature, Nurture or Both?" *New England Journal of Medicine* 343 (2000):78–85, 135–136.

Hurston, S.D. et al., "Types of Dietary Fat and the Incidence of Cancer at Five Sites." *Preventive Medicine* 9 (1990):242–253.

Hutchins, A.M. et al., "Flaxseed Consumption Influences Endogenous Hormone Concentrations in Postmenopausal Women." *Nutrition and Cancer* 39 (2001):58–65.

Institute of HeartMath. *Emotional Energetics, Intuition and Epigenetics Research.* Boulder Creek: Institute of HeartMath, 2003.

Institute of Medicine of the National Academies. *Crossing the Quality Chasm: A New Health System for the 21st Century.* Washington, D.C.: National Academy Press, 2001.

Ip, C. and H. Ganther. "Activity of Methylated Forms of Selenium in Cancer Prevention." *Cancer Research* 50 (1996):1206–1251.

Islami, F. et al., "Tea Drinking Habits and Esophageal Cancer in High Risk Area in Northern Iran: Population Based Control Study." *British Medical Journal* 338 (March 2009): b929.

Issels, Josef. *Cancer—A Second Opinion.* Garden City Park, NY: Avery Publishing Group, 1999.

Jankum, J. et al., "Why Drinking Green Tea Could Prevent Cancer." *Nature* 387 (1997):561.

Jenski, L.J. et al., "Omega-3 Fatty Acid Modification of Membrane Structure and Function. Dietary Manipulation of Tumor Cell Susceptibility to Cell and Complement Mediated Lysis." *Nutrition and Cancer* 19 (1993):135–146.

Ji, Sayer. "Further Characterization of Wheat Germ Agglutinin Interaction with Human Platelets: Exposure of Fibrinogen Receptors." *Journal of Thrombosis and Haemostasis* 56, no. 3 (1986):323–7.

———. "Wheat Germ Agglutinin Induces NADPH-Oxidase Activity in Human Neutrophils by Interaction with Mobilizable Receptors." *Infection and Immunity* 67, no. 7 (1999): 3461–8.

———. "Wheat Germ Agglutinin-Induced Platelet Activation via Platelet Endothelial Cell Adhesion Molecule-1: Involvement of Rapid Phospholipase C Gamma 2 Activation by Src Family Kinases." *Biochemistry* 40, no. 43 (2001):12992–3001.

———. "Wheat Germ Lectin Induces G2/M Arrest in Mouse L929 Fibroblasts." *Journal of Cell Biochemistry* 91, no. 6 (2004):1159–73.

———. "The Dark Side of Wheat-New Perspectives on Celiac Disease & Wheat Intolerance." *Journal of Gluten Sensitivity* (Winter 2008).

John, E.M. et al., "Vitamin D and Breast Cancer Risk: The NHANES I Epidemiologic Follow-up Study: 1971–1975 to 1992." *Cancer Epidemiology, Biomarkers and Prevention* 8 (1999): 399–406.

Johnstone, P. A. S. et al., "Lack of Survival Benefit of Post-Operative Radiation Therapy in Prostate Cancer Patients with Positive Lymph Nodes Post-Operative Radiation Therapy." *Prostate Cancer and Prostatic Diseases* 10 (2007):185–188.

Kate, M. et al., "Influence of Proinflammatory Cytokines on the Adhesion of Human Cancer Cells." *International Journal of Cancer* 112, no. 6 (December 2004): 943–50.

Katz, D.L. *Nutrition in Clinical Practice: A Comprehensive Evidence-Based Manual for the Practitioner* Philadelphia, PA: Lippincott Williams & Wilkins, 2000.

Kennedy, A.R. and N.I. Krinsky. "Effects of Retinoids, Beta-Carotene and Canthaxanthene on UV And X-Ray-Induced Transformation of C3H10T 1/2 Cells In Vitro." *Nutrition and Cancer* 22 (1994):219–232.

Khafif, A. et al., "Quantitation of Chemoprotective Synergism Between (–) Epigallocatechin-3-Gallate and Curcumin in Normal, Premalignant and Malignant Human Oral Epithelial Cells." *Carcinogenesis* 19 (1998):419–424

Kiecolt-Glaser, J.K. and Glaser, R. "Psychological Influences on Immunity." *Psychosomatics* Vol. 27, No. 9 (1986): 621–624.

Kim, K.P. et al., "Coronary Artery Calcification Screening: Estimated Radiation Dose and Cancer Risk." *Archives of Internal Medicine* 169, no. 13 (2009):1188–1194.

King, W.D. and L.D. Marrett. "Case Control Study of Bladder Cancer and Chlorination Byproducts in Treated Water (Ontario Canada)." *Cancer Causes and Control* 7, no. 6 (1996):596–604.

Lipkin, M. et al., "Diet of Young Girls May Increase Their Risk of Breast Cancer: Inadequate Levels of Dietary Calcium and Vitamin D May Increase the Risk of Breast and Other Cancers for Young Females and the Elderly." *Primary Care and Cancer* 14, no. 2 (1994):8.

Kleid, J. "Not All Nutraceuticals Are Created Equal." *Journal of the American Neutraceutical Association* 2, no. 1 (1999):60.

Klenner, F. "Observations on the Dose and Administration of Ascorbic Acid When Employed Beyond the Range of a Vitamin in Human Pathology." *Journal of Applied Nutrition* Vol. 23, nos. 3 & 4 (1971):61–88.

Kneki, P. et al., "Dietary Antioxidants and the Risk of Lung Cancer." *American Journal of Epidemiology* 134 (1991):471–479.

Knight, J.A. et al., "Vitamin D and Reduced Risk of Breast Cancer: A Population Based Case Control Study," *Cancer Epidemiology Biomarkers and Prevention* 16, no. 3 (2007): 422–429.

Komiyama, K. et al., "Studies on the Biological Activity of Tocotrienols." *Chemical and Pharmaceutical Bulletin* 37 (1989):1369–1371.

Kromhout, D. "Essential Micronutrients in Relation to Carcinogenesis." Supplement *American Journal of Clinical Nutrition* (1987): 1361–1367.

Kuijten, R.R. et al., "Gestational and Familial Risk Factors for Childhood Astrocytoma: Results in a Case Controlled Study." *Cancer Research* 50 (1990):2608–2612.

Lappe, Joan M. et al., "Vitamin D and Calcium Supplementation Reduces Cancer Risk: Results of a Randomized Trial." *American Journal of Clinical Nutrition* 85 (2007):1586–1591.

Larsson, S. C. et al., "Vitamin A, Retinol, and Carotenoids and the Risk of Gastric Cancer: A Prospective Cohort Study." *American Journal of Clinical Nutrition* 85, no. 2 (2007):497–503.

Lasne, C. et al., "Transforming Activities of Sodium Fluoride in Cultured Syrian Hamster Embryo and BALB/3T3 Cells." *Cell Biology and Toxicology* 4 (1988):311–324.

Lawson, M. et al., "Gene Expression in the Fetal Mouse Ovary Is Altered by Exposure to Low Doses of Bisphenol A." *Biology of Reproduction* 10 (2010): 1095.

Leape, L. L. "Error in Medicine." *Journal of the American Medical Association* 272, no. 23 (1994):1851–1857.

Lee, D.H. et al., "Dietary Iron Intake and Breast Cancer: The Iowa Women's Health Study." *Proceedings of the American Association of Cancer Research* 45 (2004):A2319.

Lee, J. et al., *What Your Doctor May Not Tell You About Breast Cancer: How Hormone Balance Can Help Save Your Life.* New York: Warner Books, 2002.

Lee, S.K. et al., "Vitamin C Suppresses Proliferation of the Human Melanoma Cell SK-MEL-2 Through the Inhibition Of Cyclooxygenase-2 (COX-2) Expression and the Modulation of Insulin-Like Growth Factor II (IGF-II) Production." *Journal of Cell Physiology* 216, no. 1 (2008):180–8.

Legerski, R.J. and Li, L. "DNA Repair Capability and Cancer Risk." *Cancer Bulletin* 46 (1994): 228–232.

Lefkowitz, E. and C. Garland. "Sunlight, Vitamin D and Ovarian Cancer Mortality Rates in U.S. Women." *International Journal of Epidemiology* 23, no. 6 (1994):1133–1136.

LeMarchland, L.M. et al., "Vegetables and Fruit Consumption in Relation to Prostate Cancer Risk in Hawaii: A Reevaluation of the Effect of Beta-Carotene." *American Journal of Epidemiology* 133 (1991):215–219.

Levenson, S.M. et al., *Nutritional Factors in the Induction and Maintenance of Malignancy.* New York: Academic Press Inc., 1983.

Levy, S. et al., "Correlation of Stress Factors with Sustained Depression of Natural Killer Cell Activity and Predicted Prognosis in Patients with Breast Cancer." *Journal of Clinical Oncology* 5, no. 3 (1987):348–53.

Li, J.Y. et al., "Nutrition Intervention Trials in Linxian, China: Multiple Vitamin/Mineral Supplementation, Cancer Incidence, and Disease Specific Mortality Among Adults with Esophageal Dysplasia." *Journal of the National Cancer Institute* 85 (1993):1492–1498.

Lin, L.I. et al., "Curcumin Inhibits SK-Hep-1 Hepatocellular Carcinoma Cell Invasion in Vitro and Suppresses Matrix Metalloproteinase-9 Secretion." *Oncology* 55 (1998):349–353.

Lipkin, M. and H.L Newmark. "Vitamin D, Calcium and Prevention of Breast Cancer: A Review," *Journal of the American College of Nutrition* 18, no. 5 (1999):3925–3975.

Loft, S. and Poulson, H.E. "Cancer Risk and Oxidative DNA Damage in Man." *Journal of Molecular Medicine* 74 (1996):297–312.

Lutgendorf, S. K. et al., "Social Support, Psychological Distress, and Natural Killer Cell Activity in Ovarian Cancer." *Journal of Clinical Oncology* (October 2005):7105–7113.

Maltz, G. "Sunlight May Protect Against Cancers and Melanoma." *Family Practice News* (February 1996): 21.

Manello, F. et al., "Role of Ferritin Alterations in Human Breast Cancer Cells." *Breast Cancer Research and Treatment* 126 (2011):63–71.

Mark, S.D. et al., "Prospective Study of Serum Selenium Levels and Incident Esophageal and Gastric Cancers." *Journal of the National Cancer Institute* 92 (2000):1753–63.

Marti, J.E. *Alternative Health & Medicine Encyclopedia.* Detroit, MI: Visible Ink Press, 1995.

MATES II (Multiple Air Toxics Exposure Study). California South Coast Air Quality Management District, 1999.

Matheu, A. et al., "Delayed Aging through Damage Protection by the *Arf/p* Pathway." *Nature* 448, no.7151 (2007):375–381.

Matrone, M.A. et al., "Microtentacles on Tumor Cells Appear to Play Role in How Breast Cancer Spreads." *Oncogene* 6 (2010):1–11

—— et al., "'Metastatic Breast Tumors Express Increased Tau, Which Promotes Microtentacle Formation and the Reattachment of Detached Breast Tumor Cells." *Oncogene* 22 (2010):3217–3227.

McKegney, F.P. "Psychoneuroimmunology: What Lies Ahead." *Drug Therapy* (August 1982): 25–35.

Meadows, A.T. et al., "Second Malignamt Neoplasims in Children: An Update from the Late Effects Study Group." *Journal of Clinical Oncology* 56 (1985):339–347.

Mendelsohn, R.S. *Confessions of a Medical Heretic.* Chicago: Contemporary Books, 1979.

Menendez, J.A., et al., "Anti-HER2 (erbB-2) Oncogene Effects of Phenolic Compounds Directly Isolated from Commercial Extra-Virgin Olive Oil (EVOO). *BMC Cancer* 8 (2008):377.

Metcalf, M. et al., "Lesson of the Week: Useless and Dangerous—Fine Needle Aspiration of Hepatic Colorectal Metastases." *British Medical Journal* 328 (2004):507–508.

Meydani, S.N. et al., "Vitamin E Supplementation Enhances Cell-Mediated Immunity in Healthy Elderly Subjects." *American Journal of Clinical Nutrition* 52 (1990):557–563.

Michaud, D.S. et al., "Intake of Specific Carotenoids and Risk of Lung Cancer in 2 Prospective U.S. Cohorts." *American Journal of Clinical Nutrition* 72 (2000):990–997.

Michels, K.B. et al., "DietaryAntioxidant Vitamins, Retinol, and Breast Cancer Incidence in a Cohort of Swedish Women," *International Journal of Cancer* 9, no. 4 (2001):563–567. "Millions in U.S. Drinking Dirty Water," *New York Times Digest*, December 8, 2009.

Miranda, T. K. et al., "Influence of Proinflammatory Cytokines on the Adhesion of Human Colon Carcinoma Cells to Lung Microvascular Endothelium." *International Journal of Cancer* 112, no. 6 (2004):943–950.

Moss, Ralph. *The Cancer Industry.* New York: Equinox Press, 1999.

——. *Questioning Chemotherapy.* New York: Equinox Press, 2000.

Mousa, S.A. et al., "Pro-Angiogenesis Action of Arsenic and Its Reversal by Selenium-Derived Compounds." *Carcinogenesis* 28, no. 5 (2007):962–967.

Murata, A. et al., "Prolongation of Survival Times of Terminal Cancer Patients by Administration of Large Doses of Ascorbate." Supplement *International Journal of Vitamin and Nutrition Research* 23 (1982):103–113.

Murray, Frank. *Sunshine and Vitamin D.* Laguna Beach, CA: Basic Health Publications, Inc., 2008.

National Academy of Science, "Low Levels of Ionizing Radiation May Cause Harm," news release, June 29, 2005, http://www8.nationalacademies.org/onpinews/newsitem.aspx?RecordID=11340

——. "Adults Need to Increase Intake of Folate; Some Women Should Take More," news release, April 7, 1998, http://www8.nationalacademies.org/onpinews/newsitem.aspx?RecordID=6015

National Cancer Institute. NCI # NO1-CN-45133, National Institutes of Health, Washington, D.C., 1977.

National Institutes of Health. "Dietary Supplements Fact Sheet: Vitamin A and Carotenoids." National Institutes of Health: Office of Dietary Supplements, 2006.

National Women's Health Network Position Paper. *Mammography in Women Before Menopause*, Washington, DC: Women's Health Network, 1993.

National Research Council of the National Academy of Sciences. *New Evidence Confirms Cancer Risk From Arsenic in Drinking Water,* 2001.

Navarro, E. et al., "The Microwave Syndrome." *Biology and Medicine* 22, no. 2&3 (2003):161–169.

Netherwood et al., "Assessing the Survival of Transgenic Plant DNA in the Human Gastrointestinal Tract." *Nature Biotechnology* 22 (2004): 2.

Nesaretnam, K. et al., "Effect of Tocotrienols and the Growth of a Human Breast Cancer Cell Line in Culture." *Lipids* 30 (1995):1139–1143.

Newman. T. B. et al., "Carcinogenicity of Lipid Lowering Drugs." *Journal of the American Medical Association* 275, no. 1 (1996):55–60.

Nison, Paul. *The Raw Life: Becoming Natural in an Unnatural World.* New York: Three Forty Three Publishing Company, 2000.

Norat, T. et al., "Meat, Fish, and Colorectal Cancer Risk: The European Prospective Investigation into Cancer and Nutrition." *Journal of the National Cancer Institute* 97, no. 12 (2005):906–16.

Norell, S.E. et al., "Diet and Pancreatic Cancer: A Case Control Study." *American Journal of Epidemiology* 124 (1986):894–902.

Noroozi, M. et al., "Effects of Flavonoids and Vitamin C on Oxidative Damage to Human Lymphocytes." *American Journal of Clinical Nutrition* 67 (1998):1210–1218.

Norrish, A.E. et al., "Prostate Cancer and Dietary Carotenoids." *American Journal of Epidemiology* 151 (2000):119–123.

Null, G. M. et al., *Death by Medicine.* Edinburg, VA: Axios Press, 2010.

Oakley, G. P. "Eat Right and Take a Multivitamin." *New England Journal of Medicine* 338 (1998), 9 April.

Oberfeld, G. at al., "The Microwave Syndrome: Further Aspects of a Spanish Study." International Conference Proceedings, Kos, Greece, 2004.

Oh, E., et al., "Calcium and Vitamin D Intakes in Relation to Risk of Distal Colorectal Adenoma in Women," *American Journal of Epidemiology* 165, no. 10 (2007):1178–1186.

Oh, S.J. et al., "Inhibition of Angiogenesis by Quercetin in Tamoxifen-Resistant Breast Cancer Cells." *Food and Chemical Toxicology* 48, no. 11 (2010):3227–3234.

Ohara, M. et al., "Inhibition of Lung Metastasis of B16 Melanoma Cells Exposed to Blue Light in Mice." *International Journal of Molecular Medicine* 10, no. 6 (2002):701–705.

"Omega-3 Fatty Acids Reduce Risk of Advanced Prostate Cancer," Science Daily, accessed March 25, 2009, http://www.sciencedaily.com/releases/2009/03/090324131444.htm

Omenn, G. S. et al., "Effects of a Combination of Beta Carotene and Vitamin A on Lung Cancer and Cardiovascular Disease." *New England Journal of Medicine* 334 (1996):1150–1155.

Padayatty, S. J., et al., "Intravenously Administered Vitamin C as Cancer Therapy: Three Cases." *Canadian Medical Association Journal* 174, no. 7 (2006):937–942.

Paez-Ribes, M., et al., "Antiangiogenic Therapy Elicits Malignant Progression of Tumors to Increased Local Invasion and Distant Metastasis." *Cancer Cell* 15 (2009):220–231.

Paganelli, G.M. et al., "Effect of Vitamin A, C and E Supplementation on Rectal Cell Proliferation in Patients with Colorectal Adenomas." *Journal of the National Cancer Institute* 32, no. 1 (1992): 47–51.

Pandey, D.K. et al., "Dietary Vitamin C and Beta-Carotene and Risk of Death in Middle-Aged Men: The Western Electric Study." *American Journal of Epidemiology* 65, no. 12 (1995):1269–1278.

Perera, F.P. "Environment and Cancer: Who Are Susceptible?" *Science* 278 (1997):1068–73.

Pert, C.B. et al., "The Psychosomatic Network: Foundation of Mind-Body Medicine." *Alternative Therapies in Health and Medicine* 4, no. 4 (1998):30–41.

Peskin, Brian Scott and Amid Habib. *The Hidden Story of Cancer.* Houston TX: Pinnacle Press, 2008.

Pickering, G. "Medicine and Society—Past, Present, and Future." *British Medical Journal* 1 (1971):191–196.

Pierce, Tanya Harter. *Outsmart Your Cancer* Stateline, NV: Thoughtworks Publishing, 2004.

Pisani, P. et al., "Cancer and Infection: Estimates of the Attributable Fraction in 1990." *Cancer Epidemiology Biomarkers and Prevention* 6 (1997):387–400.

Plant, Jane. *Your Life in Your Hands.* New York: Virgin Books, 2006.

Prasad, K.N. "Modulation of the Effect of Tumor Therapeutic Agents by Vitamin C." *Life Science* 27 (1980):275–280.

Prasad, K.N. et al., "Vitamin E and Cancer Prevention: Recent Advances and Future Potentials." *Journal of the American College of Nutrition* 11 (1992):487–500.

———. "High Doses of Multiple Antioxidant Vitamins: Essential Ingredients for Improving the Efficacy of Standard Cancer Therapy." *Journal of the American College of Nutrition* 18 (1999):13–25.

President's Cancer Panel. U.S. Department of Health and Human Services Annual Report "Reducing Environmental Cancer Risk: What Can We Do Now?" 2008–2009.

Prizment, A. E. et al., "Use of Permanent Hair Dyes and Bladder Cancer Risk." *International Journal of Cancer* 120, no. 5 (2007):1093–1098.

Pusztai, Arpad. "Genetically Modified Foods: Are They a Risk to Human/Animal Health?" http://www.actionbioscience.org/biotech/pusztai.html. June 2001.

Pusztai, Arpad et al., "Antinutritive Effects of Wheat-Germ Agglutinin and Other N-Acetylglucosamine-Specific Lectins." *The British Journal of Nutrition* 70, no. 1 (1993):313–21.

Quillin, Patrick. *Beating Cancer with Nutrition.* Tulsa, OK: The Nutrition Times Press, 1994.

———. *Beating Cancer with Nutrition* Carlsbad, CA: Nutrition Times Press, 2005.

362   Bibliography

Raimondi. S. et al., "Diet and Prostate Cancer Risk with Specific Focus on Dairy Products and Dietary Calcium: A Case-Control Study." *Prostate* 70, no. 10 (2010):1054–1065.

Ramon, J. M. et al., "Nutrient Intake and Gastric Cancer Risk: A Case Control Study in Spain." *International Journal of Epidemeology* 22 (1993):983–988.

Rath, M. "Plasmin Induced Proteolysis and the Role of Apoprotein(A), Lysine and Synthetic Lysine Analogs." *Journal of Orthomolecular Medicine* 7 (1992):17–23.

Reed, Kristin et al., *Health Grades Hospital Quality and Clinical Excellence Study.* Denver, CO: Health Grades, Inc., 2011.

Reeves, M. J. "Healthy Lifestyle Characteristics Among Adults in the United States." *Archives of Internal Medicine*165 (2005):854–857.

Riordan H. D., et al., "Case Study: High-Dose Intravenous Vitamin C in the Treatment of a Patient with Adenocarcinoma of the Kidney." *Journal of Orthomolecular Medicine* 5 (1990):5–7.

———. "Intravenous Vitamin C as a Chemotherapy Agent: A Report on Clinical Cases." *Puerto Rico Health Sciences Journal* June, 23, no. 2 (2004):115–118.

Riordan, N.H., et al., "Intravenous Ascorbate as a Tumor Cytotoxic Chemotherapeutic Agent." *Medical Hypotheses* March 44, no. 3 (1995):207–213.

———. "Intravenous Vitamin C in a Terminal Cancer Patient." *Journal of Orthomolecular Medicine* 11 (1996):80–82.

Ripoli, E.P.A. et al., "Vitamin E Enhances the Chemotherapeutic Effects of Adriamycin on Human Prostate Carcinoma Cells In Vitro." *Journal of Urology* 136 (1986):529–531.

Rose, D.P. and M.A. Hatala "Dietary Fatty Acids And Breast Cancer Invasion And Metastasis." *Nutrition and Cancer* 21 (1994):103–111.

Rose, D. P. and J. M. Connolly. "Antiangiogenesity of Docosahexaenoic Acid and Its Role in the Suppression of Breast Cancer Cell Growth in Nude Mice." *International Journal of Oncology* 15 (1999):1911–1915.

Saad, F. et al., "Cancer Treatment—Induced Bone Loss in Breast and Prostate Cancer." *Journal of Clinical Oncology* Nov 20 (2008):5465–5476.

Sadetzki, S. et al., "Cellular Phone Use and Risk of Benign and Malignant Parotid Gland Tumors—A Nationwide Case-Control Study." *American Journal of Epidemiology* 167, no. 4 (2008):457–467.

Samet, J. M. et al., "Do Airborne Particles Induce Heritable Mutations?" *Science* 304 (2004):971–972.

Sasano, H. "Analysis of Lectin Binding in Benign and Malignant Thyroid Nodules." *Archives of Pathology and Laboratory Medicine.* 113, no. 2 (1989):186–9.

Scheibner, Viera. *Vaccination.* Blackheath, NSW. Australian Print Group, 1993.

Servan-Schreiber, David. *Anticancer* .New York: Penguin Group, 2008.

Seyfried, Thomas N. et al., "Cardiolipin and Electron Transport Chain Abnormalities in Mouse Brain Tumor Mitochondria: Lipidomic Evidence Supporting the Warburg Theory of Cancer." *Journal of Lipid Research* 49, no. 12 (2008):2545.

Shahinian, V. B. et al., "Reimbursement Policy and Androgen-Deprivation Therapy for Prostate Cancer." *New England Journal of Medicine* 363, no. 19 (2010):1822–32.

Shealy, Norman and Dawson Church. *Soul Medicine.* Santa Rosa, CA: Energy Psychology Press, 2008.

Simone, C. B. *Cancer and Nutrition.* Garden City Park, NY: Avery Publishing, 1992.

Sloan, E. K. et al., "The Sympathetic Nervous System Induces a Metastatic Switch in Primary Breast Cancer." *Cancer Research* 70, no. 18 (2010):7042

Smith-Bindman, Rebecca "Projected Cancer Risks from Computed Tomographic Scans Performed in the United States 2007." *Archives of Internal Medicine* 169, no. 22 (2009).

Smith, Jeffery. *Seeds of Deception* Portland, ME: Yes! Books, 2003.

———. *Genetic Roulette: The Documented Health Risks of Genetically Engineered Foods.* White River Junction, VT: Chelsea Green, 2007.

"Exposure to Low Doses of BPA Alters Gene Expression in the Fetal Mouse Ovary," Science Daily, accessed August 28, 2010, http://www.sciencedaily.com/releases/2010/08/100825093249.htm.

Somers, Suzanne. *Knockout.* New York: Crown Publishing Group, 2009.

Sorensen, G. et al., "Working Well: Results from a Work Site Based Cancer Prevention Trial." *American Journal of Public Health* 86 (1996):939–947.

Spencer, M. D. et al., "Association Between Composition of the Human Gastrointestinal Microbiome and Development of Fatty Liver With Choline Deficiency." *Gastroenterology* 11.049 (2010).

"Stanford Research Builds Link Between Sleep, Cancer Progression." Science Daily October 1, 2003, http://www.sciencedaily.com/releases/2003/10/031001060734.htm

Steinmetz, K.A. and Potter, J.D., "Vegetables, Fruit and Cancer Prevention: A Review." *Journal of the American Dietetic Association* 96 (1996):1027–1039.

Strum, S. et al., "Modified Citrus Pectin Slows PSA Doubling Time: A Pilot Clinical Trial."

Presentation: International Conference on Diet and Prevention of Cancer, Tampere, Finland. May 28-June 2, 1999.

Studzinski, G.P. and D.C. Moore. "Sunlight: Can't It Prevent as Well as Cause Cancer?" *Cancer Research* 55 (1995):4014–4922.

Swanson, C.A. et al., "Fruits, Vegetables and Cancer Risk: The Role of Phytochemicals." *Phytochemicals* 1–12 (1998).

Ten Raa, S. et al., "The Influence of Reactive Oxygen Species on the Adhesion of Pancreatic Carcinoma Cells to the Peritoneum." *International Journal of Cancer* 112, no. 6 (2004): 943–50.

Tchemychev, B. "Natural Human Antibodies to Dietary Lectins." *FEBS Letter* 18; 397, no. 2–3 (1996):139–42.

Theriaul, A. et al., "Tocotrienol: A Review of Its Therapeutic Potential." *Clinical Biochemistry* 32 (1999):309–19.

Trosko, J. E. et al., "Inhibition of Cell-Cell Communication by Tumor Promoters." *Carcinogenesis* 7 (1982):565–585.

United States Department of Agriculture. Agriculture Fact Book (2001–2002).

Van der Bij, G. J. et al., "The Perioperative Period is an Underutilized Window of Therapeutic Opportunity in Patients with Colorectal Cancer." *Annals of Surgery* 249, no. 5 (2009): 727–34.

Varis, K. et al., "Gastric Cancer and Premalignant Lesions in Atrophic Gastritis: A Controlled Trial on the Effects of Supplementation with Alpha-Tocopherol and Beta Carotene." *Scandinavian Journal of Gastroenterology* 33 (1998):294–300.

Vilchez, R.A. et al., "Association Between Simian Virus 40 And Non-Hodgkin Lymphoma." *Lancet* 359 (2002): 817–23.

Voisin, A. S. et al., "Infant Swimming in Chlorinated Pools and the Risks of Bronchiolitis, Asthma and Allergy." *European Respiratory Journal* 36 (2010):41–47.

Walford, R. L. and L. Walford. *The Anti-Aging Plan: The Nutrient-Rich, Low-Calorie Way of Eating for a Longer Life—The Only Diet Scientifically Proven to Extend Your Healthy Years.* New York: Marlowe & Company, 2005.

"Walnuts Slow Prostate Tumors in Mice, Study Finds," Science Daily, accessed March 23, 2010, http://www.sciencedaily.com/releases/2010/03/100322153953.htm

Wang, G. Q. et al., "Effects of Vitamin/Mineral Supplementation in the Prevalence of Histologic Dysplasia and Early Cancer of the Esophagus and Stomach: Results from the General Population Trial in Linxian, China." *Cancer Epidemiology Biomarkersand Prevention* 3 (1994):161–166.

Wang, Z. et al., "Mammary Cancer Promotion and MAPK Activation Associated with Consumption of a Corn Oil-Based High Fat Diet." *Nutrition and Cancer* 34 (1999):140–146.

Warburg, Otto. "The Metabolism of Carcinoma Cells." *Journal of Cancer Research,* Vol. 9: (1925)148–163.

———. "On the Origin of Cancer Cells." *Science* 123 (1956):3139.

Warburg, Otto, et al., "The Metabolism of Tumors in the Body." *Journal of General Physiology,* 8 (1928):519–530.

Wei, Q. et al., "DNA Repair: A Potential Marker for Cancer Susceptibility." *Cancer Bulletin* 46 (1994):233–237.

Welch, H. Gilbert, et al., "Are Increasing 5-Year Survival Rates Evidence of Success Against Cancer?" *Journal of the American Medical Association,* 283 (2000):2975–2978.

Williams, R. J. *Nutrition Against Disease: Environmental Prevention.* New York: Bantam Books, 1973.

Wolf, R. and D. Wolf. "Increased Incidence of Cancer Near a Cell-Phone Transmitter Station." *International Journal of Cancer Prevention* 2 (2004).

World Cancer Research Fund "Food, Nutrition, Physical Activity and the Prevention of Cancer: A Global Perspective." Washington, DC: American Institute for Cancer Research, 2007.

Wyllie, S. and J.G. Liehr. "Release of Iron from Ferritin Storage by Redox Cycling of Stilbene and Steroid Estrogen Metabolites: A Mechanism of Induction of Free Radical Damage by Estrogen." *Archives of Biochemistry and Biophysics* 346 (1997):180–186.

Xiaohua Xu et al., "Diesel Exhaust Is Linked to Cancer Development via New Blood Vessel Growth." *Toxicology Letters* 191, no. 1 (2009):57–68.

Xu, Y.X. et al., "Curcumin Inhibits IL-1 alpha and TNF-alpha induction of AP-1 and NF-kB DNA— Binding Activity in Bone Marrow Stromal Cells." *Hematopathological Molecular Hematology* 11 (1997–1998):49–62.

Yu, W. et al., "Induction of Apoptosis in Human Breast Cancer Cells by Tocopherols and Tocotrienols." *Nutrition and Cancer* 33 (1999):26–32.

Ziegler, R. G. et al.,. "Migration Patterns and Breast Cancer Risk in Asian-American Women." *Journal of the National Cancer Institute* 85 (1993):1819–27.

Zhang, S. et al., "Dietary Carotenoids and Vitamins A, C, and E and Risk of Breast Cancer." *Journal of the National Cancer Institute* 91, no. 6 (1999):547–556.

Zhang, Y. et al., "Geographic Variation in the Quality Of Prescribing." *New England Journal of Medicine* 363, no. 21 (2010):1985–8.

Zhu. X. et al., "Growth-Promoting Effect of Bisphenol A on Neuroblastoma In Vitro and In Vivo." *Journal of Pediatric Surgery* 44, no. 4 (2009):672–680.

Index

Abel, Ulrich, 23
Acetaldehyde, 77–78
acidosis, 70–79, 84, 346
acrylamide, 175, 177, 204
adenosine triphosphate (ATP), 43, 85
adrenaline, 225
advanced glycation end-products (AGEs), 127
affirmations, 229–231
aflatoxin, 79, 166, 184, 264
air filters, 97, 198, 200
air pollution, 193–200
airborne particles, 197–198
alcohol, 76–78, 92, 179
alkaline diet, 345–347
alkalinity, 70–71, 158, 251, 322, 345–347. *see also* pH ranges
allergens
   avoiding, 344–345
   food sources, 76, 131–132, 142–145, 157–158
   in personal care products, 205–206
allopathic medicine, 298–299. *see also* conventional medicine
alternative treatment. *see also specific categories*; supplements
   overview, 4–7
   case histories, 20–21, 32–33, 113–114, 144–145
   Gerson anti-cancer therapy, 216, 347
aluminum, 295
Alzheimer's disease, 29, 38, 75, 246
American Cancer Society, 22, 26, 28, 235, 309, 332
American Medical Association (AMA), 329, 332
Ames, Bruce, 87
anesthetics, 278, 296–298
angiogenesis, 95–97, 115–117, 121, 225, 279
animal feeding studies, 156–157
animal feedlots, 140
animal protein, 78–79, 141–150, 340
antibiotic-resistant bacteria strains, 293
antibiotics, 290–293

anticancer diet, 161–170
anti-fibrin enzymes, 90–91
anti-inflammatories, 73–73, 80, 82, 139, 318–319, 345
antioxidants, 58–60, 116–117, 178–179, 314–322. *see also specific antioxidants*
apoptosis, 31, 54, 81, 93–95, 115–117
apples, 110
appliances, 195–196, 243, 250
arachidonic acid, 147
arsenic, 96, 186
artificial colors, 109–111, 204–205
artificial sweeteners, 129–130
Asian women, 145
aspartame, 129
attention and intention, 228–230
autoimmune diseases, 81, 134, 289–290
Avastin, 281
avocados, 149

B vitamins, 265, 307
bacteria, 156–157, 290–291, 293
basal cell carcinoma, 311
bathrooms, toxic exposure and, 198
Becker, Robert, 249
bee death, 157
beef consumption, 140
belly breathing, 239–240
benzopyrene, 263–264
beta-carotene, 117–118, 316
beverage containers, 97, 127, 175–177, 181
Bieler, Henry, 298
birth control pills, 287–288
bisphenol-A (BPA), 97, 127, 175–177, 181, 192
black tea, 165
bladder cancer, 167, 185, 205
Blanc, Bernard, 120
blenders, 163
blood clots, 88–91
blood sugar levels, 77, 129, 130, 214, 235. *see also* insulin
bloodletting, 25–26